CONGENITAL MALFORMATIONS
Antenatal Diagnosis, Perinatal Management, and Counseling

John W. Seeds, MD
Director of Prenatal Diagnostic Services
Associate Professor
Departments of Obstetrics and
Gynecology and Radiology

Richard G. Azizkhan, MD
Chief of Pediatric Surgery
Associate Professor of
Surgery and Pediatrics

University of North Carolina
Chapel Hill, North Carolina

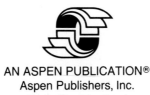

AN ASPEN PUBLICATION®
Aspen Publishers, Inc.
Rockville, Maryland
1990

Library of Congress Cataloging-in-Publication Data

Seeds, John W.
Congenital malformations : antenatal diagnosis, perinatal
management, and counseling / John W. Seeds, Richard G. Azizkhan.
p. cm.
"An Aspen publication."
ISBN: 0-8342-0140-2
1. Fetus—Abnormalities. 2. Prenatal diagnosis. 3. Genetic counseling.
I. Azizkhan, Richard G. II. Title.
[DNLM: 1. Abnormalities—diagnosis. 2. Abnormalities—therapy. 3.
Prenatal Diagnosis.   WQ 209 S45lc]
RG626.S44   1990
618.3'2—dc20
DNLM/DLC
for Library of Congress
89-18541
CIP

Aspen Publishers, Inc., grants permission for photocopying , such as
copying for general distribution, for advertising or promotional purposes,
for creating new collective works, or for resale. For information, address
Aspen Publishers, Inc., Permissions Department, 1600 Research
Boulevard, Rockville, Maryland 20850.

The authors have made every effort to ensure the accuracy of the information
herein, particularly with regard to drug selection and dose.   However,
appropriate information sources should be consulted, especially for new or
unfamiliar drugs or procedures. It is the responsibility of every practitioner
to evaluate the appropriateness of a particular opinion in the context of
actual clinical situations and with due consideration to new developments.
Authors, editors, and the publisher cannot be held responsible for any
typographical or other errors found in this book.

Editorial Services: Jane Coyle Garwood

Library of Congress Catalog Card Number: 89-18541
ISBN: 0-8342-0140-2

Printed in the United States of America

1 2 3 4 5

Dedicated to
our deceased brothers
Asa E. Seeds, Jr., MD
and
Karl C. Azizkhan, MD
for the love and inspiration
their lives offered us all

Table of Contents

Preface

As the technologies of prenatal diagnosis have developed over the past 20 years, the clinical coordination of these technologies and the appropriate perinatal management of pregnancies complicated by congenital disease have been slow to keep pace. Critical components of a successful prenatal diagnosis effort include appropriate identification of patients with pregnancies at risk for congenital disease, coordination of available diagnostic techniques, and accurate counseling about fetal prognosis and perinatal management. These critical components of prenatal diagnosis form the basis for this book.

Our goal is to provide both primary providers and referral specialists with a single "first reference" for the answers to questions asked after the diagnosis of congenital disease. Accurate answers can not only facilitate correct medical management but also ease the emotional adaptation to such a diagnosis. Inaccuracies of diagnosis or counseling can lead to inappropriate management, delayed or pathological emotional adjustment, and even unnecessary pregnancy termination.

The accurate diagnosis and counseling of patients with pregnancies complicated by congenital disease require the attention of a variety of clinical specialists. The synthesis of a reference text that includes both prenatal diagnostic techniques and postnatal surgical principles of care, including probable outcome, is intended to provide an efficient source of information for the frontline practitioner.

After reviewing general principles, including the organization of such a service, patient risk assessment, and the various methodologies of prenatal diagnosis, we will examine certain specific categories of congenital disease in greater detail. In each case, clinical signs or symptoms associated with the condition will be outlined and illustrative sonographic examples of the malformation will be presented along with technical suggestions for optimal imaging. In each case perinatal management, neonatal care, pediatric surgical intervention (if appropriate), and ultimate prognosis will be discussed.

These discussions do not substitute for the coordinated efforts of a well-organized prenatal diagnostic service. They will provide concise, accurate information about congenital disease that will facilitate accurate diagnosis and accurate answers to a patient's first anxious questions. We have tried to maintain a practical, informative style throughout. Tables are used to streamline data presentation, the illustrations provided are from contemporary equipment and are carefully labeled for clarity, and selected bibliographies provide relevant further reading sources.

Once a congenital malformation has been detected, accurate information is critical. Postnatal survival with or without disabilities may be impossible or possible only with specialized care. The inevitable pain for the parents can be unnecessarily amplified by misinformation. It is the goal of this book to help prevent that.

JWS, RGA

Part I

General Considerations

Chapter 1

Organization of a Multidisciplinary Antenatal Diagnosis Program

In beginning our examination of antenatal diagnostic techniques, counseling issues, and neonatal care, it is appropriate that we begin with a discussion of the basic organization of the multidisciplinary team that delivers such services, describe the facilities necessary to deliver them, and finally review the process of antenatal diagnosis itself.

Although many patients might prefer that their care be provided by a single individual, no single provider can offer such a broad range of skills, among them antenatal diagnosis, counseling, perinatal and neonatal care, and follow-up. Inevitably, in the course of antenatal diagnosis, care and consultation are required from a variety of specialists. The provision of appropriate and optimal care requires thoughtful coordination of the necessary consultations. In this chapter we will review some principles of prenatal diagnosis that should be viewed as suggestions offered to guide an institution in the development of a successful prenatal diagnosis and treatment center.

Three categories essential to consider in the development of a successful antenatal diagnosis service include the personnel and their demonstrated level of skill, the facilities available, and the proper coordination and sequencing of the process itself, from low-risk screening through final referral and resolution. Undertaking antenatal diagnostic services without careful attention to each of these elements significantly increases the probability of error, inappropriate diagnosis, inappropriate intervention, and incomplete or inaccurate counseling.

PERSONNEL

Those individual specialists who may contribute to the care of a patient undergoing antenatal diagnosis are found in Table 1-1. Certainly, not all of the individuals on this list will be appropriate in every case, and in unique cases additional special interests may be required, but these individuals constitute a core of specialists upon which to build a successful program.

Table 1-1 Members of the Perinatal Diagnosis Team

Maternal-fetal medicine subspecialist
Pediatric surgeon
Medical geneticist
Genetic counselor
Neonatologist
Pediatric neurosurgeon
Disabled children specialist
Pediatric urologist
Sonologist experienced with antenatal diagnosis
Social worker

Coordinator

If, at the beginning of development, an antenatal diagnosis service lacks an individual or individuals willing to be or assigned to be the primary coordinator of care in the case of a patient undergoing antenatal diagnosis, then the institution of antenatal diagnostic services should be reconsidered. It is very important for the patient to identify with a coordinator or "quarterback," from the pretesting counseling and the selection and planning of testing through the evaluation of test results. The coordinator may be a perinatologist, genetic counselor, or social worker with special experience. He or she must be knowledgeable in the principles of genetic disease, have some understanding of technical diagnostic procedures, be completely familiar with local facilities and services, and ideally possess considerable interpersonal counseling skills. The specific type of specialist is not as important as the commitment to be the focal point for the patient's questions and anxiety.

Each of the following specialists plays a unique role in the coordination and efficient function of an antenatal diagnostic service. Not all referral centers will have on staff every type of specialist mentioned, but access to this expertise is considered important.

Perinatologist

The participation of a maternal-fetal medicine specialist in the antenatal diagnosis process is pivotal to the success of such a program. First, it is usually the perinatologist who is trained to perform many of the invasive tests upon which the antenatal diagnosis is based. Second, prenatal diagnosis raises many clinical management issues apart from simply the accurate detection of congenital disease. Obstetrical implications of the diagnosis of a congenital malformation include potential complications of pregnancy for the mother and the method, timing, and location of delivery. It is the perinatologist who is often identified by the patient as her primary physician during the pregnancy and birth of the child with congenital disease, and who is often seen by the patient as the coordinator of clinical care. Such a central role does not exclude the possibility of a genetic counselor or social worker serving also in a focal role as patient coordinator or advocate.

Sonologist

The sonologist is often, but not always, the same person as the perinatologist. Whether the sonologist is a perinatologist or a radiologist, this individual is a key participant in any successful antenatal diagnostic service. Ultrasound is the primary technique for the diagnosis of a broad variety of structural anomalies, and the accuracy and sensitivity of the technique are critically dependent on the skill and experience of the sonologist. It is fundamental to patient counseling that an accurate and honest evaluation of the skill and accuracy of this test be given to the patient. Further, if the opinions and advice of all other consultants are to be of optimal accuracy and relevance, it is critical that they also be aware of the skill and accuracy of the sonologist and his or her level of confidence regarding the specific diagnosis.

It is important that if this individual is not himself or herself a perinatologist, that he or she work closely and easily with the perinatal team in the provision of the whole spectrum of antenatal diagnostic services. The inherent discoordination of sonographic services offered in a physical location different from that of the perinatal and other consultative services must be overcome if a smooth sequence of services is to be provided.

Pediatric Surgeon

In the case of the diagnosis of a congenital malformation that is potentially remediable, a pediatric surgeon is a vital source of information for the patient and the rest of the antenatal health care team. Regardless of the gestational age at the time of diagnosis, the personal consultation of a pediatric surgeon forms the basis for most management decisions for both the parents and the perinatologist. Questions of prognosis, types of corrective surgery, likelihood of morbidity or mortality during or after corrective surgery, and likelihood of permanent disabilities come up immediately upon the diagnosis of such a condition and benefit from the input of a pediatric surgeon.

If the diagnosis is made at a gestational age below the legal limit for elective termination, consultation with the pediatric surgeon is a rational basis for a decision regarding the continuation of the pregnancy. If the diagnosis of a nonlethal malformation is made late in pregnancy, accurate information about prognosis and neonatal care is important both for obstetrical planning and the parents' emotional adaptation. It is critical that this input be sought before the birth of the infant, not only to allow the parents to become familiar with the surgeon but also to anticipate the possible surgical management decisions that they will likely have to deal with before the anxiety of the postnatal period develops.

Ideally, the pediatric surgeon is consulted early after the diagnosis of the condition and has the opportunity to meet with the parents and discuss issues of prognosis, surgical care, and follow-up. The pediatric surgeon becomes a primary consultant to the obstetrician on issues of timing of delivery. Is the condition in question likely to benefit from preterm delivery or not? Is the condition in question likely to deteriorate in utero and therefore require frequent sonographic surveillance to ensure that deterioration is not occurring unrecognized? Is it likely that the condition in question will lead to an immediate neonatal emergency? For these questions and many more, the pediatric surgeon should be a primary member of the team involved with antenatal diagnosis.

Genetic Counselor

During the past 2 decades, genetic counseling has developed as a unique career within medical genetics. The role of genetic counselor in understanding issues of inheritance, congenital disease, and patient education can be central to the success of a comprehensive antenatal diagnosis program. Genetic counselors are trained professionals with expertise in patient education, grief counseling, and appropriate follow-up. It is often the genetic counselor who puts a human face on a process that for many patients is an overwhelmingly unfamiliar experience. In many programs, it is the genetic counselor who is the central coordinator mentioned above.

Initial consultation usually involves a preliminary discussion of the specific congenital abnormality in question and the availability, risks, nature, and accuracy of antenatal testing relative to that abnormality. The counselor introduces the patient to the process and sequence of decisions that she will be asked to make. The counselor next arranges access to the appropriate antenatal testing if desired by the patient, collects and organizes the results, and evaluates for the patient the accuracy and meaning of those results. Additional consultation with a perinatologist, pediatric surgeon, or medical geneticist can then be planned.

The genetic counselor, as the central coordinator of many successful programs, is also in the best position to provide primary grief and adjustment counseling to both the mother and the father. Follow-up telephone conversations, hospital visits, and coordination of late follow-up visits all contribute to the completion of the experience for the patient. The last consultation, with an explanation of the abnormality, its etiology, and the risk of recurrence that is as complete as possible, can be critical to the final emotional resolution of an experience that might otherwise be destabilizing to an individual and a family.

Medical Geneticist

In the case of a genetic condition that is known to be based on Mendelian allelic inheritance, or a cytogenetic abnormality involving structural chromosomal abnormalities of greater complexity than simple trisomy, consultation with a trained medical geneticist is important to ensure complete and accurate information for the patient.

Neonatologist

Regular consultation with the neonatologist who will be directing the neonatal medical care of the disabled infant is important early in the planning of clinical care of such a pregnancy. This expert becomes an advocate of the infant from a slightly different viewpoint and often argues effectively for issues of maximum maturity and development prior to delivery that contribute significantly to long-term survival. Coordination of immediate neonatal care is fundamental to optimal outcome even in cases requiring pediatric surgical intervention, and therefore the neonatologist must be included in all discussions of perinatal care of the nonlethal congenital malformation.

It is equally important that the neonatologist be included in discussions regarding the birth of infants with typically lethal malformations. Prenatal discussions with the parents of such an infant may allow the team to avoid heroic or misguided efforts to resuscitate an infant with an anomaly likely to be lethal, such as pulmonary hypoplasia in the case of renal agenesis. Such heroic efforts in the case of a hopeless situation are often extremely upsetting to the parents.

Pediatric Neurosurgeon, Pediatric Crippled Children Specialist

One of the more commonly diagnosed fetal anomalies is the neural tube defect, such as anencephaly, encephalocele, or spina bifida. Other commonly diagnosed anomalies of the central nervous system include Dandy-Walker cyst of the posterior fossa, hydrocephalus, holoprosencephaly, porencephaly, hydranencephaly, and iniencephaly. If the diagnosis is made prior to viability, the expert evaluation and advice of both a pediatric neurosurgeon and a pediatrician with special experience in the care of disabled children assist the parents to make an informed decision with regard to the pregnancy. The long-term functional prognosis for many infants with central nervous system malformations, when appropriate neonatal neurosurgical intervention is provided, is rapidly changing. The informed consultation of a pediatric neurosurgeon should be available anytime management decisions are made for pregnancies with these diagnoses.

Parents deliberating the fate of a pregnancy complicated by the discovery of a nonlethal defect of the central nervous system also should be given access to the experience of a pediatrician familiar with the care of children with analogous disabilities.

Pediatric Urologist

The fetal urinary tract is among the most frequent sites of antenatally diagnosed malformation. From agenesis/dysgenesis, to ureteropelvic junction obstruction, to bladder outlet obstruction, the management of pregnancies complicated by such diagnoses clearly benefits from the consultation of a urologist specially trained and experienced in the care of neonates with such anomalies. Both for the planning of perinatal management and the rare consideration of antenatal intervention, the special knowledge of the pediatric urologist is important in providing appropriate care. Often, parents of a fetus with a urinary tract anomaly are reassured regarding the ultimate prognosis for most children with similar anomalies by a prompt antenatal consultation.

Social Worker

Congenital disease does not respect socioeconomic strata. The diagnosis of a congenital malformation, whether lethal or nonlethal, is equally tragic for the poor and the affluent. Unfortunately, both antenatal testing and the special perinatal and neonatal care these infants can require are not inexpensive. A specialized social worker, knowledgeable in the identification of community resources and the alternative funding opportunities available to some patients can significantly improve the quality of the medical care available to individual patients, as well as contribute to the financial health of the antenatal diagnostic service.

HEALTH CARE FACILITIES

The majority of the techniques used for contemporary antenatal diagnosis are available in an outpatient setting. The coordinated operation of an antenatal diagnostic service in a comfortable outpatient clinic, with access to the variety of consultants reviewed above and access to any inpatient services required, including intrauterine intervention, neonatology, pediatric surgery, pediatric neurosurgery, and intensive perinatal surveillance, offers the patient both the flexibility of services and the desired continuity of care. The diagnosis made at such a comprehensive center is more likely to be made with a level of confidence known to all the consultants, and their advice therefore will be given with optimal confidence. The coordination of inpatient services may be accomplished with a minimum of confusion, and there is less opportunity for error.

An isolated freestanding antenatal diagnostic service, on the other hand, often suffers severe impairment of overall quality of service for many patients with a positive diagnosis. Without the ability to offer the entire spectrum of consultative services, such a service increases the probability that the patient with a positive diagnosis of a nonlethal anomaly will make a management decision based on incomplete or inaccurate information. If such a decision is made, and the patient later becomes aware of more accurate or more detailed information that might have altered her decision, then a significant liability risk will exist for such a service.

TECHNICAL SERVICES

A comprehensive antenatal diagnostic service should offer the technical services listed in Table 1-2. Many of the services listed are more complex than might be immediately obvious to individuals not involved with them on a daily basis.

Maternal serum alpha-fetoprotein (MSAFP) screening is reviewed in detail elsewhere (Chapter 2). But it bears repeating that MSAFP assays demonstrate sufficient interlaboratory variability that optimal service requires each laboratory to accumulate a large statistical sample before attempting to estimate risk from their results. No quantitative result from one laboratory can be extrapolated to the database and risk estimates of another laboratory, even if they are using identical assay procedures. The risk of fetal anomaly is proportional to the degree of elevation or depression of the MSAFP, and therefore, it is not sufficient to report only that the result was high or low. A fully informative screening service also provides patient-specific relative risk information. The patient must often decide whether to proceed with an invasive and potentially morbid procedure (amniocentesis) based on estimated risk of malformation. Therefore, the provision of imprecise risk information because the test is performed in a laboratory with an insufficient database or a system of reporting that offers imprecise risk estimation significantly impairs the quality of the patient's decision.

High-resolution ultrasound is one of the fundamental services of antenatal diagnosis. As noted above, the sensitivity and accuracy of this service is dependent on the skill and experience of the operator. Certainly the quality of the equipment is important also, but the skill and experience of the operator have a far greater impact on the overall quality of the service. Each institution must carefully and honestly evaluate the accuracy and sensitivity of sonographic diagnosis in its clinic in order to offer the patient a fair assessment of the confidence level in the case of her diagnosis.

Chorionic villus sampling is a relatively recent addition to the list of accepted antenatal diagnostic techniques. Discussed in some detail in Chapter 4, this technique offers the patient considerable temporal advantages. There continues to be the caution that there appears to be a greater risk of pregnancy loss after chorionic villus sampling compared with traditional amniocentesis, but that increase in risk may disappear with greater operator experience. Chorionic villus sampling remains a useful but primarily elective alternative to the more traditional amniocentesis.

Amniocentesis is the standard technique for obtaining fetal cells from which a karyotype may be derived. Traditionally performed between 15 and 18 weeks, the accepted risk of pregnancy loss ranges from 0.4% to 1.2%. In addition to this proven level of safety, another advantage of traditional amniocentesis is the greater sensitivity of the accompanying ultrasound for noncytogenetic structural anomalies.

Fetal blood sampling is an important antenatal diagnostic technique that was first reported in 1982 and has since become an accepted and useful tool in antenatal diagnosis for late registrants at risk for congenital disease. The risk of pregnancy loss after fetal blood sampling appears similar to that of amniocentesis, though the technical difficulty is somewhat greater. Most contemporary services offer fetal blood sampling in selected circumstances.

Table 1-2 Services of a Contemporary Antenatal Diagnosis Service

Maternal serum alpha-fetoprotein screening
High-resolution ultrasound (both transabdominal and transvaginal)
Fetal echocardiography, including Doppler
Chorionic villus sampling
Amniocentesis from 13 weeks
Fetal blood sampling from 16 weeks
Intrauterine transfusion
Magnetic resonance imaging
Computed tomography
Pediatric surgery
Neonatal intensive care
Pediatric anesthesia
Pediatric neurosurgery
Pediatric urology

The probability of success and the likelihood of complications are logically related to the degree of experience of the individual providing the service.

Magnetic resonance imaging (MRI) and computed tomography (CT) should be available to any comprehensive antenatal diagnosis program for selected cases where other more traditional techniques cannot provide a confident diagnosis and where the diagnosis is of sufficient significance that major management decisions hang in the balance. Occasionally, sonography clearly demonstrates abnormal fetal anatomy, but due to either acoustic artifact or other considerations, ultrasound cannot provide a conclusive diagnosis. Under such circumstances, MRI or CT might provide additional diagnostic data and allow a more confident diagnosis. Therefore, it is recommended that access to such services be investigated by any institution contemplating the organization of a comprehensive antenatal diagnostic service.

THE ANTENATAL DIAGNOSTIC PROCESS: COORDINATION AND SEQUENCING

A patient referral for antenatal diagnosis may be based on biochemical, clinical, historical, or sonographic screening. The patient might be referred with no knowledge about her condition, inaccurate or misleading information about her condition, or considerable but incomplete knowledge about her condition. The patient may be referred with only the generic risk of malformation associated with an abnormality of MSAFP, or for confirmation and care of a specific malformation detected by her local physician. An appropriate sequence of counseling and diagnostic testing should guide the patient through the prenatal testing process in a logical manner, resulting in the use of the least invasive testing procedures that provide a reliable diagnosis (Table 1-3).

Historical Review

The first step, optimally, is a review of previous records accompanying the patient and an interview to learn the patient's understanding of the basis for the referral. If the basis for the referral is a risk for a specific or nonspecific genetic disease, the subsequent discussion should include a review of genetic principles of inheritance on a level understood by the patient.

Mendelian principles such as autosomal recessive, autosomal dominant, or sex-linked recessive inheritance, if relevant to a specific patient, should be discussed. Principles of chromosomal structure and replication should be discussed if relevant. If the referral is based on exposure to environmental

Table 1-3 Sequence of Antenatal Diagnosis

1. Clinical screening
   Historical
   Physical
   Biochemical
   Sonographic
2. Initial referral interview
   Family history
   Review of records
   Patient education
3. Initial testing
   Ultrasound
4. Discussion of risk/benefit of further invasive testing: informed consent
5. Invasive testing if requested
   Chorionic villus sampling
   Amniocentesis
   Fetal blood sampling
6. Evaluation of test results
   Assessment of accuracy and precision
   Access to specialized consultation
   Evaluation of prognosis
7. Perinatal planning
   Timing, location, and method of delivery
8. Postnatal care
   Follow-up counseling

---

toxins, principles of teratology would be important to share with the patient to facilitate an understanding of the nature of any malformation detected.

Review of Relevant Tests

At some point during the process, a discussion of the risk, if any, and the accuracy and precision of the testing offered should take place. The patient should understand the limits of confidence of the diagnosis of a malformation or congenital condition, as well as the limits of confidence of exclusion of the diagnosis by a normal test. Rarely if ever does any antenatal test offer 100% confidence of either a specific positive diagnosis or a perfectly normal final outcome.

Invasive Testing: Informed Consent

Informed consent prior to invasive testing such as chorionic villus sampling, amniocentesis, or fetal blood sampling requires a fair and honest assessment of the risk of the procedure and the proposed benefit. The counseling that precedes any invasive test with potential morbidity (or mortality in the case of the fetus) must be neutral to be ethical. Antenatal diagnosis is rarely medically indicated and almost always elective. Truly informed consent is based on the provision of the necessary knowledge to allow the patient to make a decision herself with regard to any invasive test. If the bias of the counselor becomes the basis for the decision, then informed consent has not been obtained.

The sequencing of testing generally follows the principle of ascending risk. That is, those tests with least risk are performed first. Taking the history and the physical exam are generally without risk. Counseling is without risk, unless as a result of counselor bias an invasive and potentially morbid test results. Ultrasound is generally considered to be without risk, but prudent advice is to use it only when some clinical benefit is expected. Chorionic villus sampling, amniocentesis, and fetal blood sampling all are associated with a defined risk of excess pregnancy loss and therefore require prior informed consent. These tests are offered only when there is a specific risk for a specific abnormality that is detectable by no other means.

Counseling and Care after Positive Diagnosis

Once a diagnosis is made, a careful, complete, and accurate assessment of the diagnosis must be given to the patient, and she should also be given access to the kinds of special expertise reviewed above. It is often the genetic counselor who is critical here to the continuity of emotional care of the patient. It can be very important for the patient to maintain communication with the counselor in order to obtain a "common language" interpretation of highly specialized advice. It can be important for the counselor or other central coordinator to provide a simple, understandable summary of the prognosis and likely outcome in the case of the term birth of an infant with a specific congenital condition.

Following the diagnosis of a congenital disease or malformation, a plan must be made and implemented for the antenatal and perinatal care of the patient and her pregnancy. Such a plan is optimally made by the perinatologist in consultation with all relevant consultants and primarily with the patient. Location, timing, and method of delivery must be discussed and planned in advance to reduce the stress on the patient and the system, and to promote optimal outcome.

AFTER THE BIRTH

Finally, following the birth of the affected child, either as the result of an early termination or at term, it is important for the central coordinator to collect and assess all available information, including postnatal examinations either in the nursery or at autopsy, and synthesize this information into as complete an explanation as possible of this event. The complete collection and synthesis of this information may require considerable time and effort but offers the patient the greatest chance of completion of the experience and a healthy emotional adaptation.

Individualized service to the patient by her central coordinator also provides vital continuity of support in the case of the survivor who requires neonatal surgery or special care. Although the health care specialist providing care changes from perinatologist to pediatric surgeon or neonatologist at the time of birth, the continuity offered by the continued interest and involvement of the genetic counselor or social worker can be very important to the patient's sense of comfort and stability.

REGULAR REVIEW OF CLINICAL ACTIVITIES

The techniques of antenatal diagnosis are constantly evolving, and much of the value of techniques such as ultrasound is based on subjective interpretation. If the diagnostic and prognostic information provided to the patient is to be accurate, each member of the team assembled must be comfortable with his or her understanding of the test upon which the diagnosis is based, and the accuracy and confidence of the diagnosis. Furthermore, upon the detection of a fetal abnormality, the patient naturally has immediate questions about prognosis and outcome. Since access to specialized consultation is rarely immediate, it is of considerable benefit that all members of the diagnostic team develop opportunities to increase their general fund of knowledge with regard to these specific questions. It is equally useful for the pediatrician or pediatric surgeon to have a clear understanding of antenatal diagnostic techniques, including their accuracy and precision, since the perinatologist or sonologist may not always be available at the time of such a collateral consultation. A clear understanding of these complex issues is difficult unless some regular team communication takes place.

Optimally, then, a comprehensive antenatal diagnostic service holds regular conferences where cases and issues of accuracy and prognosis can be discussed and the general level of knowledge and understanding of all members of the team increased. Such prenatal diagnosis conferences provide a forum for the discussion of issues of importance to all team members listed in Table 1-1. Other colleagues within the health care system not directly involved with antenatal diagnosis often find such discussions useful as well. It is strongly recommended that any institution contemplating the organization of a comprehensive antenatal diagnostic service include a regularly scheduled review conference and encourage regular attendance by all concerned individuals.

Chapter 2

Patient Selection: Risk Assessment and Screening

Accurate and effective identification of patients at risk for congenital disease requires both historical and clinical sensitivity to detail. Risk identification is based on a combination of history, physical examination, and antenatal screening tests. A careful personal and family history about the birth of previous children with malformations or disabilities should be taken from each couple as they enter prenatal care. The initial physical examination should include attention to any subtle indications of parental malformation including stature. Ongoing care should pay careful attention to the growth of the uterus since certain malformations may lead to altered fetal growth and/or altered amniotic fluid volume. Finally, screening low-risk patients for certain malformations may be performed using either MSAFP screening or ultrasound, or both.

HISTORY

Historical factors that suggest an increased risk of fetal malformation or disease include the previous birth of a malformed child or a child affected by congenital disease; repetitive previous pregnancy losses, especially if accompanied by dysmorphology; and exposure to environmental factors known to be capable of causing fetal malformation (Table 2-1).

Although the majority of human malformation occurs without benefit of previous history, an understanding of the etiological basis of human congenital disease can be helpful. Etiologies of human malformation include Mendelian factors, which refer to congenital disease that results from defective genetic information associated with allelic genetic determinants that demonstrate consistent patterns of inheritance described as autosomal recessive, autosomal dominant, or sex-linked recessive. Mendelian factors are known to account for about 20% of human congenital disease, multifactorial/polygenic influences are blamed for another 15%, 10% is believed to result

Table 2-1 Historical Indications for Consideration of Antenatal Diagnosis

Maternal age over 35 years at the time of delivery
Previous birth of an infant with aneuploidy
Known parental balanced translocation
Multiple pregnancy losses
Previous stillbirth with unknown karyotype
Previous congenital malformation
Sonographic dysmorphology
Parents identified carriers for recessive condition
Mother identified carrier for X-linked condition
Close family history of congenital malformation or undiagnosed mental retardation

from environmental causes, and 5% is associated with aneuploidy. The remaining 50% results from unknown causes.

Autosomal Recessive Conditions

In the case of autosomal recessive disease, in the absence of consanguinity the risk for the birth of an affected child is very low in any family with no previous history of an affected infant (Table 2-2). After the birth of the proband (the first affected family member), the recurrence risk is 25%. Most often such congenital disease involves an incorrect gene determinant, resulting in the nonproduction or inadequate production of a critical metabolic enzyme or the production of a defective enzyme. For the expression of the disease, the defective gene must be present at both allelic sites of respective paired chromosomes. Sickle cell disease is an example of such an autosomal recessive condition.

Autosomal Dominant Conditions

In the case of autosomal dominant inheritance, the defective gene is required at only one of the two gene sites to result in expression of the disease

Table 2-2 Selected Autosomal Recessive Conditions

Cystic fibrosis
Sickle cell disease
Tay-Sachs disease
Osteogenesis imperfecta types II and III
Infantile polycystic kidney disease
Congenital adrenal hyperplasia
Phenylketonuria
Homocystinuria
Hepatolenticular degeneration

(Table 2-3). Examples of autosomal dominant inheritance are provided by many of the long bone dysplasias, such as achondroplasia. Although 50% of the offspring of an individual with an autosomal dominant condition would be expected to be affected, these conditions often occur in normal families as acute mutations, and therefore within that sibship (siblings of the proband) the risk of recurrence is often not increased.

Sex-Linked Recessive Conditions

The defective gene in the case of a sex-linked recessive condition is located on an X chromosome, and 50% of the male children of a mother carrying such a trait will be affected by the condition (Table 2-4). Hemophilia is an example of a sex-linked recessive condition. Carrier status may be ascertained by the previous birth of a hemophiliac child or by the identification of such a condition in a sibling coupled with carrier testing of the mother. It is interesting to note that a small percentage of heterozygous carrier mothers will be affected due to random inactivation in those few individuals of a majority of the X chromosomes carrying the normal allele for factor VIII.

Polygenic/Multifactorial Conditions

A large number of congenital malformations are considered to be the result of the interaction of several different influences and are designated as

---

Table 2-3 Autosomal Dominant Conditions

Achondroplasia
Osteogenesis imperfecta types I and IV
Porphyria: five of six types
Ehlers-Danlos syndrome
Marfan's syndrome
Myotonic dystrophy
Neurofibromatosis
Tuberous sclerosis
Noonan's syndrome
von Willebrand's disease

Table 2-4 Sex-Linked Recessive Conditions

Hemophilia A (factor VIII)
Hemophilia B (factor IX)
Duchenne muscular dystrophy
Glucose-6-phosphate dehydrogenase deficiency

polygenic or multifactorial. Certain epidemiologic patterns of expression characterize congenital malformations associated with multifactorial/ polygenic influences. First, such malformations typically affect single organ systems, such as the heart, central nervous system, gastrointestinal tract, or urinary tract. The initial incidence of each of these malformations is usually less than 1 to 2 in 1000, but the recurrence within a sibship is more than 10-fold greater, or closer to 3% to 5%. Furthermore, there is no family history in 95% of cases. These patterns of recurrence do not suggest Mendelian influences, but the 10-fold higher recurrence risk after the birth of such a child nevertheless suggests some genetic influences at work, even if only in a facilitative role.

Teratogenic Influences

Environmental or toxic factors are associated with 10% of human malformations (Table 2-5). These might be the rare but powerful influence of substances such as thalidomide or isotretinion, or the common but often more subtle influence of maternal alcohol ingestion. The result may be obvious and severe, as in the case of tetraphocomelia associated with thalidomide, or more subtle, as in the case of the vague facial dysplasia and learning disabilities often associated with fetal alcohol syndrome.

Aneuploidy

Finally, cytogenetic abnormalities such as trisomy, triploidy, or unbalanced translocations are potential causes of unexpected fetal congenital disease that receive considerable attention in the lay press. Fetal aneuploidy is, however, the cause of only 5% of human malformation of known etiology. Trisomies 21, 13, and 18 are the most common cytogenetic abnormalities identified in liveborn aneuploid fetuses. Although other trisomies undoubtedly occur, live birth is rare if not unknown. After the birth of an infant with a pure trisomy,

---

Table 2-5 Known Teratogens

Alcohol
Hydantoins
Folic acid antagonists
Lithium
Sex steroids
Tetracyclines
Thalidomide
Warfarin derivatives

the recurrence within that family of another such infant is estimated empirically to be between 1% and 2%, and prenatal diagnosis with subsequent pregnancies is usually offered. Trisomies 2 and 6 are commonly seen in karyotypes of early spontaneous abortions but not in liveborn or late pregnancy losses, as these apparently do not allow any significant development of a fetus.

Sex chromosome deletions or redundancies account for a large number of aneuploid live births but result in perhaps less severe disabilities, such as short stature or sterility. Intelligence is not typically impaired unless X chromosome counts exceed two. About 5% of cases of Down syndrome are the result not of pure trisomy but of unbalanced translocation (i.e., a balanced translocation present in the karyotype of a phenotypically normal parent that is transmitted unbalanced to a conceptus). In the case of a maternal balanced translocation, the risk of birth of an infant with an unbalanced translocation is 8% to 10%, whereas if the father is the carrier, the risk is only about 2%. The reasons for this discrepancy in risk are not clear.

Triploidy (3N chromatin material) or tetraploidy (4N chromatin material), designating conditions with duplication of entire sets of chromosomes, are rare causes of congenital disease that are incompatible with survival and often incompatible with development even beyond the first trimester. Significant fetal dysmorphology such as severe ventral wall defects, holoprosencephaly, and severe early intrauterine growth retardation have been associated with these conditions.

Unknown Etiology

Approximately half of all human congenital disease is without known cause. Undoubtedly the vast majority, if the cause were known, would fall into one of the above-mentioned categories, and in fact, family counseling must often be done without knowledge of the specific inheritance pattern involved. If the proband did not undergo an autopsy, or the autopsy was performed by a pathologist who was inexperienced in examining infants or fetuses with dysmorphology, accurate information necessary to establish a confident diagnosis and appropriate family counseling may have been lost.

Congenital metabolic disease is often counseled as autosomal recessive. The birth of an infant with a condition known to be autosomal dominant may have been the result of acute mutation, with a very low probability of recurrence. Isolated single organ system malformations are usually attributed to multifactorial or possibly environmental factors. In many instances, there is a history of the birth of an infant with congenital malformations or disease that was subsequently not carefully examined, so that the exact nature of the condition cannot be known at the time of counseling or prenatal encounter. Therefore, the estimated probability of recurrence may range from near zero to as high as 25% if the condition might have a recessive character. In cases where there is a history of congenital disease of unknown etiology, prenatal diagnosis in the form of both ultrasound and karyotype determination should be considered. Fetal visualization with ultrasound, amniocentesis, and fetal blood sampling must be discussed with the patient in light of their potential for detecting a recurrence of the previous condition.

CLINICAL CLUES FOR CONGENITAL DISEASE

Amniotic Fluid Volume Abnormalities

A uterus that is larger or smaller than expected for gestational age may be the result of inaccurate clinical dates, abnormal fetal growth, or an abnormality of amniotic fluid volume. Amniotic fluid is the result of a complex equilibrium between sources of amniotic fluid and pathways for its removal. The fetus is both the source of amniotic fluid in the form of urine and active in its removal, by swallowing. A fetal malformation may cause either increased or decreased production of urine or, conversely, impaired removal and either abnormality would result in a clinically detectable abnormality of fluid volume.

Polyhydramnios

Normally, the curvilinear measurement of the pregnant uterus in centimeters above the pubic symphysis between 20 and 35 weeks is approximately equal to the gestational age in weeks. Relatively few studies have been done to document the precision of this relationship, but those that are available suggest that the limits of normal variation are about 4 cm above or below this standard. Therefore, if a uterus measures 4 cm more than expected, or 4 cm less, it is reasonable to request an ultrasound examination to determine the basis for the discrepancy.

Polyhydramnios complicates between 0.5% and 1.0% of pregnancies. Although the standard definition of polyhydramnios is a volume of 2000 mL or more, such a definition is both inappropriate for the whole range of gestational ages and clinically irrelevant since no safe method is available to accurately estimate the volume of fluid. This standard is the product of studies that established normal volumes and limits of normal using double amniocentesis techniques and dye dilution. Since a double amniocentesis procedure carries a risk of complication, it is rarely justified. The clinical definition of polyhydramnios, therefore, becomes the more practical approach and is based on a uterus large for dates, ballotable fetal parts, a distant fetal heart, and ultrasonic confirmation of appropriate fetal dimensions, with the excess uterine volume visibly the result of amniotic fluid excess.

Polyhydramnios is not a unique disease itself but the result of a variety of influences. Approximately one third of cases are the result of either diabetes or Rh disease, and another third are idiopathic, without detectable maternal or fetal disease. The final third result from congenital fetal malformation or malfunction. The fetal malformations that might cause polyhydramnios include craniospinal malformations, thoracic or abdominal malformations, or abdominal and urinary tract malformations. The majority of these are detectable with ultrasound and will be reviewed in greater detail in later chapters. In general, these malformations affect amniotic fluid equilibrium by increasing fetal urine production or by decreasing the efficiency of fetal ingestion or absorption of the fluid.

Many craniospinal malformations result in increased intracranial pressure and decreased secretion of fetal antidiuretic hormone, with increased fetal urine production. Esophageal obstruction may occur either from congenital atresia or extrinsic compression from either hydrothorax or cardiomegaly. Duodenal or proximal small bowel obstruction, either from intrinsic malformation or extrinsic compression, is also associated with polyhydramnios, and large bowel obstruction, especially when perforation and meconium peritonitis result, is also associated with polyhydramnios. Small bowel functional obstruction and polyhydramnios may also complicate fetal ventral wall malformations. Urinary tract malformations can be seen to cause increased amniotic fluid. Complete ureteropelvic junction obstruction will result in severe hydronephrosis and enlargement of the renal pelvis or a large retroperitoneal urinoma that can achieve sufficient size to cause significant bowel compression and resulting polyhydramnios. Prune-belly syndrome with megacystis, bilateral hydroureter, and bilateral hydronephrosis, but without physical urinary tract obstruction, can also be associated with polyhydramnios. Finally, many congenital short limb dysplasias are associated with polyhydramnios. Most, but not all, of the short limb conditions with polyhydramnios also demonstrate significant fetal thoracodystrophy (very small chest with compression of intrathoracic soft tissues) and presumably cause the increased amniotic fluid by esophageal compression within a very small chest. A few mild types of limb dysplasias without thoracodystrophy may also be seen with polyhydramnios, and the explanation for the amniotic fluid excess in these cases is unclear.

The majority of fetal malformations associated with polyhydramnios are detectable by ultrasound. It is reasonable to conclude that if a fetal malformation is the cause of the excess fluid, the malformation will in the majority of cases be detectable with careful high-resolution ultrasound.

Oligohydramnios

A uterus that is significantly small for the gestational age can result from an error in clinical dates, severe intrauterine growth retardation, or deficiency of amniotic fluid. A patent, functional fetal urinary tract is not necessary for amniotic fluid prior to 20 weeks' gestation, but after 20 weeks little amniotic fluid will be seen without fetal urine production. Lack of fetal urine contribution to the amniotic cavity can result from renal agenesis, dysplasia, obstruction, or even unrecognized leakage of amniotic fluid. Renal agenesis or bilateral dysplasia would cause oligohydramnios, with no visible fluid accumulation within the uterus or fetus. Urethral obstruction or bilateral complete ureteropelvic junction obstruction (rare) will result in severe oligohydramnios but also in accumulation of urine and visible dilatation of the system above the obstruction within the fetal trunk. Each of these conditions is explored in greater detail in later chapters.

The prognosis for the fetus in cases of severe oligohydramnios is largely determined by the specific malformation or condition that is the cause of the decreased fluid. It is, however, often impossible to confidently diagnose the specific lesion, due to the impaired clarity of the images in the case of oligohydramnios. Severe oligohydramnios, however, even in the absence of a specific diagnosis, carries a very poor empiric prognosis. Sustained fetal development in an environment of severely decreased amniotic fluid is associated with a high incidence of fetal pulmonary hypoplasia, as well as skeletal and facial deformities. The pulmonary hypoplasia results in an inability to ventilate and oxygenate the infants, and most often neonatal death occurs shortly after birth.

MATERNAL SERUM ALPHA-FETOPROTEIN SCREENING

In addition to a careful history and careful physical screening for clues to the possibility of a fetal malformation, maternal screening based on the concentration of alpha-fetoprotein in maternal serum can be an important source of information that may lead to the detection of fetal malformations.

Alpha-fetoprotein is a major fetal serum protein similar to albumin but immunologically distinct. It is produced initially in the yolk sac and later in the fetal liver and peaks in fetal serum at about 14 weeks, decreasing thereafter. Its concentration slowly increases in both amniotic fluid and maternal serum between 15 and 20 weeks' gestation, but at much lower levels than in fetal serum. Alpha-fetoprotein is 50,000 times more concentrated in fetal serum than in maternal serum at 16 weeks.

Alpha-fetoprotein may be measured in maternal serum by radioimmunoassay in picograms per mL; however, most reference laboratories report results in multiples of the median (MOM) because this value is statistically more normally distributed, making analysis and clinical correlation easier.

The potential benefit of MSAFP screening is that the MSAFP levels in the case of pregnancies complicated by certain fetal malformations are often higher than in uncomplicated pregnancies. The average level of MSAFP values from pregnancies complicated by open neural tube defects, ventral wall defects, and severe oligohydramnios is significantly elevated. However, since there is substantial overlap between the MSAFP distribution curves of the abnormal pregnancies and those of normal pregnancies, the test is not diagnostic of an abnormality, only suggestive of increased risk.

The level of MSAFP chosen as a cutoff between "normal pregnancy" and a pregnancy needing further diagnostic testing is arbitrary. A low cutoff would result in a larger proportion of abnormalities being selected for further evaluation (higher sensitivity), but also a much larger proportion of those selected would be normal since a greater portion of the normal curve would lie above the chosen cutoff. Furthermore, the normal curve contains so many more pregnancies than the distribution curve describing affected infants that a larger proportion of those above the cutoff would be unaffected. This would result in a lower predictive value. A high cutoff would result in a higher proportion of those selected as abnormal actually having an abnormality (higher predictive value), but a lower proportion of the total number of pregnancies complicated by the targeted fetal malformations will be detected (lower sensitivity).

Each MSAFP screening program must establish its own database and cutoff values because of assay variability and population risk variability. The laboratory assay for MSAFP is very sensitive to minor procedural variation. Quality control procedures, including the processing of blinded control samples, are mandatory to maintain reasonable accuracy, but even with such measures, results from one specific laboratory are not interchangeable with another laboratory. Each program must accumulate an individual database of MSAFP values, calculate medians, and establish clinical relevance through experience. Furthermore, the incidence of some malformations varies with geographic area. Open neural tube defects, for instance, decrease in incidence from North to South and from East to West. Since the general population risk is used to calculate relative risk estimates from MSAFP values, an MSAFP database accumulated from one geographic area cannot be used to evaluate assay results from another.

The appropriate cutoff for MSAFP will vary depending on maternal race, medical condition, previous history, and weight. Each of these can either influence the basic risk of an open neural tube defect, and therefore alter the relative risk estimate, or alter the MSAFP levels. No single cutoff is accurate or appropriate for a specific screening program or a specific patient, but some generalities are at least descriptive of the process. The cutoffs chosen for each program and group of patients are typically intended to provide for the detection of at least 80% of cases of open neural tube defects. This is a compromise, as mentioned above, between sensitivity and predictive value. This means that perhaps one out of five cases of open neural tube defect will have an MSAFP value within the normal range. A higher sensitivity is possible, but only at the expense of a much higher number of cases being selected for further testing when there is not, in fact, a fetal malformation.

It is estimated that given a cutoff for a program that provides this level of sensitivity for open neural tube defects, the positive predictive value for an elevated MSAFP test result is about 5%. This means that only about 1 out of 20 cases with an elevation actually is a case complicated by an open neural tube defect. Another 1 to 2 infants out of the 20 will have another congenital malformation, such as severe oligohydramnios or a ventral wall defect.

In the case of an elevated MSAFP, the most appropriate next step is to repeat the test. The MSAFP level is elevated in about 5% of cases, and about a third of these will be normal upon repeat. Such a transient elevation can result from a small fetomaternal bleeding episode. The MSAFP concentration is about 50,000 times higher in fetal compared with maternal blood, so even a small leakage can result in a transient elevation. On occasion, testing of maternal blood (Kleihauer-Betke test) can reveal the presence of fetal red cells. If the MSAFP is elevated on repeat, targeted high-detail ultrasound is indicated. In about one third of these cases, the elevated MSAFP is explained by correction of gestational age, diagnosis of twins, or the diagnosis of fetal death. Fetal malformations are detected in about 10% of cases (the sum of neural tube defects and the others). The sensitivity of high-detail ultrasound for neural tube defects, ventral wall defects, and severe oligohydramnios should exceed 95% if adequate images are possible. Maternal obesity and fetal position can, however, influence the adequacy of the examination.

In the event of an elevated MSAFP with an adequate and normal high-detail ultrasound examination, amniocentesis should be considered for further evaluation. Analysis of amniotic fluid for alpha-fetoprotein offers a sensitivity of over 99% for neural tube defects. Analysis of the fluid for acetylcholinesterase, if the amniotic fluid alpha-fetoprotein is elevated, offers a final confirmation of the presence of an open neural tube defect. Amniocentesis is not, however, without risk. Estimates of excess pregnancy loss following amniocentesis vary from 0.5% to 1.2%. In considering the decision, the patient should consider the adequacy of the ultrasound and balance the risk of amniocentesis against a revised estimate of relative risk of malformation, using the 90% to 95% sensitivity of ultrasound. In other words, whatever the relative risk for an open neural tube defect based on the MSAFP alone, it may be reduced by at least 90% if an adequate high-detail ultrasound examination is performed by an experienced examiner (see Chapter 6). The decision regarding amniocentesis should be based on the revised relative risk estimate compared with the risk of amniocentesis.

ULTRASOUND SCREENING

Routine ultrasound screening of low-risk pregnancy is not advocated in the United States by any national public organization. The basis for this is at least in part the product of a National Institutes of Health Consensus Development Conference that in 1984 published a review of the then-current literature that failed to find sufficient evidence of benefit from low-risk screening to justify such a recommendation. The report of the conference did not prohibit routine screening; it only concluded that there was insufficient evidence of benefit to promote it. The report did cite 28 recognized clinical indications for ultrasound screening. It has been estimated that diligent application of these approved indications would result in ultrasound examination of at least half of most prenatal populations. In other countries, particularly in Western Europe, routine ultrasound screening is advocated, and sonographic screening is performed in up to 80% of pregnancies.

Although no documented reproducible evidence exists that diagnostic ultrasound causes any effect, harmful or otherwise, to the human pregnancy, it remains the obligation of the clinician to justify any proposed ultrasound examination on the basis of proposed benefit. The most likely benefits proposed by proponents of routine ultrasound include confirmation of gestational age, early diagnosis of multiple gestation, early confirmation of placental location, and the provision of baseline data for later fetal growth evaluation. The detection of fetal malformations by routine ultrasound screening in a historically and clinically low-risk population is the least likely benefit of the procedure. Campbell, in 1984, in fact, reported the detection of 34 out of only 39 possible fetal malformations during the screening of 11,684 low-risk pregnancies.

However, a great many fetal malformations will be found at the time of ultrasound examination for clinical indications. The careful historical screening of prenatal patients for risk for genetic disease is not universally practiced, and therefore a great many patients with some increase in risk go unexamined.

REFERRAL

When a patient is identified as being potentially at increased risk for the birth of an infant with congenital disease, the nature of the risk, the degree of risk, and the appropriate procedures necessary to further evaluate the pregnancy should be explained carefully to her. In most cases it will be appropriate to refer the patient to a comprehensive antenatal diagnostic service where appropriate genetic counseling and diagnostic testing are offered.

The choice of referral resource for the practicing physician is not only based on an assessment of the quality and accuracy of the services offered to the patient but often also turns on his or her assessment of the quality of feedback. The referring physician benefits most from a service that offers prompt and complete referral feedback in the form of a letter of summary, as well as direct feedback in the case of referrals made after the local detection of sonographic dysmorphology. The failure to provide good follow-up information to the referring physician despite excellent services to the patient should result in the referring physician's researching the availability of alternative referral services that do provide such follow-up.

FURTHER READING

Bakketeig LS, Jacobsen G, Brodkorb CJ, et al. Randomised controlled trial of ultrasonographic screening in pregnancy. *Lancet.* 1984; 2:207.

Belfrage P, Fernstrom I, Hallenberg G. Routine or selective ultrasound examinations in early pregnancy. *Obstet Gynecol.* 1987; 69:747.

Diagnostic Ultrasound Imaging in Pregnancy. NIH Publication No. 84–667. Washington: Government Printing Office; 1984.

Hill LM, Breckle R, Gehrking WC, et al. Prenatal detection of congenital malformations by ultrasonography. *Am J Obstet Gynecol.* 1985; 151:44.

Hook EB, Cross PK, Schreinemachers DM, et al. Chromosomal abnormality rates at amniocentesis and in live born infants. *JAMA.* 1983; 249:2034.

Main DM, Mennuti MT. Neural tube defects: Issues in prenatal diagnosis and counseling. *Obstet Gynecol.* 1986; 67:1

Persson PH, Kullander S. Long-term experience of general ultrasound screening in pregnancy. *Am J Obstet Gynecol.* 1983; 146:942.

Royal College of Obstetricians and Gynecologists. *Report of the RCOG Working Party on Routine Ultrasound Examination in Pregnancy.* December 1984. Available from The Royal College, 27 Sussex Place, Regent's Park, London NW 1 4RG.

Simpson, JL. Genetic counseling and prenatal diagnosis. In: Gabbe SG, Niebyl JF, Simpson JL, eds. *Obstetrics: Normal and Problem Pregnancies.* New York: Churchill-Livingstone; 1986.

Simpson JL, Elias S, Gatlin M, Martin AO. Genetic counseling services in obstetrics and gynecology. *Am J Obstet Gynecol.* 1981; 140:70.

Simpson JL, Golbus MS, Martin AO, Sarto GE. *Genetics in Obstetrics and Gynecology.* New York: Grune & Stratton; 1982

Vintzileos AM, et al. Antenatal evaluation and management of ultrasonically detected fetal anomalies. *Obstet Gynecol.* 1987; 69:640.

Chapter 3

Ultrasound and Doppler

Real-time ultrasound imaging plays a central role in any contemporary antenatal diagnosis program. The ability to visualize fetal anatomy with high-detail resolution allows not only the recognition of normal and abnormal anatomy but also the precise guidance of invasive instruments for the relatively safe acquisition of amniotic fluid, fetal blood, and chorionic villi. The common use of ultrasound in pregnancy is a relatively recent development. Although the human medical use of ultrasound first occurred over 40 years ago, real-time ultrasound equipment (ultrasound images showing movement in real time) first became commercially available in 1977, and widespread usage of real-time ultrasound only became a reality in the early 1980s.

The analysis of Doppler frequency changes in echoes of ultrasound pulses reflected from moving red blood cells within fetal blood vessels allows precise examination of blood flow velocity patterns that can lead to the antenatal diagnosis of fetal malformations, as well as monitor fetal condition.

Ultrasound is physically noninvasive and painless. There is no documented, reproducible effect, harmful or otherwise, on human pregnancy. In this chapter we briefly review the technology of ultrasound and Doppler velocity analysis, as a basis for much of what follows in this book.

ULTRASOUND

Sound energy is kinetic energy in the form of physical agitation of the molecules of a medium resulting in the temporary distortion of intermolecular spatial relationships that is transmitted through a medium by the resilience of intermolecular forces. Typically, sound is depicted as alternate phases of high and low pressure or density, radiating from the surface of a sound source (Figure 3-1). As the generating surface compresses or rarifies the layer of medium in immediate proximity, intermolecular forces act to re-establish the norm and thereby transmit the energy of the initial distortion event to the next adjacent area of the medium. The alternate phases of high and low pressure or density within the transmission medium are usually depicted by a graphic

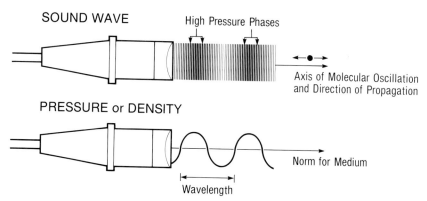

Figure 3-1 Illustrated here is the pressure waveform generated from the surface of a single-crystal ultrasound transducer. Although the molecular movement occurs in a horizontal axis, the graphic representation of the molecular pressure or density rises or falls in the vertical plane. *Source*: Reprinted from *Practical Obstetrical Ultrasound* (p 4) by JW Seeds and RC Cefalo, Aspen Publishers Inc, © 1986.

sine curve that shows wavelength, frequency, and amplitude. Sound with a frequency between 20 and 20,000 cycles per second is within the human audible range. Sound with frequencies above 20,000 cycles per second (20,000 Hz) is called ultrasound. Ultrasound used in medical imaging applications uses frequencies between 2.5 million and 10 million cycles per second (2.5 to 10 MHz), usually between 2.5 and 5.0 MHz in obstetrical applications.

The physical source for the production of sound of such high frequency is the piezoelectric crystal. Piezoelectric crystals have the natural quality of

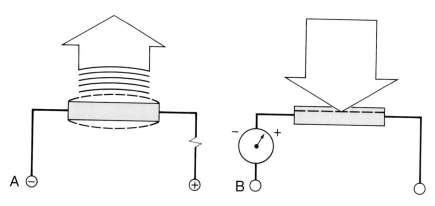

Figure 3-2 The piezoelectric crystal alters its shape in response to electrical stimulation and generates a small electric potential if exposed to incoming sound energy. *Source*: Reprinted from *Practical Obstetrical Ultrasound* (p 5) by JW Seeds and RC Cefalo, Aspen Publishers Inc, © 1986.

changing their shape and vibrating at very high frequencies when stimulated with a brief electric potential (Figure 3-2), thus providing the basis for the production of ultrasound. Conversely, when such a crystal is in the path of sound energy, alternately exposed to high- and low-pressure peaks and troughs, the crystal produces a tiny electric potential. Piezoelectric crystals, therefore, represent both the source and sensitive detectors for ultrasound. Quartz is a naturally occurring piezoelectric crystal, but the majority of ultrasound machines use synthetic piezoelectric crystals.

Contemporary real-time ultrasound machines produce high-resolution images that depict movement in real time. Piezoelectric crystals are positioned within the ultrasound transducer in a very precise linear order. The linear alignment of the crystals and the precise sequencing of their electronic stimulation produces rapid, repetitive parallel pulses of sound energy that

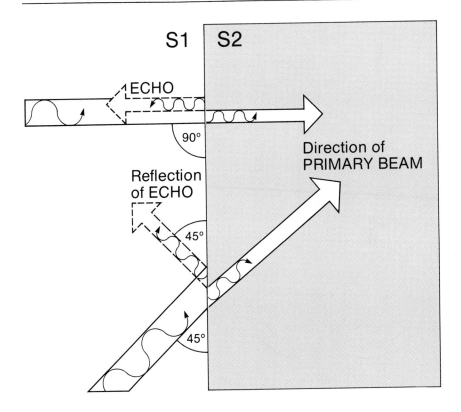

Figure 3-3 When sound pulses encounter surfaces between tissues of different acoustical impedance, echoes are created. The upper echo is reflected back to the source, with the amplitude of the echo being subtracted from the amplitude of the incoming pulse. The lower echo is reflected at an angle equal to the angle of incidence. *Source*: Reprinted from *Practical Obstetrical Ultrasound* (p 7) by JW Seeds and RC Cefalo, Aspen Publishers Inc, © 1986.

provide the echo information required for imaging. Imaging systems are not based on the production of continuous sound from each crystal element but rather on the production of brief sound pulses. In a typical system, a given crystal would generate a microsecond of sound energy every millisecond. This pulse-echo technique allows each crystal to be both transmitter and receiver.

Sound pulses interact with tissue surfaces by either passing through them or reflecting from them (Figure 3-3). Since energy is not created at the surface encountered, the amplitude of the echo generated at the surface must be subtracted from the amplitude of the through-transmitted pulse. Older static picture ultrasound machines created composite images from a large number of such echoes generated by a single moving crystal contacting the surface of the patient (Figure 3-4).

The feature of sound transmission through human tissue that allows the construction of images is the reflection of sound at surfaces between unlike

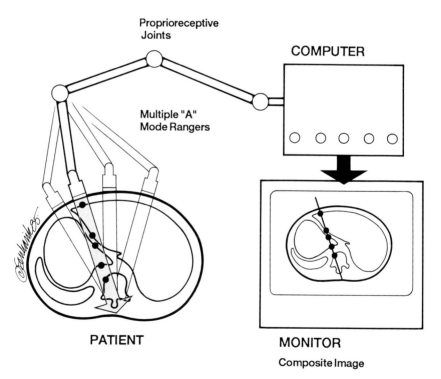

Figure 3-4 The first ultrasound imagers produced composite images constructed from echoes along a series of scan pulses produced as a single transducer was moved across the surface of the patient. All of the echoes were geometrically referenced to the starting point. If movement occurred during the construction of the image, clarity was lost. *Source*: Reprinted from *Practical Obstetrical Ultrasound* (p 9) by JW Seeds and RC Cefalo, Aspen Publishers Inc, © 1986.

tissues, which produces the echoes. Each tissue demonstrates a unique resistance to intermolecular spatial distortion, called acoustical impedance or "intermolecular stiffness." Adjacent tissues of identical acoustic impedance produce no echoes from incident sound at the surface separating them (interface). But as adjacent tissues begin to differ in acoustic impedance, a portion of an incident sound will be reflected as an echo. The greater the discrepancy between the two tissues, the stronger the echo.

If a sound pulse encounters an echo-producing surface at a right angle, the echo will return to the source, and the detection of that echo along with accurate temporal analysis of the interval between original pulse generation and time of echo reception will provide important information for the construction of an image. If, however, the pulse encounters a surface at any angle other than 90°, the echo is reflected at an equal angle, and it is lost in

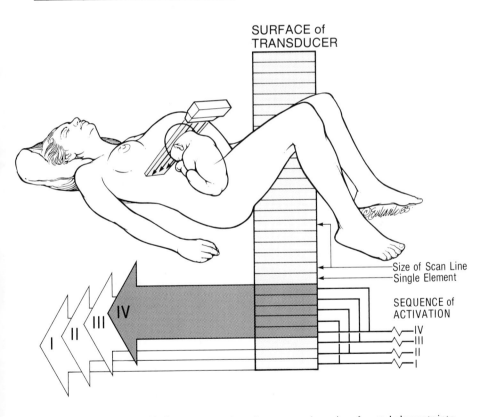

Figure 3-5 The linear array real-time transducer incorporated a series of crystal elements into the surface of the transducer with a fixed relationship to one another. Teams of crystals were stimulated in overlapping sequence to produce scanlines that were integrated into images showing movement in real time. *Source*: Reprinted from *Practical Obstetrical Ultrasound* (p 10) by JW Seeds and RC Cefalo, Aspen Publishers Inc, © 1986.

terms of contributing to an image. The distance between the surface of the transducer and the surface producing the echo is precisely estimated using the time of generation of the primary pulse, the time of detection of the echo, and the speed of sound in soft tissue, which is an agreed international convention of 1540 m/sec. An image of soft tissue may therefore be constructed using the echo information accumulated from each of the crystal elements within a transducer and updated many times a second, producing an image with real-time movement.

The linear array transducer provides for a field of view that is rectangular in shape, with a useful depth of penetration that will vary with the complexity of the tissue within the field (Figure 3-5). Another type of transducer is the mechanical sector transducer, which produces a wedge-shaped field of view, generated by a rotating or oscillating crystal within the transducer head. The moving crystal is stimulated only within a 90° arc or sector, producing a field of view that is divergent, with a small near field or aperture. A third type of transducer is the convex array or curvilinear transducer. It is a nonmechanical phased array, similar to a linear array but with a convex contact surface that

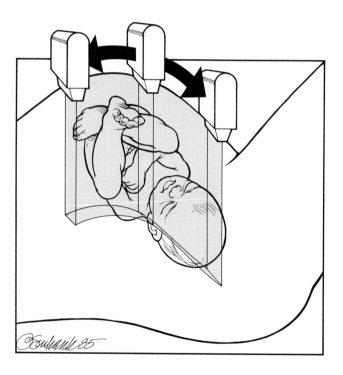

Figure 3-6 One of the three cardinal movements of a real-time ultrasound transducer is the sliding movement. *Source*: Reprinted from *Practical Obstetrical Ultrasound* (p 24) by JW Seeds and RC Cefalo, Aspen Publishers Inc, © 1986.

gives a trapezoidal shape to the field of view, with divergent sides. The convex array transducer has a broader near field than the older mechanical sector transducer and no noticeable loss of image quality in the far field, which was typical of the mechanical sector transducer.

All of the real-time transducers are freely mobile in the hand of the examiner. This freedom of movement, while greatly increasing the flexibility of image construction, can create confusion unless the operator exercises discipline in the movement of the transducer. The three basic movements possible with the transducer are a sliding movement (Figure 3-6), an angling movement (Figure 3-7), and a rotating movement (Figure 3-8). The experienced examiner usually makes movements that are complex combinations of all three of these, but it is recommended that the inexperienced operator try to use each movement individually until greater confidence is gained in image construction.

It is further recommended that the image display on the viewscreen be formatted in a consistent manner with each examination. The generally

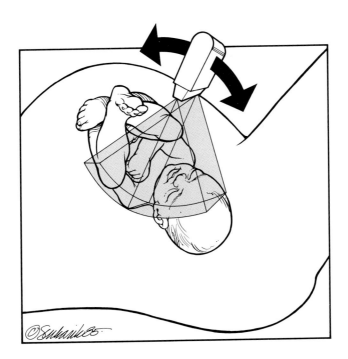

Figure 3-7 The angulation movement is another basic transducer movement often useful in constructing precisely the scanplane required for specific anatomic visualization. *Source*: Reprinted from *Practical Obstetrical Ultrasound* (p 26) by JW Seeds and RC Cefalo, Aspen Publishers Inc, © 1986.

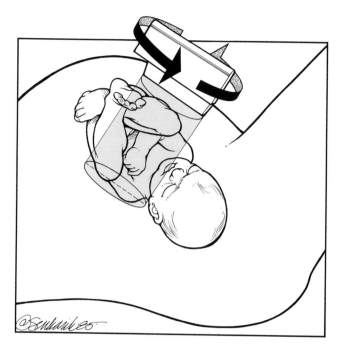

Figure 3-8 The rotational movement is the third of the basic movements possible with a real-time freehand ultrasound transducer. *Source*: Reprinted from *Practical Obstetrical Ultrasound* (p 25) by JW Seeds and RC Cefalo, Aspen Publishers Inc, © 1986.

accepted format in the longitudinal orientation is that the lower uterus be displayed to the right of the screen and the fundus to the left (Figure 3-9). In the transverse orientation, the accepted convention is for the patient's right to appear on the left of the screen (Figure 3-10).

The nature of the ultrasound image is unique, compared with other imaging systems. Although tissue density is related to echogenicity, the relationship between density and echogenicity is not direct, and it is strongly influenced by the complexity of the tissue surface. Since echoes are produced at surfaces between dissimilar tissues, a soft tissue organ such as lung or liver will appear echodense because of the many closely mingled internal surfaces, without necessarily implying great density or calcification. Fat tissue typically appears echodense because of the many internal surfaces, though quite soft in physical texture. One characteristic of truly calcified structures that is missing from ultrasound images of echodense soft tissues is acoustical shadowing. An acoustical shadow is essentially a black, echo-free (anechoic) area distal to the bone or calcified structure. The shadow simply indicates that the machine detects no echoes from that area and therefore depicts it as black. So even a very echodense structure that produces no shadowing is likely to be complex soft tissue, not bone.

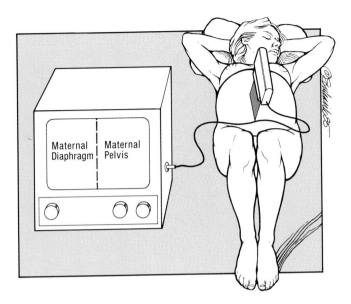

Figure 3-9 The accepted convention for image format in the longitudinal scanplane is to depict the maternal diaphragm to the left of the viewscreen and the pelvis to the right. *Source*: Reprinted from *Practical Obstetrical Ultrasound* (p 23) by JW Seeds and RC Cefalo, Aspen Publishers Inc, © 1986.

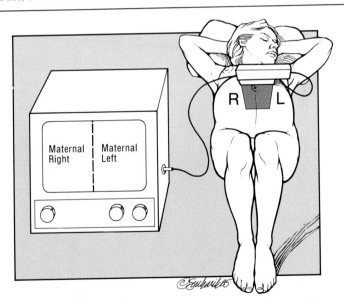

Figure 3-10 On transverse scanning, the viewscreen should be arranged to show the maternal right on the left side of the screen and the maternal left on the right side of the screen. *Source*: Reprinted from *Practical Obstetrical Ultrasound* (p 22) by JW Seeds and RC Cefalo, Aspen Publishers Inc, © 1986.

Another important characteristic of ultrasound images is that any homogeneous fluid of whatever composition appears anechoic (black). The absence of surfaces within fluid results in the absence of echoes from that area. The viewscreen therefore depicts that area as black. The fluid may be maternal or fetal urine, amniotic fluid, blood, or ovarian cyst fluid. In the case of the nonpregnant patient or the very early pregnancy, a full bladder offers advantages, such as displacing gas-containing maternal small bowel out of the pelvis to allow imaging of deep pelvic anatomy. Amniotic fluid nicely outlines the fetal surface and allows the diagnosis of malformations that alter or distort fetal shape. Cerebrospinal fluid allows the evaluation of anatomy such as cerebral ventricles. Fetal blood highlights intracardiac anatomy, and fetal urine outlines both normal and abnormal fetal urinary tract anatomy. The echocontrast between all of these normal fluids and adjacent soft tissue is a cornerstone of ultrasonic diagnosis.

Clinical Applications of Ultrasound

Real-time ultrasound provides a tomogram of anatomy. Anatomy on either side of the image onscreen is not seen. The quality of an ultrasound examination, therefore, is uniquely subjective. If the examiner does not specifically produce an image of the relevant anatomy by the proper positioning of the transducer, it is not seen. Furthermore, if the relevant anatomy is not imaged, it will not likely be captured in any permanent image documentation, such as still pictures or even videotape.

Each obstetrical ultrasound examination must include a minimum amount of information in order to minimize missed or inaccurate clinical information. Content may be divided into three categories, including a uterine survey, fetal biometry, and a review of fetal anatomy (Table 3-1). The survey should document fetal number, position, viability, amniotic fluid volume, and placental location. The list of possible fetal measurements is large, but each examination should measure at least a biparietal diameter and a long bone, usually a femur, and abdominal circumference or mean diameter if indicated. The review of fetal anatomy should include craniospinal anatomy and thoracoabdominal anatomy, including the urinary tract. Careful and methodical attention to these elements will avoid most errors of omission. The ultrasound examination of the obstetrical patient at low risk for fetal malformation is intended to provide relevant clinical information, not primarily a high-detail anatomic examination. If the patient offers historical or clinical indications of increased risk status for a fetal malformation, then the clinician should consider referral for evaluation by a unit experienced with the detection of fetal anomalies. Everyone performing obstetrical ultrasound, however, should follow a careful plan in order to avoid obvious management errors.

Table 3-1   Components of Standard Obstetrical Ultrasound Examination

Uterine survey
- Fetal number
- Fetal viability
- Fetal position
- Amniotic fluid volume
- Placental location and appearance

Fetal biometry
- Biparietal diameter (average of three)
- Abdominal circumference or mean diameter
- Femur length

Fetal anatomic survey
- Craniospinal anatomy
  —Lateral ventricles
  —Posterior fossa including cerebellum
  —Longitudinal and transverse spinal views
- Thoracoabdominal anatomy
  —Four-chamber cardiac view
  —Stomach
  —Umbilical insertion site
- Urinary tract
  —Kidneys
  —Bladder

DOPPLER

Sound reflected from an object moving toward or away from the sound source is altered in frequency. If the object is moving toward the source, the frequency is higher, and if the object is moving away from the source, the frequency is lower (Figure 3-11). The degree of change in frequency is proportional to the speed of the object and to the angle between the direction of propagation of the sound and the direction of movement of the object (angle of insonation or interrogation). If these quantities are known, the speed of the object may be calculated. If the object is a red cell within a deep vessel, such as the umbilical artery, the velocity of flow may be determined. If the size of the vessel is known, the quantity of flow may be calculated.

Unfortunately, the angle of insonation is often difficult to determine, and the cross-sectional area of the umbilical artery and many other arteries is constantly changing in response to the pressure waves, making accurate calculation of volume flow difficult. However, there are characteristics of blood velocity that may have clinical value both in the evaluation of high-risk pregnancies and in prenatal diagnosis.

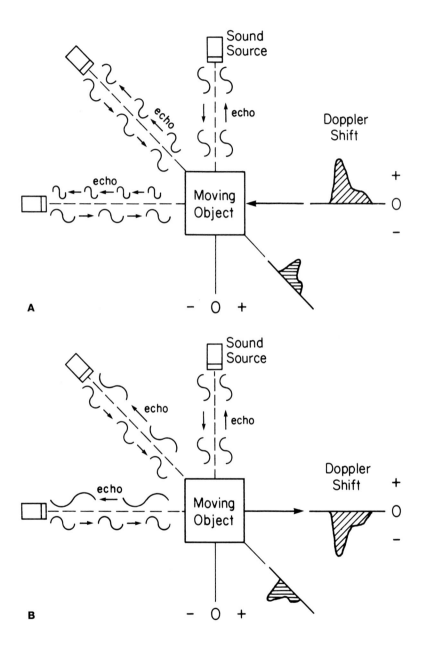

Figure 3-11 A, Illustrated here is the relationship of an object moving toward a sound source, resulting in a positive frequency shift (positive Doppler shift) for the echoes. The Doppler shift is less if the angle of insonation is anything but zero degrees, and the shift is zero if the angle is 90°. **B,** This drawing is similar to A but with the object moving away from the sound source. Note the longer wavelength and the negative Doppler frequency shift, which is similarly less when the angle of insonation is anything but zero degrees.

There are two types of Doppler devices available for clinical use. The continuous wave (CW) Doppler device uses at least two crystals in the transducer (Figure 3-12). One is continuously producing sound while the other is listening for echoes. Clear disadvantages of such a system include an inability to accurately estimate the angle of insonation, the inability to isolate the signal from a specific depth, and the interference of any movement occurring between the vessel of interest and the transducer.

CONTINUOUS WAVE DOPPLER

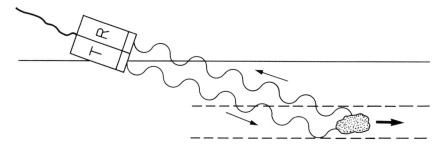

Figure 3-12 The continuous wave Doppler transducer uses both a transmitting crystal and a receiving crystal to interrogate the moving red cells within a vessel.

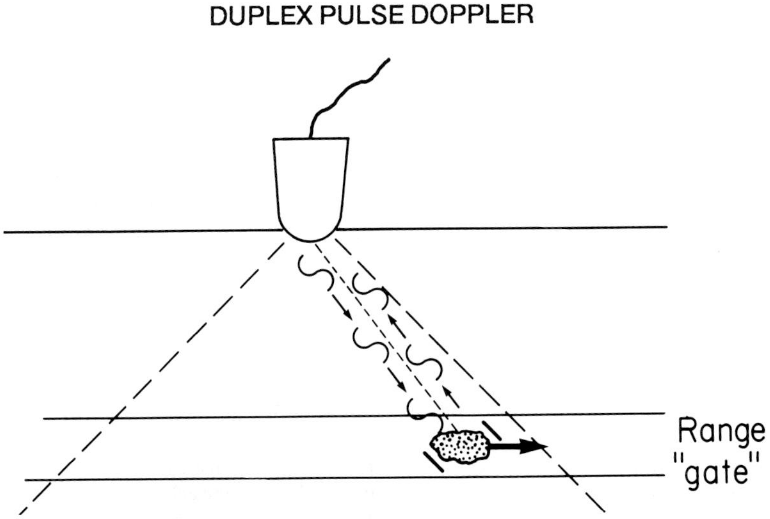

DUPLEX PULSE DOPPLER

Range "gate"

Figure 3-13 The duplex pulse Doppler system integrates Doppler capabilities with two-dimensional imaging, which allows identification of the specific vessel being examined and a reasonable estimation of the angle of insonation.

The other type is the duplex pulse Doppler, which incorporates the Doppler signal into the transducer of a two-dimensional imaging system (Figure 3-13). Most duplex systems allow the isolation of signals from selected depths, which eliminates interference from proximal movement and allows the analysis of velocity waveforms from deep fetal vessels such as the aorta and the middle cerebral artery, in addition to the umbilical artery. Duplex systems, however, are expensive, and although they produce pulsed signals, they use considerably greater acoustical power than continuous wave systems.

Regardless of the type of equipment used, if the sound beam is aimed at the umbilical artery, a typical pulsatile velocity waveform is seen. The waveform includes the velocities of all the red cells within the field. The edge of the waveform is called the maximum velocity envelope and typically assumes a predictable pattern (Figure 3-14). The systolic peak (S) is the highest velocity, and the diastolic trough (D) is the lowest.

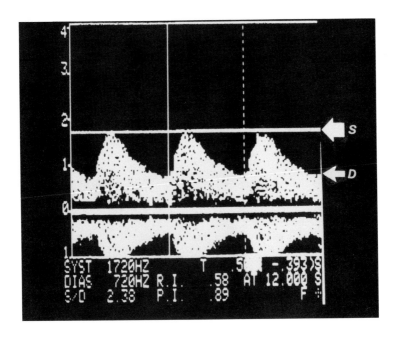

Figure 3-14   The typical Doppler velocity waveform shows a pulsatile pattern with a systolic peak (S) and a diastolic minimum (D). The S/D ratio allows at least a qualitative analysis of vascular resistance distal to the point of insonation.

Clinical Applications of Doppler

The clinical value of continuous wave Doppler appears to lie in the analysis of the ratio of systolic peak to diastolic velocities, or the S/D ratio. The S/D ratio bears a proportional relationship to downstream vascular resistance. If resistance is high, the peak is raised and the trough lowered, raising the ratio. Such an observation in the umbilical artery would suggest increased resistance within the placental vascular bed.

In a normal pregnancy, the S/D ratio from the umbilical artery is about 3.4 early, dropping to 2.5 by term. This suggests a progressive drop in placental vascular resistance in the normal case. In high-risk pregnancies, however, the ratio is often higher to begin with and either rises or does not drop as expected. High S/D ratios are associated with growth retardation and a higher perinatal mortality rate.

Many observers have noted an association between high S/D ratio in early pregnancy and malformations of the fetal cardiovascular system and trisomies. The exact nature of this relationship is not entirely clear but may arise from abnormalities of villus vascular development, leading to increased resistance. The sensitivity and specificity of Doppler detection of aneuploidy is not established.

FURTHER READING

Campbell S, Bewley S, Cohen-Overbeek TE. Investigation of the uteroplacental circulation by Doppler ultrasound. *Semin Perinatol.* 1987;11:362.

Diagnostic Ultrasound Imaging in Pregnancy. NIH Publication No. 84-667. Washington: Government Printing Office, 1984.

Gill RW. Doppler ultrasound: Physical aspects. *Semin Perinatol.* 1987;11:311.

Perone N, Carpenter RJ, Robertson JA. Legal liability in the use of ultrasound by office-based obstetricians. *Am J Obstet Gynecol.* 1984; 150:801.

Royal College of Obstetricians and Gynecologists. Report of the RCOG Working Party on Routine Ultrasound Examination in Pregnancy. December 1984. Available from The Royal College, 27 Sussex Place, Regent's Park, London NW 1 4RG.

Schulman H, Fleischer A, Stern W, Farmakides G, Jaqani N, Blahner P. Umbilical velocity wave ratios in human pregnancy. *Am J Obstet Gynecol.* 1984;148:985.

Trudinger BJ, Cook CM. Umbilical and uterine artery flow velocity waveforms in pregnancy associated with major fetal abnormality. *Br J Obstet Gynaecol.* 1985;92:666.

Trudinger BJ, Giles WB, Cook CM. Flow velocity waveforms in the maternal uteroplacental and fetal umbilical placental circulations. *Am J Obstet Gynecol.* 1985; 152:155.

Chapter 4

Tissue Acquisition Techniques

The methods by which antenatal diagnosis of congenital disease or malformation might be made require either visualization of an anatomic abnormality or the acquisition of fetal tissue or other material that manifests the fetal abnormality. Visualization of fetal anatomic abnormality is most often accomplished using ultrasound and is reviewed in this chapter.

Transcervical or transabdominal chorionic villus sampling (CVS) may be performed between 9 and 11 weeks' gestation and is the earliest technique for the acquisition of fetal tissue. Transabdominal amniocentesis is possible from 12 weeks' gestation through term and provides both fluid and amniocytes for analysis for a variety of purposes. Between 15 and 20 weeks' gestation maternal serum forms the basis for early screening for fetal malformation or dysfunction in the form of MSAFP assay. Biopsies of fetal skin have been obtained using fetoscopic guidance for the antenatal diagnosis of certain congenital ichthyoses. Amniocentesis involves the placement of a narrow-gauge needle percutaneously into the amniotic fluid surrounding the fetus and the aspiration of a sample of that fluid. The amniotic fluid may be analyzed for the presence of diagnostic fetal substances, and fetal fibroblasts suspended in the fluid may be cultured to provide either a fetal karyotype or genetic material for more sophisticated analysis. Finally, ultrasonically guided funipuncture (cordocentesis or percutaneous umbilical blood sampling [PUBS]) now provides direct access to the fetal circulation for both diagnostic and therapeutic purposes.

CHORIONIC VILLUS SAMPLING

The transcervical placement of a narrow-gauge catheter into the uterus and the aspiration of trophoblastic villi in early pregnancy have relatively recently achieved popularity. The technique was first introduced 20 years ago in China and the Soviet Union without visual sonographic guidance and was associated with a fairly high rate of pregnancy loss. The procedure method developed in Great Britain and the United States in the late 1970s and early 1980s utilized ultrasound guidance to minimize the number of catheter passes and therefore trauma to the pregnancy. It is likely that the innovation of sonographic guidance is responsible for a significantly lower rate of pregnancy loss and therefore a higher rate of acceptance.

Chorionic villus sampling provides a sample of trophoblastic material with a chromosomal complement identical in most cases to that of the fetus. Fetal karyotype may be prepared directly from the material obtained, or later from cultured cells. A wide variety of congenital metabolic disorders are detectable using DNA fragmentation analysis of the chromatin of cultured villi.

Indications

Any patient who is determined to be at increased risk for the birth of an aneuploid infant, either on the basis of increased maternal age, previous birth of an aneuploid infant, presence of a parental balanced translocation, or other historical information, is a candidate for CVS. Furthermore, any patient at risk for the birth of an infant with congenital metabolic disease that is detectable using restriction fragment length polymorphism (RFLP) analysis is a potential candidate for CVS. In general, candidates for CVS demonstrate risk that is definable prior to pregnancy or in very early pregnancy. Such early identification is necessary since the procedure is possible only through the 11th postmenstrual week.

Technique

The majority of CVS procedures are performed transcervically using a narrow-gauge catheter with a curved stylet. The patient is placed in the dorsal lithotomy position, and the introitus and vagina are swabbed with an antiseptic. Through a sterile speculum, the cervix is swabbed with an antiseptic. Using transabdominal ultrasonic guidance, a 16-gauge Silastic catheter with a flexible stylet is advanced through the endocervical canal to the thickened echogenic area of the peripheral gestational sac. Optionally, the cervix may be grasped with a tenaculum to provide traction. Typically, little discomfort is associated with the placement of the catheter, but some considerable discomfort may be associated with the use of a tenaculum.

Once well within the echogenic thickening of the peripheral gestational sac, the stylet is removed, and a 20-mL syringe containing 7 mL of holding medium is attached to the catheter. Full aspiration suction from the syringe is applied as the catheter is slowly removed. Once removed, the syringe contents—holding medium, villi, and usually some decidual material—are emptied through the catheter into a petri dish and examined under a dissecting microscope. Villi are easily distinguished visually from decidua and blood, appearing as fine branching structures of semitransparent tissue. An adequate sample amounts to 30 to 50 mg. In experienced hands, most often only one passage of the catheter is required to obtain an adequate sample. Most laboratories limit themselves to two or at most three catheter placements to minimize trauma and pregnancy loss.

Transabdominal CVS may be accomplished using a fine-gauge needle advanced through an aseptic field under ultrasonic guidance into the thickened area of echogenicity targeted above. Aspiration is accomplished in much the same manner, and evaluation of the sample is identical. Transabdominal CVS is often preferred when the uterus is sharply anteflexed with an anterior placenta, as these conditions require a transcervical catheter to follow a very difficult course. Some investigators prefer the transabdominal approach for most procedures because it provides better aseptic conditions. The transabdominal approach would not be an appropriate choice for the retroflexed uterus or the posterior placenta, however, and therefore most successful laboratories offer both techniques.

Benefits

The benefits of CVS accrue mainly from the early gestational age at which diagnostic material may be obtained or a fetal karyotype produced. The direct karyotype may be available within 48 hours of the procedure, and the cultured karyotype within 7 days. In the case of an abnormal result, the patient may then exercise management options privately, before it is physically apparent that she is pregnant. Moreover, termination of pregnancy at 12 to 13 weeks' gestation is in most cases much simpler and safer than termination at 19 to 20 weeks. In cases requiring tissue culture and referral of diagnostic material to a reference laboratory, the time required for processing may exceed the usual interval between amniocentesis and the legal limit for pregnancy termination in some states. Therefore, CVS may provide the only practical means for antenatal diagnosis.

Complications

Excess pregnancy loss is the most common complication associated with CVS. Until recently, the loss associated with the procedure was difficult to assess since the natural rate of pregnancy loss associated with a normal-appearing pregnancy at 9 to 11 weeks was not well known. Recent reports suggest that this natural rate of loss in the case of a pregnancy that is viable and normal in appearance on ultrasound between 9 and 11 weeks' gestation is approximately 2%. The overall rate of pregnancy loss following CVS as reported and compiled by the International Registry for Chorionic Villus Sampling is 4% to 4.5%. Simple comparison of these data would suggest that the excess loss attributable to the procedure is 2% to 2.5%. Inevitably, institutional and individual differences in technique cannot be critically evaluated in the compiled data of an international registry. It is likely that the rate of loss bears some relationship to the experience and talents of individual investigators. It has been shown, for instance, that there is a direct relationship between the number of catheter passes and the risk of pregnancy loss. Physician experience very likely plays an important role in the number of passes required to obtain an adequate sample. In experienced hands, therefore, the rate of excess pregnancy loss after CVS may be considerably lower than 2% to 2.5%.

It seems apparent, however, that the pregnancy loss associated with CVS in most cases is substantially higher than the rate of loss associated with amniocentesis (see below), and this difference must be clearly explained to any potential candidate prior to the procedure.

Another possible complication of CVS is inaccuracy of results. Inappropriately abnormal results are not seen from cultured preparations but have been reported to occur in 1% to 2% of cases from the direct preparations. The nonrepresentative aneuploidies reported in this case have been very unusual in character and not consistent with a normally developing pregnancy. Therefore, patients are usually advised to wait and undergo amniocentesis for confirmation of the diagnosis prior to making any management decisions. The probability of a karyotype not representative of the fetus is much less from the cultured CVS tissue, as mentioned above. Inaccurate results from the cultured material reportedly occur at a rate of about 1 in 3000. This is similar to the rate of inaccuracy seen with cultured fibroblasts obtained at amniocentesis.

Very rarely, delayed maternal sepsis has been reported following CVS. Such sepsis can be serious and life threatening but is very rare. It has often been recommended that a maternal cervical culture be obtained for gonococcus or beta streptococcus prior to the procedure, with treatment of patients with positive culture results to minimize the risk of septic complications.

Informed Consent

If a patient is referred for prenatal diagnosis for appropriate indications at a gestational age that would allow for CVS, complications including the rate of pregnancy loss must be carefully discussed. She must be willing to accept the estimated risk of pregnancy loss as well as the less likely risks of inaccuracies and sepsis. Chorionic villus sampling remains in most cases an elective alternative to amniocentesis as a means of antenatal diagnosis. The benefits are largely those associated with a greater degree of privacy and convenience derived from the earlier gestational age at diagnosis.

AMNIOCENTESIS

Amniocentesis is the more traditional method of antenatal diagnosis. First introduced in the late 1950s and performed without visual guidance for decades, a recent refinement of the technique involves continuous ultrasound guidance. Traditionally, amniocentesis is performed between 16 and 18 weeks of gestation and provides a sample of amniotic fluid for either component analysis or cell culture for karyotype.

Technique

Immediately prior to amniocentesis, a careful ultrasound examination is performed to establish gestational age, fetal viability, and placental location and to exclude visible fetal structural anomalies. An antiseptic skin preparation and sterile drape of the puncture site are performed; optionally, infiltration of the puncture site with local anesthetic may be performed. A narrow-gauge (often 20-gauge) needle is advanced through the maternal skin into the uterus, a sample of fluid aspirated, and the needle removed. If a large area of fluid was identified with ultrasound immediately prior to needle placement, with the fetus well away from the area, many clinicians will not use direct ultrasonic guidance. However, if no such clear, large area of fluid is seen, direct ultrasonic guidance of the needle is recommended to ensure correct placement with a minimum number of punctures and therefore a lower rate of complication or failure. Ultrasonic guidance of the needle is easily accomplished by either using a sterile plastic cover designed and marketed by the ultrasound machine manufacturer or covering the transducer with a sterile glove. The transducer is coated with transmission gel, inserted into the sterile cover, and covered with sterile surgical lubricant as a transmission coupling agent.

If the amniocentesis is being performed prior to a gestational age reasonably associated with neonatal survival, no postprocedural evaluation of fetal well-being is normally performed. A postprocedure real-time scan may be done for maternal reassurance if requested, but no intervention would be appropriate at such an early gestational age if immediate complications were identified. After 24 to 26 weeks' gestation, however, follow-up fetal evaluation is indicated to exclude the possibility of complications that might require intervention or delivery. Laceration of a blood vessel by the amniocentesis needle can be visually identified with real-time ultrasound as the hemorrhaging produces a typical echogenic cascade from the site of the tear. Fetal heart rate monitoring is typically recommended for 30 to 60 minutes following amniocentesis once the age of fetal viability is passed, if sonographic examination after the puncture is not performed.

Complications

The risk of excess pregnancy loss associated with amniocentesis is typically reported to be approximately 0.5%, based on collaborative perinatal data. Published data suggest that the risk of pregnancy loss after 17 weeks without amniocentesis is about 3%, and that this risk rises to 3.5% if amniocentesis is performed. Thus it is concluded that amniocentesis introduces an additional risk of about 0.5%. In fact, studies that use sonographically normal patients as a control group have not been done, suggesting that the background rate of loss may be significantly lower than 3%. If so, the risk from the procedure may be higher than 0.5%. In fact, relatively small studies from individual investigators report that the risk of pregnancy loss following amniocentesis ranges from 0.5% to 1.4%. However, the relatively recent technique of using ultrasound to guide the amniocentesis needle into the fluid and avoid the fetus and placenta, if possible, probably results in a lower risk of loss. The majority of data published to date regarding pregnancy loss after amniocentesis reviewed amniocentesis procedures that did not use direct sonographic guidance.

Several investigators report a significantly higher rate of pregnancy loss if the amniocentesis needle traverses the placenta. The rate of loss in one relatively small study was increased by 75% (0.8% to 1.4%) if transplacental needle passage occurred. This emphasizes the possible benefits of careful search for a puncture site free of placenta. Often no placenta-free area is present, and therefore if the procedure is to be performed the placenta must be traversed. In such a case, the altered probability of complications may be important information for the patient.

Early Amniocentesis

The traditional time interval for genetic amniocentesis is 16 to 18 weeks. The time interval required for preparation of a fetal karyotype is 10 to 21 days. The patient will receive her results, therefore, by 21 weeks' gestation. The development of CVS offers considerable temporal advantage since results are available by 12 to 13 weeks' gestation. The disadvantage is a significantly higher risk of pregnancy loss. Many investigators have recently reported experience with early amniocentesis as an alternative to CVS. Amniocentesis using sonographic guidance is technically possible with a high degree of success from 12 weeks onward and can therefore provide results prior to 16 weeks. The likelihood of culture failure is small, and the reported risk of pregnancy loss appears to be similar to that for later amniocentesis, or considerably lower than with CVS. The volume in milliliters of fluid removed should be limited to an amount about equal to the gestational age in weeks.

Early amniocentesis, therefore, offers similar though not identical advantages to CVS but with a lower apparent rate of complications.

Informed Consent

In choosing CVS, early amniocentesis, or later amniocentesis, the patient must consider the probability of the condition in question and the risk of complication from the procedure chosen. It is important that the information be presented in a nondirective manner and that the information be complete.

FETAL BLOOD SAMPLING

A sample of fetal blood would enable the preparation of a karyotype from fetal lymphocytes, the analysis of chromatin material by fragmentation techniques, or component analysis including hemoglobin electrophoresis and coagulation factor assay. Early attempts to sample fetal blood were made using placentocentesis, which involved the repeated puncture of the chorionic plate with a needle, followed by the aspiration of amniotic fluid near the site of puncture. Placentocentesis produced a sample almost always contaminated by maternal blood and amniotic fluid.

In 1973 fetoscopy was reported for the aspiration of a pure sample of fetal blood, and the procedure enjoyed considerable popularity for the next 10 years. Fetoscopy involved the puncture of the uterus with a 2 x 3-mm trocar, then the placement of a small needlescope through the cannula into the amniotic cavity. Using ultrasound guidance and direct visualization, a fine-gauge needle threaded through a side port on the fetoscope was then advanced into the umbilical vein at its insertion on the chorionic plate. Although fetoscopic fetal blood sampling provided a pure sample of fetal blood, the technique was hampered by limited availability and a relatively high rate of pregnancy loss of about 5%.

In 1982 Beng first reported successful percutaneous fetal blood sampling and intravascular transfusion using only a sonographically guided needle. Daffos, in 1983 and 1985, reported his experience with percutaneous fetal blood sampling for a variety of indications in 606 cases. He reported a high rate of success and a pregnancy loss rate of only 0.8% in pregnancies under 24 weeks at the time of sampling.

Technique

Percutaneous fetal blood sampling is most often accomplished from the umbilical vein at its insertion on the chorionic plate. The insertion may be anterior or posterior (Figure 4-1). In the case of an anterior insertion, the needle is guided through the substance of the placenta into the base of the

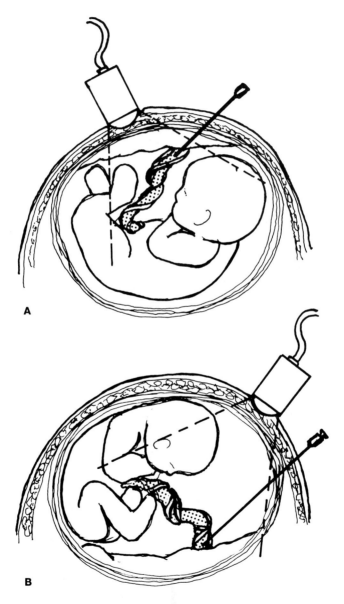

Figure 4-1 A, This drawing illustrates the fetal blood sampling needle approaching the umbilical vein at its insertion on the anterior placenta. **B,** Here, the aspiration needle approaches the umbilical insertion on a posterior placenta. Note that the needle crosses the amniotic cavity and is vulnerable to fetal movement.

cord. In the case of a posterior insertion, the needle is guided transamniotically to the vein (Figure 4-2). Alternatively, a free loop of cord, the cord at the umbilicus (Figure 4-3), or the umbilical vein within the substance of the fetal liver may be chosen. Since fetal movement during the procedure may result in laceration of the vein or dislodgement of the needle, temporary arrest of fetal movement may be desired and may be accomplished with either intramuscular or intravenous pancuronium bromide or d-tubocurare.

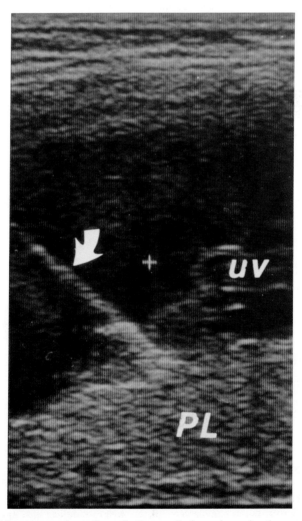

Figure 4-2 This sonogram shows the aspiration needle (arrow) crossing the amniotic cavity to puncture the umbilical vein (UV) at its insertion on a posterior placenta (PL).

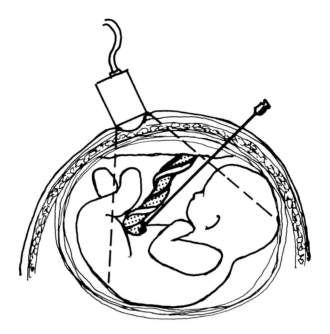

Figure 4-3 Here, the needle approaches the umbilicus of the fetus.

Following a preliminary ultrasound examination to confirm gestational age, locate the cord insertion and a probable aspiration site, and exclude visible fetal malformations, the abdomen is prepared with an antiseptic, and a sterile drape is applied. Skin infiltration with local anesthetic is recommended to minimize maternal movement. The ultrasound transducer is covered with a sterile cover and is therefore available on the field. The aspiration needle is advanced through maternal tissues using direct sonographic guidance to the umbilical vein at the chosen aspiration site. Once the vein is punctured, fetal blood is aspirated in the required amount. A long (12 to 17 cm) 22-gauge needle facilitates the procedure because it allows an assistant plenty of room to affix and replace syringes. One-mL syringes are used as they allow for the easy aspiration of fetal blood through the narrow-gauge needle. The syringes may be anticoagulated with heparin, citrate, or nothing at all, depending on the requirements of the test planned for the blood.

After the blood is obtained, it is often necessary to confirm that the blood is of fetal origin, since often the needle tip is quite close to maternal tissues. Confirmation of fetal origin may be accomplished by cell size analysis (since fetal red cells are significantly larger than adult), by staining techniques that highlight the high rate of basophilia and nucleation in fetal blood, or by an alkali denaturation technique known as the Apt test. In the latter, a few drops of the blood are added to a test tube of tap water, the cells lyse, and a dilute hemoglobin solution is produced. When a few drops of 10% potassium hydroxide are added to the solution, adult blood turns green-yellow but fetal blood remains pink. This is based on the relative resistance of fetal hemoglobin to alkali denaturation. This test can be done at the bedside and yields results within minutes.

Indications

A pure sample of fetal blood may be necessary to make or exclude the diagnosis of hemophilia, sickle cell disease, fragile X syndrome, or a variety of other congenital conditions. The ability to obtain a rapid karyotype may be useful in the case of the mother at risk for an aneuploid fetus who is identified or presents for antenatal evaluation after 19 weeks' gestation. The availability of a fetal karyotype in 1 week instead of 3 can be a substantial advantage under these circumstances.

In the case of a mother with isoimmunization, fetal blood sampling can serve several purposes. First, if the father is determined to be heterozygous for the red cell antigen in question, fetal blood sampling can provide a fetal blood type and in 50% of cases avoid multiple amniocenteses for bilirubin studies. Later, in a severe isoimmunization case, direct fetal blood sampling provides direct hematologic data and even access to the fetal circulation for direct transfusion.

Fetal blood sampling can provide prompt karyotype information in the case of the fetus with sonographic dysmorphology. Such information can be important in planning obstetrical management. Finally, fetal blood sampling can provide tissue for karyotype and blood for respiratory gas analysis in the case of severe fetal growth retardation discovered late in gestation that might be the result of either aneuploidy or uteroplacental insufficiency.

FURTHER READING

Elias S, Simpson JL, Martin AO, Sabbagha RE, Gerbie AB, Keith LG. Chorionic villus sampling for first trimester prenatal diagnosis. *Am J Obstet Gynecol*. 1985; 152:204.

Simpson JL. Genetic counseling and prenatal diagnosis. In: Gabbe SG, Niebyl JF, Simpson JL, eds. *Obstetrics: Normal and Problem Pregnancies*. New York: Churchill-Livingstone, 1986.

Simpson JL. Low fetal loss rate after normal ultrasound at eight weeks gestation: Implications for chorionic villus sampling (CVS). *Am J Hum Genet*. 1984; 36 (suppl): 197S.

Simpson JL, Elias S, Gatlin M, Martin AO. Genetic counseling services in obstetrics and gynecology. *Am J Obstet Gynecol*. 1981; 140:70.

Simpson JL, Golbus MS, Martin AO, Sarto GE. *Genetics in Obstetrics and Gynecology*. New York: Grune & Stratton, 1982.

Chapter 5

Perinatal Management Considerations

During the past decade the ability to visualize the fetus has been dramatically enhanced by the development of high-resolution real-time ultrasound. Both normal and abnormal fetal anatomy can be imaged in great detail, and the accumulation of clinical experience has improved the sensitivity and accuracy of antenatal diagnosis. Certain specific clinical abnormalities, such as polyhydramnios or oligohydramnios, that may be directly linked to a fetal malformation are more often recognized early and result in referral for fetal malformation screening. Routine sonographic screening of low-risk obstetric patients, although not uniformly accepted, is often performed and can result in the early detection of fetal malformations.

The antenatal diagnosis of a significant fetal malformation offers a variety of clinical opportunities to improve the management of the affected pregnancy. Aside from pregnancy termination, the detection of a fetal malformation, particularly a potentially correctable one, can result in an altered method of delivery, altered time or place of delivery, and possibly even consideration of prenatal therapeutic intervention (Table 5-1).

A thorough evaluation of the fetus, including precise anatomic definition of the anomaly in question, is required prior to any therapeutic decisions and parental counseling. The identification of one malformation increases the risk of other associated fetal malformations (Figure 5-1). The observation of subtle abnormalities may lead to further diagnostic tests, such as karyotype analysis, which might not otherwise have been done (Figure 5-2). Furthermore, real-time sonography may yield important information about vital fetal functions, including fetal breathing movements, trunk or limb movement, micturition, and cardiac rhythm.

In addition to imaging techniques, methods for fetal tissue sample acquisition have undergone significant evolution during the past 10 years. Amniocentesis and chorionic villus sampling, discussed in Chapter 4, permit detection of fetal chromosomal defects and many inheritable metabolic conditions. With minimal risk, fetal blood sampling and fetal skin biopsies are useful for diagnosing hemoglobinopathies and other congenital conditions. Fluid col-

Table 5-1 Potential Clinical Impact of Antenatal Diagnosis

1. *Decision to reproduce*: The patient at high risk for a malformation might not choose to reproduce unless antenatal diagnosis were available.
2. *Decision to terminate*: Most malformations do not increase maternal medical risk. Some patients would choose to continue pregnancy even with a lethal diagnosis.
3. *Anticipatory grief*: With the knowledge of a lethal anomaly, the emotional adaptation can begin. With knowledge of a nonlethal but disabling anomaly, adaptation and preparation can begin.
4. *Preparation*: Preparation by both the medical providers and the family for the birth of a child with serious disabilities can greatly facilitate final adaptation and optimal outcome.
5. *Remote referral*: Early referral to a center prepared for the disabled neonate improves patient comfort and confidence.
6. *Tertiary delivery*: Even the late detection and referral for tertiary delivery of the fetus with congenital disease improve outcome.
7. *Timing of delivery*: At term in most cases, but early in selected individuals.
8. *Method of delivery*: Vaginal or cesarean.
9. *Antenatal treatment*: In selected cases.
10. *Anticipatory counseling*: Regarding probable neonatal care.

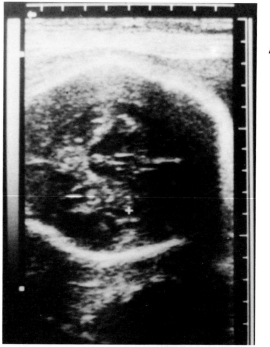

Figure 5-1 A, This occipitofrontal scanplane shows the unusually angular cranial outline and brachycephaly associated with Down syndrome. **B,** These sonograms of the same fetus show the ascites on the left (short arrows) and the atrioventricular defect on the right (long arrow) that were present. Trisomy 21 was confirmed by amniocentesis.

lection within fetal organs, including cerebrospinal fluid, urine, and ascitic fluid, can be readily identified and aspirated under sonographic guidance for both diagnostic and therapeutic purposes.

For some patients, antenatal diagnosis and extensive fetal evaluation will not alter perinatal management. Many parents would choose not to intervene but would benefit from the added preparation for the birth of the nonviable or disabled infant. For many parents the management of the pregnancy and delivery would be significantly altered. Therefore, prenatal diagnosis has assumed significant practical clinical importance. The diagnostic and therapeutic alternatives for management of a variety of fetal anomalies are outlined in this chapter.

FETAL MALFORMATIONS CONSIDERED LETHAL OR INCOMPATIBLE WITH A REASONABLE QUALITY OF LIFE

The early diagnosis of serious malformations that are either incompatible with life or incompatible with a reasonable quality of life often results in consideration of termination of pregnancy (Table 5-2). If the diagnosis is made at a gestational age that is below the statutory limit for elective

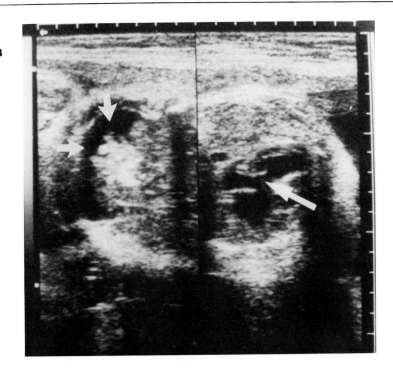

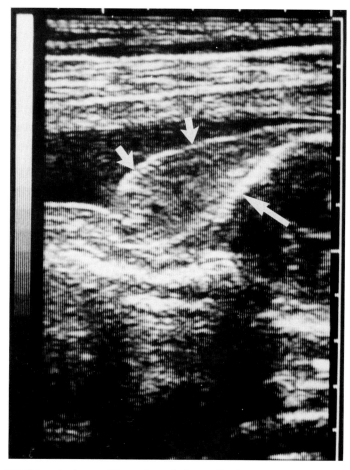

Figure 5-2 This sagittal scan of the occiput of a fetus with trisomy 21 shows the skin thickening (short arrows) dorsal to the occipital skull (long arrow). This skin thickening has been seen with trisomy 21 but its diagnostic sensitivity and specificity are unclear.

Table 5-2 Malformations Often Leading to Pregnancy Termination

Trisomies 21, 13, and 18
Untreatable inherited metabolic disorders, such as Tay-Sachs disease, adrenoleuko-
    dystrophy, Lesch-Nyhan syndrome
Anencephaly, hydranencephaly, alobar holoprosencephaly, complete craniospinal
    rachischisis
Bilateral renal agenesis, infantile polycystic renal disease
Lethal cartilage-bone dysplasias, thanatophoric dwarfism, recessive osteogenesis
    imperfecta
Multiple congenital anomaly complexes detected with ultrasound

termination, such a decision may be made by the parents purely on the basis of the diagnostic and prognostic information available and private considerations. On the other hand, in the case of a fetus with the diagnosis of a confidently lethal malformation, such as anencephaly or renal agenesis, the legal gestational age limit for elective termination may not strictly limit the individual's access to termination. After any legal limit for elective termination is passed, termination might still be available in some institutions if a lethal diagnosis is made. If serious but nonlethal malformations are recognized too late for legal elective pregnancy termination, the family can be carefully informed about the expected outcome and appropriate intrapartum and postnatal care arranged. Anticipatory discussions about the risk or benefit of cesarean delivery should be held. Many inherited chromosomal, metabolic, and anatomic malformations will fall into this category.

MALFORMATIONS BEST FOLLOWED TO FULL TERM

The majority of infants with potentially repairable malformations diagnosed in utero are best treated after term delivery, as opposed to either preterm delivery or intrauterine therapy (Table 5-3). In general, the term infant is a significantly better surgical and anesthetic risk than the preterm neonate. Antenatal diagnosis allows for careful planning of appropriate perinatal and postnatal care and referred delivery at a center prepared for the special needs of such an infant. When necessary, the delivery can be planned so that important personnel, such as a neonatologist, pediatric surgeon, or pediatric anesthesiologist, are immediately available.

FETAL MALFORMATIONS THAT MAY BENEFIT FROM EARLY DELIVERY

Premature delivery may be warranted for infants with a few fetal malformations that might benefit from the earliest possible correction or in whom

---

Table 5-3 Common Malformations Best Delivered at Term

Small anterior abdominal wall defects, omphalocele/gastroschisis
Small, intact spina bifida
Intestinal atresias
Meconium ileus
Unilateral renal anomalies: hydronephrosis, ureteropelvic junction obstruction,
    multicystic dysplasia
Small sacrococcygeal teratoma
Benign cysts: ovarian, enteric, urachal, choledochal
Craniofacial malformations
Chest wall anomalies
Cystic hygroma

in utero deterioration is noted (Table 5-4). The principal basis for early delivery is that continued in utero existence would lead to progressive damage to the fetus. For each of these specific cases, the risk of delivery and prematurity must be balanced against the risk of continuing the pregnancy. The rationale for early delivery and corrective surgery is unique for each type of anomaly. In each case, it is concluded that progressive deterioration of specific organ function will occur until the lesion is repaired or the process reversed. In each case, the complications of prematurity must be balanced against the perception of progressive deterioration. In obstructive hydrocephalus, for example, high intraventricular pressure compresses the developing cerebral cortex. Early delivery and ventricular decompression might improve subsequent brain development and avoid a potentially difficult delivery of an infant with an extremely large head. An early urinary tract obstruction (bilateral congenital hydronephrosis) may result in progressive deterioration of renal function. Premature delivery and decompression of the urinary tract may stabilize renal function and permit adequate renal growth and improved function.

Some anomalies may be associated with progressive tissue ischemia and require early correction to promote survival of the infant. In utero volvulus associated with meconium ileus or malrotation is such an anomaly. This type of intestinal disorder may lead to perforation, meconium peritonitis, or fetal death. Surgical correction of this anomaly is intended to reverse the ischemic process and promote the preservation of functional intestine.

Advances in the management of preterm infants, including improvements in ventilatory support, the stimulation of surfactant production with maternally administered steroids, and the use of exogenous surfactant, have dramatically improved survival and decreased the morbidity for preterm infants. However, although such advances have added some flexibility to these management decisions, prematurity remains a formidable problem, and no preterm delivery of the fetus with a malformation should be considered lightly.

FETAL MALFORMATIONS THAT MAY BENEFIT FROM CESAREAN DELIVERY

Elective cesarean delivery is indicated for malformations that would cause maternal/fetal dystocia or when there is reasonable cause to expect fetal trauma from the vaginal delivery process (Table 5-5). Cesarean delivery may be indicated for the rare situation in which an infant has a malformation that requires immediate neonatal surgical correction in a sterile environment. In such cases, a planned cesarean facilitates coordination of neonatal surgical services. Furthermore, if preterm delivery is considered necessary in the case

Table 5-4 Malformations That Might Require Preterm Delivery

Severe or progressive hydrops fetalis
Intestinal ischemia (i.e., volvulus)
Progressive obstructive hydrocephalus
Progressive bilateral hydronephrosis

Table 5-5 Malformations That Might Benefit from Cesarean Delivery

Large omphalocele
Gastroschisis with dilated, obstructed external bowel
Severe hydrocephalus, large encephalocele
Large cervicofacial tumors, large teratoma, cystic hygroma
Large or ruptured myelomeningocele
Large sacrococcygeal teratoma
Conjoined twins
Any anomaly potentially leading to dystocia

---

of a maternal cervix that is unfavorable to induction, or there is evidence of fetal distress, cesarean delivery may be required.

CONGENITAL CONDITIONS THAT MAY BENEFIT FROM PRENATAL THERAPY

Liley in 1963 reported the first successful transperitoneal fetal blood transfusion for hemolytic disease. Since then, a number of fetal conditions have been successfully treated in utero by both medical and surgical means (Table 5-6). Fetal transfusions have been refined to the point that direct cannulation and infusion into umbilical cord vessels can be readily accomplished with sonographic guidance. Fetuses with persistent supraventricular tachycardia and hydrops have been successfully treated with maternally administered digoxin. Recent reports of the successful prevention of the stigmata of adrenogenital syndrome with maternally administered steroids are encouraging. In the few cases reported, the typical phenotypic masculinization of affected female infants has been minimized by this therapy. It is of interest that since the fetus continuously swallows significant volumes of amniotic fluid, administering medications or nutrients to the fetus through the amniotic fluid appears feasible, but this potential remains unexplored.

The concepts and technology required to surgically correct an anatomic malformation in utero are substantially more complicated than providing medications or hormones to a fetus by administering them to the mother. Anatomic malformations that have been considered for prenatal therapy include those that cause progressive damage to an organ, arrest vital growth

Table 5-6   Malformations That Might Benefit from Antenatal Treatment

1. Anatomic
    Urethral obstruction with bilateral hydronephrosis and severe oligohydramnios
    Unilateral renal obstruction with consequent polyhydramnios and preterm labor
    Severe fetal hydrothorax with consequent polyhydramnios and preterm labor
    Diaphragmatic hernia
2. Metabolic conditions
    Intrauterine growth retardation
    Erythroblastosis fetalis
    Hypothyroidism
    Pulmonary surfactant deficiency
    Methylmalonic acidemia
    Biotin-dependent multiple carboxylase deficiency
    Adrenogenital syndrome, 21-hydroxylase deficiency
    Nonimmune hydrops
    Cardiac dysrhythmias

and development of an organ system, or produce damage to an organ that cannot be satisfactorily remedied following delivery.

Malformations that might be considered candidates for antenatal intervention must not only be ultimately correctable but also should be detectable at a gestational age sufficiently remote from term that reasonable time for in utero recovery and benefit yet remains. Generally, the diagnosis and in utero therapy of a condition after 32 weeks' gestation offers no clear advantage over delivery and neonatal treatment. Currently three anatomic malformations—urethral obstruction with severe oligohydramnios and progressive bilateral hydronephrosis, diaphragmatic hernia, and obstructive hydrocephalus—have been considered severe enough to interfere with fetal development to the extent that in utero treatment has been offered under investigational protocols.

Congenital Urethral Obstruction with Bilateral Hydronephrosis

Fetal bladder outlet obstruction is currently recognized with increasing frequency because fluid-filled masses within the fetus are relatively easy to visualize by sonography and because the associated oligohydramnios is a common obstetric indication for sonography (Figure 5-3). Hydronephrosis secondary to urethral obstruction provides an excellent example of a potentially life-threatening abnormality that interferes with normal fetal development. These infants not only have significant functional renal damage but typically also suffer severe pulmonary hypoplasia that is usually the immediate cause of death. Other anomalies, such as limb and joint deformities, may be reversible with appropriate neonatal therapy. Although there have been several reported alternatives for decompressing the obstructed fetal urinary

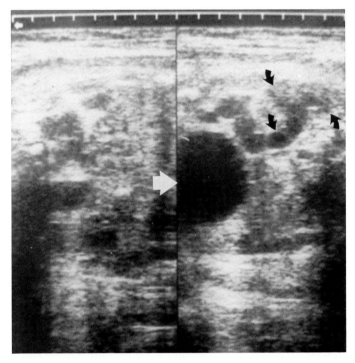

Figure 5-3 These sonograms from a 26-week fetus with bladder outlet obstruction due to posterior urethral valves show a distended bladder (white arrow) and hydronephrosis and hydroureter (black arrows). This fetus might be a suitable candidate for antenatal diversion catheterization.

tract, current concepts of management entail the suprapubic drainage of fetal urine into the amniotic fluid space and continued gestation. Sonographically guided percutaneous placement of a double pigtail catheter into the fetal bladder, permitting drainage into the amniotic cavity, has been successfully employed in a number of centers for several years. Recently, hysterotomy and surgical vesicostomy in the fetus have been successfully performed, but the number of patients who have undergone this procedure is too few at this time to allow confident conclusions to be drawn regarding clinical efficacy. However, these pioneering procedures have clearly opened avenues of correction for other anomalies.

Congenital Diaphragmatic Hernia

Congenital diaphragmatic hernia typically carries a 50% to 90% mortality when treated at birth. Repair of the diaphragmatic hernia in the neonatal period is technically not difficult but many of these children succumb because of severe pre-existing pulmonary hypoplasia.

Investigators have demonstrated in a sheep model that compression of fetal lungs produces fatal pulmonary hypoplasia; removal of pulmonary compression allows the lungs to develop sufficiently so that the animal survives at birth. Harrison and his colleagues have pioneered in developing experimental techniques that may be applied to diaphragmatic hernia repair in humans in utero. Although repair of a diaphragmatic hernia has been attempted in utero in a few human patients, to date there has been only one reported survivor. Correction of the diaphragmatic hernia in utero is by far the most ambitious of all the prenatal surgical procedures undertaken. It requires hysterotomy and exteriorization of the fetus, then repair, replacement, and continuation of the pregnancy. It remains to be seen whether this type of intervention would have any advantage over the current accepted practice of postnatal repair. It is likely that larger defects, which are more likely to be discovered in early gestation, are least likely to benefit from any intervention. However, it is quite remarkable that several exteriorization procedures have been performed with successful continuation of pregnancy.

Congenital Hydrothorax

Congenital pleural effusion can occur at any gestational age and can be isolated or part of the greater syndrome of hydrops fetalis. Isolated pleural effusions seen early in gestation may resolve spontaneously or progress to hydrops and are often associated with cytogenetic or cardiac abnormalities. Isolated pleural effusion later in gestation often results from thoracic duct leakage and may interfere with fetal esophageal function, causing polyhydramnios and preterm labor. In such a clinical context, several isolated cases as well as a small series of cases appear to support the benefit of antenatal intervention.

The aspiration of the effusion or the placement of an indwelling catheter draining the pleural effusion from the pleural cavity to the amniotic cavity can decompress the chest and improve the amniotic fluid volume equilibrium. Such intervention should be undertaken only by an experienced team and is not without risk, but it may be of considerable benefit in prolonging pregnancy.

The fetal chest fluid is essentially intestinal lymph and in the fetus is serous in consistency, containing many lymphocytes from which fetal karyotype is easily obtained.

Congenital Obstructive Hydrocephalus

Hydrocephalus secondary to obstruction of the aqueduct of Sylvius has been an attractive target lesion for antenatal therapy. Antenatal treatment of congenital hydrocephalus was considered in light of both the historically poor outcome for infants with congenital hydrocephalus overt at birth and the general neurosurgical axiom that the earlier hydrocephalus is treated, the better. Animal studies included the induction and subsequent treatment of fetal hydrocephalus in both primates and sheep and appeared to show a benefit. In both types of animals, following the induction of fetal hydrocephalus either surgically or with pharmacological agents, the in utero relief of the ventriculomegaly resulted in arrest of growth of the hydrocephalus and improved survival, compared to untreated animals. No functional conclusions could be drawn from these studies, however.

The human experience is limited, but there has been no demonstrated clinical advantage in more than 80 fetal patients who have had a ventriculoamniotic shunt placed, when compared with infants who were managed with conventional postnatal shunting procedures. Furthermore, a disturbing number of infants treated in utero for isolated progressive hydrocephalus ultimately had a variety of associated or alternative diagnoses made after birth that had been missed prior to treatment. More recent reports of outcome in the case of infants with isolated congenital hydrocephalus overt at birth and managed for best outcome have shown dramatically improved results over previous experience, and there appears to be no significant benefit from in utero treatment compared to appropriate neonatal treatment. This experience has been consistent in many centers, and currently prenatal intervention for obstructive hydrocephalus has been abandoned by most investigators.

Assessing the Risks and Benefits

Antenatal diagnosis and therapy have raised complex medical and ethical issues about the rights of the mother and the fetus as patients. Most of the severe fetal anatomic malformations and deficiency states that have been treated prenatally have been treated with the knowledge that nonintervention would likely result in either fetal death or permanent disability. A number of important diagnostic and therapeutic procedures can be performed with relatively low risk to the mother and an acceptable risk to the fetus, such as fetal blood and fluid sampling, fetoscopy, amniography, intravascular cannulation, and even placement of indwelling diversion catheters. The risk to the human fetus and mother of more extensive manipulation, as occurs in hysterotomy and open surgical vesicostomy or repair of diaphragmatic hernia, is not known because of limited clinical experience. However, the possibility of misdiagnosis, poor patient selection, and ill-advised therapy remain significant risks and must be considered prior to any intervention.

As our ability to diagnose and treat the fetal patient achieves greater technical sophistication, the maternal/fetal ethical issues will also be brought into sharper focus. We must weigh the woman's right as a competent adult to manage her own well-being as well as that of her fetus, even when these two considerations may conflict. In a few cases women may not appear to act in the best interests of their unborn babies. The responsibility of the physician is to present a balanced and objective medical and moral case for acting in the best interests of both the mother and the fetus, whether those interests appear to favor cesarean delivery or in utero therapy. The final decision regarding management is the patient's. Only in the case where a proven medical therapy that is required for fetal survival or health is declined by the patient is there any basis for seeking legal intervention in any court system.

FURTHER READING

Bensen JT, Dillard RG, Burton BK. Open spina bifida: Does cesarean section delivery improve prognosis? *Obstet Gynecol.* 1988;71:532.

Carpenter MW, Curci MR. Dibbins AW, Haddow JE. Perinatal management of ventral, wall defects. *Obstet Gynecol.* 1984; 64:646.

Chervanak FA, Duncan C, Ment LR, et al. Perinatal management of meningomyelocele. *Obstet Gynecol.* 1984; 63:376.

Kirk EP, Wah RM. Obstetric management of the fetus with omphalocele or gastroschisis: A review and report of one hundred twelve cases. *Am J Obstet Gynecol.* 1983; 146:512.

Main DM, Mennuti MT. Neural tube defects: Issues in prenatal diagnosis and counseling. *Obstet Gynecol.* 1986; 67:1.

Simpson, JL. Genetic counseling and prenatal diagnosis. In: Gabbe SG, Niebyl JF, Simpson JL, eds. *Obstetrics: Normal and Problem Pregnancies.* New York: Churchill-Livingstone; 1986.

Simpson JL., Golbus MS, Martin AO, Sarto GE. *Genetics in Obstetrics and Gynecology.* New York: Grune & Stratton, 1982.

Vintzileos AM, Campbell WA, Nochimson DJ, Weinbaum PJ. Antenatal evaluation and management of ultrasonically detected fetal anomalies. *Obstet Gynecol.* 1987; 69:640.

Vintzileos AM, Campbell WA, Weinbaum PJ, Nochimson DJ: Perinatal management and outcome of fetal ventriculomegaly. *Obstet Gynecol.* 1987; 69:5.

Part II

Antenatal Diagnosis and Perinatal Management of Specific Congenital Disorders

Chapter 6

Neural Tube Defects

The neural tube is the embryonic precursor to the central nervous system, including the cranium and spinal cord. The neural tube begins to form in the dorsal midline of the early disk-shaped embryo by about 20 days after conception, with the dorsal growth toward the midline of two parallel paramedian neural ridges. Fusion of the ridges in the central region to form a tube is followed by continued sequential fusion both caudally and cephalically. By 26 days postconception the caudal neuropore closes, completing the formation of the neural tube. Failure of fusion at either terminus or at any intervening segment during this process produces clinically a family of related congenital birth defects called neural tube defects, which include anencephaly, iniencephaly, encephalocele, craniospinal rachischisis, and thoracic or lumbosacral spinal dysraphism (spina bifida) with or without myelomeningocele (Table 6-1). Roughly half of the number of cases of open neural tube defects are spinal defects, and half are cranial defects, including anencephaly and encephalocele.

Table 6-1 Types of Neural Tube Defects

1. *Anencephaly:* Absence of cranium, variable brain formation
2. *Cephalocele:* Cranial meningocele, protrusion of sac with no neural elements
3. *Encephalocele:* Sac with neural elements
4. *Craniospinal rachischisis:* Absent cranium, completely open spine
5. *Spina bifida occulta:* Skin-covered dysraphic bone defect of spine
6. *Meningocele:* Dysraphic spinal defect with dorsal meningeal sac with no neural elements
7. *Myelomeningocele:* Spinal defect with dorsal meningeal sac containing neural elements
8. *Iniencephaly:* Dysraphic defect of cervical spine, fusion of occipital skull to spine

The incidence of open neural tube defect (ONTD) varies within the United States and around the world. Nationally, ONTDs occur at a rate of about 1.2 per 1000 live births, but in some areas such as North Carolina the incidence is closer to 1.7 per 1000. The incidence in the United Kingdom approaches 4 per 1000, while in Japan the rate is only 0.6 per 1000. These geographic variations as well as the epidemiology of recurrence of ONTDs suggest at least an element of genetic influence in the etiology of these malformations. For a couple who have delivered a child with a neural tube defect, the risk of conceiving another is roughly 10 times the original risk, or 2% to 4%. Furthermore, the second child with such a defect may have any variety of neural tube defect, not necessarily a copy of the malformation seen in the first child. The calculated risk of conception of a child with a neural tube defect based on related family history shows a declining risk as the relationship to the malformed child becomes more distant. On the other hand, the risk increases as the familial proximity increases. These are typical epidemiological observations common to many different types of congenital malformations thought to result from polygenic or multifactorial influences and describe the case in which multiple gene loci interact with usually unidentified environmental factors to result in a malformation.

CLINICAL PROGNOSIS

The potential for influencing the course of pregnancy and the final clinical outcome for infants with ONTDs vary both with the location and size of the defect and with the clinical care given.

A pregnancy with an anencephalic fetus may deliver prematurely or late, related to the unique evolution of clinical events in a particular patient. About 30% of such pregnancies are complicated by polyhydramnios secondary not to defective ingestion of amniotic fluid, as once thought, but to decreased antidiuretic hormone secretion and secondary fetal polyuria. Premature labor is a common consequence of the polyhydramnios. Delayed labor, or postdatism, sometimes complicates the anencephalic pregnancy that does not develop polyhydramnios, perhaps because the unstimulated fetal adrenal gland does not support the usual level of gestational estrogen production, and therefore the uterine myometrium is not properly prepared for labor and is less responsive to normal maternal oxytocin secretion at term.

Since the majority of infants with spina bifida will develop some degree of hydrocephalus, polyhydramnios and premature labor can also complicate these pregnancies. Furthermore, all varieties of ONTDs are predisposed to obstetrical malpresentation, including breech presentation and transverse lie, either because of the absence of an appropriate vertex to engage in the normal pelvis or possibly due to decreased motor tone in the lower extremities. Therefore, any pregnancy complicated by malpresentation or polyhydramnios should be carefully evaluated for the presence of congenital malformation, especially neural tube defects.

NEONATAL OUTCOME

The majority of infants with anencephaly will not survive more than a few days or weeks, though rarely a victim of anencephaly will survive several months. Neonates with occipital encephalocele or frontal cephalocele have a variable prognosis that depends on the severity of damage to the central nervous system. Interestingly, frontal cephaloceles have a somewhat better prognosis than occipital encephaloceles. An occipital encephalocele containing fluid only and not associated with microcephaly may be resected and reasonably good clinical outcome achieved. But encephaloceles containing significant neural tissue and associated with microcephaly are not consistent with successful repair and normal functional survival.

Spinal dysraphism (spinal bifida) can occur anywhere along the spine or include the entire spine. Craniospinal rachischisis describes the case of anencephaly and a completely unfused or open spine. Survival with craniospinal rachischisis is not possible.

Both the likelihood of survival and the degree of permanent disability as a result of spina bifida are roughly dependent on the level of the defect and its size. Survival is less probable with large thoracic lesions than it is with small sacral defects. The majority of cases, however, involve lumbosacral defects that are most often survivable but with significant permanent disabilities such as motor paralysis and mental retardation. Often the child with a successfully closed lumbosacral spina bifida can ambulate as a child with the assistance of braces but by early adulthood becomes confined to a wheelchair. On the other hand, in the case of a small sacral lesion, survival is expected, and the preservation of sufficient motor control to allow unassisted ambulation is the rule, although even here loss of bowel or bladder control is probable. With appropriate neurosurgical repair and decompression of hydrocephalus, if needed, the majority of victims of lumbosacral or lower spina bifida demonstrate intellectual function within the normal range. It is, of course, impossible to know if these individuals would have enjoyed a higher level of function in the absence of the malformation.

PRENATAL DETECTION

Clinical Detection

The relatively limited clinical indications of the presence of a fetus with a neural tube defect arise either from the palpable nature of the defect or disruption of the normal physiology of pregnancy (Table 6-2).

Table 6-2 Clinical Indicators of Neural Tube Defect

Failure to palpate a fetal cranium by third trimester
Polyhydramnios
Fetal malpresentation
Elevated MSAFP
Visualization on ultrasound done for other indications

During the second half of a normal pregnancy, the fetal vertex becomes transabdominally palpable in the majority of cases. This is not necessarily true in the case of the obese patient, but it is true of most others. Certainly, the failure to palpate a fetal cranium by the third trimester in the patient of normal size could indicate the possibility of a problem. The identification in late pregnancy or in labor of a breech presentation in a few cases also provides the opportunity to palpate the defect transcervically. This obviously requires a sufficiently dilated cervix and an appropriately positioned fetus to allow palpation of the lower fetal spine.

Altered fundal growth can also lead to the detection of a neural tube defect. A common cause of increased fundal growth is excess amniotic fluid, which can be associated with both anencephaly and severe hydrocephalus complicating spina bifida. A careful sonographic examination of both intracranial and spinal anatomy should be undertaken in every case of polyhydramnios.

Screening Tests

Screening for neural tube defects can be accomplished by both biochemical and imaging techniques. An ONTD results in increased amniotic fluid alpha-fetoprotein and increased MSAFP. Large populations can therefore be screened with a blood sample, and those individuals with elevated MSAFP can be referred for further evaluation. It is important to remember that MSAFP testing is not diagnostic. There is considerable overlap between the distributions of MSAFP levels in normal and affected pregnancies, and therefore the threshold for abnormal is arbitrary, with a majority of those individuals with levels above the cutoff not affected by ONTDs (Table 6-3). Furthermore, other causes for an apparently elevated MSAFP include twins, incorrect gestational age, fetal death, and other malformations such as urinary tract defects and ventral wall defects. Finally, about one third of the cases in which MSAFP is elevated on one occasion show a normal result upon subsequent evaluation, with no observed poor outcome associated with the single elevation. Such a transient single elevation may result from a small leakage of fetal serum into the maternal circulation. Therefore, the appropriate follow-up for a single elevation of MSAFP is to repeat the test. If the

Table 6-3 Diagnostic Assessment of Increased MSAFP

Incorrect gestational age	20%
Twins	11%
Fetal death	3%
Malformation	9%
Unknown after level II scan	56%

repeat result is still elevated, ultrasound examination is indicated to confirm gestational age, exclude multiple gestation, and establish fetal viability. If none of these observations resolves the apparent elevation, then referral for targeted high-detail evaluation of the fetal neural axis is appropriate, along with consideration of amniocentesis (see below).

Routine ultrasound screening of low-risk populations for clinical reasons has been undertaken at many centers. In the course of such screening, fetal malformations may be detected, including neural tube defects. However, the low incidence of ONTDs suggests that at least 1000 examinations must be done for every defect detected. Also, the skill and experience level required to ensure maximum sensitivity of the highly subjective ultrasound technique is not widely available. It is not likely, therefore, that routine ultrasound screening will become an effective method for neural tube defect detection, although there may be other clinical reasons for consideration of routine ultrasound examination.

ULTRASOUND EVALUATION OF THE
FETAL NEURAL AXIS

An imperfect nomenclature has evolved to describe the two types of ultrasound relevant to the detection of ONTDs in association with an MSAFP screening program. The two types of ultrasound are designated level I and level II. The designations can be somewhat confusing because they do not describe the location of the examination, only the content and goals.

A level I scan may be performed in an obstetrician's office or a referral hospital. The level I scan may be done with any quality of equipment and has the limited goals of determining the number, viability, position, and gestational age of the fetus or fetuses. It is not the specified goal of level I ultrasound to exclude the presence of a neural tube defect to the limit of the technique. Although experience among investigators varies, the fraction of cases of elevated MSAFP that may be explained by a level I ultrasound examination is near one third, based on the identification of incorrect gestational dates, twins, and fetal death. Furthermore, a level I examiner would expect to detect some of the 9% of fetuses with malformations among pregnancies with elevated MSAFP.

Level II ultrasound could as well be termed "targeted," "high detail," "high resolution," "referral," or any other designator to indicate that the goal of the examination is to specifically search for malformations in addition to the basic screening goals of a level I scan. Careful, organ system-targeted, high-detail fetal anatomic evaluation with ultrasound, as we will shortly see, should lead to the detection of 95% or more of all open neural tube defects.

Ultrasound therefore complements MSAFP screening for neural tube and other malformations, at two levels. First, a good-quality screening ultrasound examination in the clinician's office in the case of an elevated MSAFP can explain up to one third of the cases on a nonanomalous basis and avoid the need for referral and prolonged anxiety for the patient. Second, at the referral facility, high-detail targeted ultrasound can detect and characterize the great majority of ONTDs before amniocentesis.

Normal Ultrasound Anatomy of the Neural Axis

Clinically meaningful sonography of the fetal neural axis may be done as early as 12 weeks' gestation, using transvaginal scanners (Figure 6-1). With good-quality transabdominal equipment and a patient of average weight, the

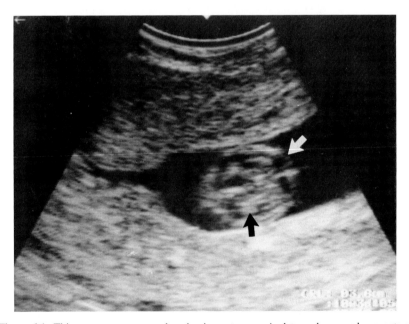

Figure 6-1 This sonogram was produced using a transvaginal transducer and presents an occipitofrontal scanplane of the fetal cranium (white arrow), with the typically prominent choroid plexuses (black arrow), at about 10 weeks' gestation.

fetal cranium and even a large part of the spine are visible by 14 to 15 weeks. In the paramedial sagittal scanplane, the horseshoe-shaped lateral ventricle is seen extending over the thalamus, with the choroid plexus arising from above the thalamus and filling the lateral ventricle behind the thalamus (Figure 6-2). The normal fetal cranium in an occipitofrontal scanplane at the level of the thalami presents a symmetrical, oval echogenic outline with frontal ventricular horns, midline, thalami, and choroid plexuses visible (Figure 6-3). By 16 weeks' gestational age both intracranial anatomic detail and spinal detail may be imaged with high-resolution ultrasound. In the standard occipitofrontal scanplane, the uniform oval shape of the cranium and intracranial details such as midline, frontal horns, cavum septum pellucidum, thalami, and choroid filling the posterior lateral ventricle are seen. At a more superficial level, the choroid plexuses dominate the hemispheres (Figure 6-4), while rotating the transducer slightly in a caudal direction will reveal the posterior fossa (Figure 6-5). The cerebellar hemispheres are symmetrical, circular echolucent structures with a faint echogenic outline just dorsal to the brainstem. The cerebrospinal fluid filling the cisterna magna

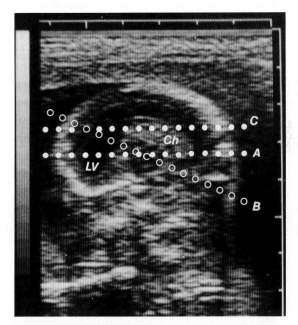

Figure 6-2 A sagittal scanplane just to one side of the midline of the cranium of a 16-week fetus shows the horseshoe-shaped lateral ventricle (LV) arched over the thalamus, with the choroid (Ch) arising from the top of the thalamus and filling the posterior ventricle. Scanplane A is appropriate for a biparietal diameter, scanplane B is best suited to imaging of the posterior fossa, and scanplane C would show mainly the choroid plexuses.

POSTERIOR   ANTERIOR

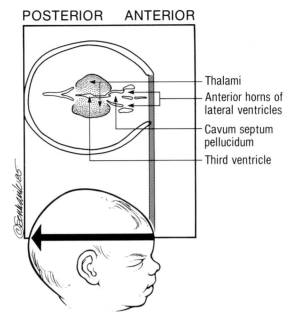

- Thalami
- Anterior horns of lateral ventricles
- Cavum septum pellucidum
- Third ventricle

Figure 6-3 This artist's drawing illustrates the approximate scanplane and the anatomy typical of the occipitofrontal orientation of scanplane A in Figure 6-2. *Source*: Reprinted from *Practical Obstetrical Ultrasound* (p 33) by JW Seeds and RC Cefalo, Aspen Publishers Inc, © 1986.

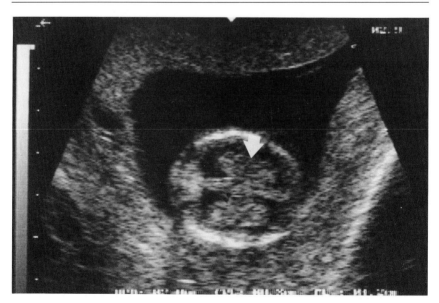

Figure 6-4 This sonogram corresponds to scanplane C of Figure 6-2, and shows the massive choroid plexuses (arrow) typical of the 14-week fetus.

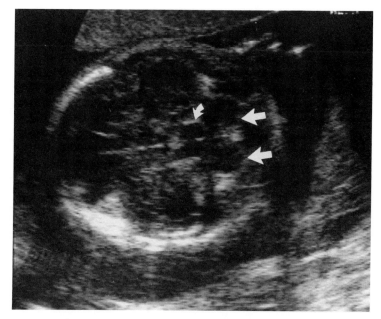

Figure 6-5 Scanplane B of Figure 6-2, illustrated here, shows the cerebellar hemispheres (straight arrows) to be symmetrical, circular structures dorsal to the brainstem (curved arrow). The dorsal interface of the hemispheres with the fluid of the cisterna magna is clear.

may be seen behind the cerebellar outline. The normal cranial outline and the above-described intracranial anatomy are important in contemporary prenatal diagnosis of neural tube defects because up to 95% of ONTDs visibly alter these features of cranial anatomy. The width of the lateral ventricles may be measured at the frontal horns, but the examination of the ventricles at a more posterior point may be more sensitive for the early detection of dilatation (Figure 6-6).

The early fetal spine may be examined both transversely and longitudinally. In transverse scanning, the normal fetal spine in early pregnancy consists of three echocenters spaced equal distances apart, as if at the points of an equilateral triangle, corresponding to the calcification centers of the vertebral body in the anterior midline and the neural arches in each dorsal, slightly paramedial area (Figure 6-7). The skin and other soft tissue dorsal to the spinal echocenters may be seen and their integrity evaluated throughout the length of the spine. The spinal echocenters in transverse views should maintain symmetrical spacing throughout the length of the spine when examined sequentially. Longitudinal scans of the fetal spine may be made in five planes (Figure 6-8): two oblique, one sagittal, and two coronal. The two coronal scanplanes are the most sensitive in the detection of spina bifida. The

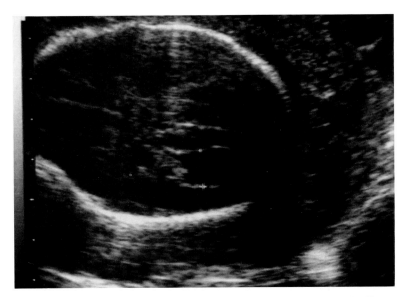

Figure 6-6 In this occipitofrontal scan of the fetal cranium, the measurement of the diameter of the posterior lateral ventricle is shown. This is the point of measurement that offers greatest sensitivity for hydrocephalus. This diameter should never exceed 1.2 cm prior to 24 weeks.

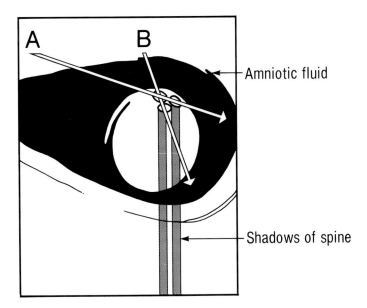

Figure 6-7 The two most popular scanplanes for the longitudinal examination of the fetal spine are illustrated here, with plane A being the more useful coronal plane. *Source*: Reprinted from *Practical Obstetrical Ultrasound* (p 34) by JW Seeds and RC Cefalo, Aspen Publishers Inc, © 1986.

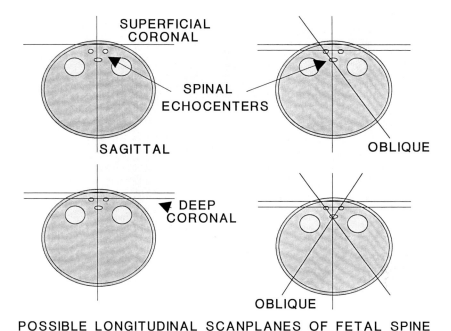

SUPERFICIAL
CORONAL

SPINAL
ECHOCENTERS

SAGITTAL

OBLIQUE

DEEP
CORONAL

OBLIQUE

POSSIBLE LONGITUDINAL SCANPLANES OF FETAL SPINE

Figure 6-8 All five possible longitudinal orientations for the examination of the fetal spine are presented here.

most superficial coronal longitudinal scanplane offers the opportunity to detect even the very small skin defect, due to the anechoic nature of the spinal fluid or amniotic fluid that would fill the area.

The longitudinal examination is typically seen as two fine parallel lines of echocenters (Figure 6-9). Longitudinal examination in one of the coronal planes offers the best sensitivity in the detection of neural tube defects.

Although it is not possible to visualize the fetal spine in high detail or to image intracranial anatomy with great clarity at 12 weeks, it is possible to clearly see the normal cranium, and therefore absence of it would be significant. Anencephaly should therefore be detectable in most cases by 12 to 14 weeks, and defects such as a large encephalocele or a large spina bifida might also be detectable. Such early detection of an ONTD offers the advantage of simpler clinical management alternatives for the patient, and therefore patients known to be at risk for the birth of a child with an ONTD should be offered early ultrasound in future pregnancies since up to half of the recurrences are in the form of anencephaly or encephalocele.

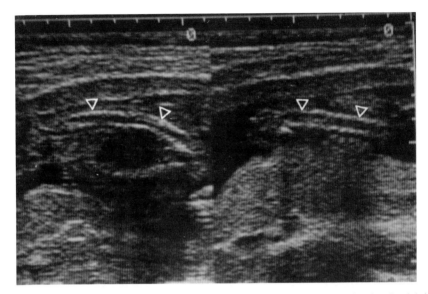

Figure 6-9 Both the oblique orientation (on the left) and the coronal orientation (on the right) are shown in this sonogram of the spine of a 17-week fetus. The coronal view is considered the most sensitive longitudinal view for the detection of spina bifida. Triangles indicate bone echocenters of fetal spine. *Source:* Adapted from *Practical Obstetrical Ultrasound* (p 35) by J W Seeds and RC Cefalo, Aspen Publishers Inc, © 1986.

Sonographic Appearance of Neural Tube Defects

Anencephaly

Failure of the rostral neuropore to close leads to anencephaly or encephalocele. Through the use of good-quality sonographic equipment (Figure 6-10), absence of the fetal cranium should be clear by 14 weeks' gestation in the patient of average size. Obesity or images of poor clarity might make the diagnosis more difficult. Confirmation by a second examiner of the absence of a fetal cranium confirms a malformation of proven lethality. Most often there is a fetal face, with orbits, nose, and mouth. Occasionally soft tissue masses are seen arising from the base of the skull that may be seen to move with fetal movement (Figure 6-11). These soft tissue masses represent incomplete fetal brain formation.

Occipital Encephalocele

Essentially a cranial meningocele (sac only) or myelomeningocele (sac containing neural elements), encephaloceles may present a variety of configurations. Encephaloceles may be sacs of variable size filled with fluid only,

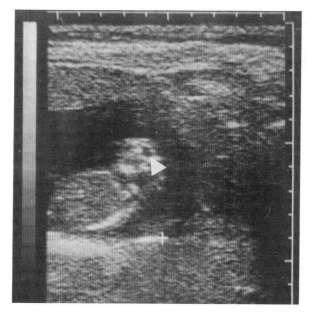

Figure 6-10 Anencephaly in a 15-week fetus is illustrated here. The face, including orbit (triangle) is seen, but the cranium is absent. *Source*: Reprinted from *Practical Obstetrical Ultrasound* (p 99) by JW Seeds and RC Cefalo, Aspen Publishers Inc, © 1986.

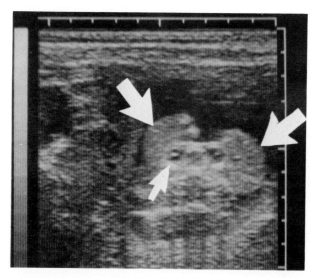

Figure 6-11 This frontal view of an anencephalic fetus is an example of the occasional case with considerable but incomplete brain formation (large arrows). Again, the orbits (small arrow) are seen. *Source*: Reprinted from *Practical Obstetrical Ultrasound* (p 98) by JW Seeds and RC Cefalo, Aspen Publishers Inc, © 1986.

arising from the occipital midline (Figures 6-12 and 6-13), or they may be filled with variable amounts of neural tissue (Figures 6-14 and 6-15). Encephaloceles might also be seen in combination with hydrops (Figure 6-16). Encephaloceles most often are located in the occipital region, but rarely may be seen frontally. Prognosis is tied to the amount of neural tissue within the sac and to the effect on brain growth. In the case of a sac filled with tissue and/ or associated with microcephaly, the prognosis is very poor. If the encephalocele is fluid filled and the cranium is of appropriate size, the prognosis can be good for repair and survival, although significant neurosurgical care may be necessary.

Spinal Dysraphism (Spina Bifida)

Neural tube failure in the thoracic, lumbosacral, or sacral areas may be associated with a simple opening of the spine (dysraphism), an empty sac (meningocele), or more often a sac with neural elements either within it or embedded in its base (myelomeningocele). Sonographic detection of spina bifida depends either on direct visualization of the defect itself or detection of secondary anatomic deformations of cranial and intracranial anatomy.

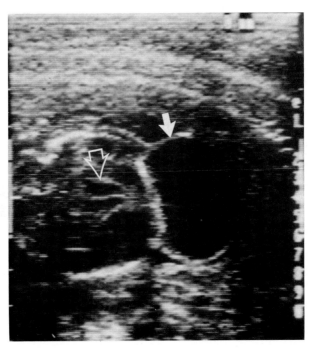

Figure 6-12 An occipital encephalocele originates in the occipital midline, as shown here. This encephalocele (solid arrow) is fluid filled (anechoic). The brainstem is also seen (open arrow).

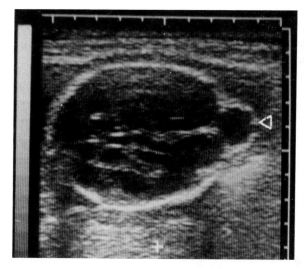

Figure 6-13   Occipital encephaloceles may be small, as seen here (triangle).   Small sacs containing only fluid have a significantly better overall prognosis. *Source*: Reprinted from *Practical Obstetrical Ultrasound* (p 106) by JW Seeds and RC Cefalo, Aspen Publishers Inc, © 1986.

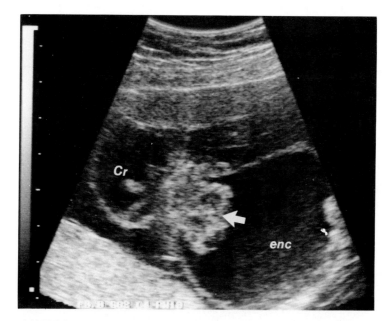

Figure 6-14 This is a large encephalocele (enc) containing both fluid and neural tissue (arrow) and associated with a microcephalic fluid-filled cranium (Cr). The prognosis in such a case is very poor.

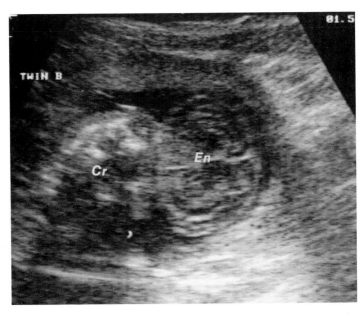

Figure 6-15 This large encephalocele (En) is completely filled with brain tissue and results in severe microcephaly of the cranium (Cr). This is essentially a nonsurvivable malformation.

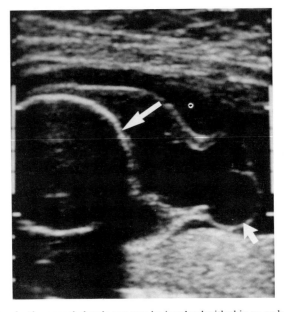

Figure 6-16 Rarely, the encephalocele sac may be involved with skin or scalp edema, as seen here. The cranium (long arrow) is to the left, and the sac (short arrow) is seen to extend through considerable scalp edema.

Table 6-4 Five Cranial Signs of Spina Bifida

Biparietal diameter 1 to 2 weeks behind dates or femur length
Mild ventriculomegaly
Frontoparietal notching (lemon sign)
Compressed cerebellar hemispheres (banana sign)
Absence of cisterna magna

As mentioned above, the cranial contour and intracranial anatomy are critical features to be examined when searching for spina bifida. There are five cranial signs of spina bifida in early pregnancy (Table 6-4). The fetal biparietal diameter is almost universally 1 to 2 weeks less than expected for both menstrual dates and femur length, in the case of spina bifida in early pregnancy. Late in gestation the reverse may be true, as developing hydrocephalus may cause expansion of the ventricles and excessive growth of the head, but before 20 weeks it is small for dates. Typically there is ventriculomegaly, but it is usually mild. The normally smooth contour of the cranium in the occipitofrontal scanplane is lost due to depressions in the frontoparietal areas (Figure 6-17). This has been referred to as the "lemon sign." In the posterior fossa, instead of clear, symmetrical, circular cerebellar hemispheres, they are compressed and distorted into more linear structures (Figure 6-18),

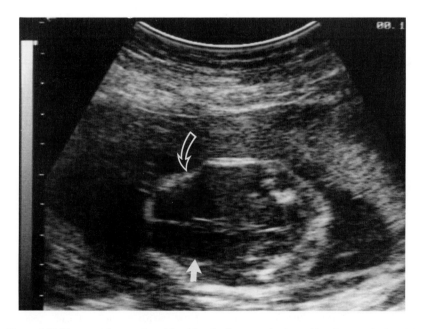

Figure 6-17 The curved arrow here identifies the frontoparietal notching (lemon sign) and the solid arrow the mild ventriculomegaly typically associated with spina bifida.

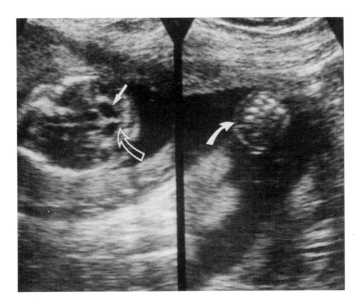

Figure 6-18 The compression of the cerebellar hemispheres associated with spina bifida is shown here. The cerebellar hemispheres (solid arrow on left) are flat instead of circular (banana sign). The cisterna magna is absent (open curved arrow). The meningomyelocele sac is clearly seen on the right (curved solid arrow).

and the normal fluid interface dorsal to them (cisterna magna) is lost. This appearance has been referred to as the "banana sign." Several investigators have shown these cranial changes to accompany over 95% of cases of spina bifida, including even the very small defects. The search for spina bifida, therefore, now begins with a careful evaluation of the fetal cranium.

Direct sonographic views of the defect in spina bifida may be longitudinal or transverse. It is possible, however, to miss a case using only one of the oblique longitudinal views (Figure 6-19). A coronal view of the dorsal spinal soft tissue combined with a sagittal view will often detect very small defects (Figure 6-20). Sonograms of spina bifida in late pregnancy show clearly the divergence of the spinous processes in the area of the defect (Figure 6-21). If present, the sac of the meningocele may be seen dorsal to the area of the defect (Figure 6-22). Dysraphic lesions can be combined with other anomalies, such as ventral wall defects (Figure 6-23), and in some cases severe spinal scoliosis may accompany the spina bifida (Figure 6-24).

Complete craniospinal rachischisis causes failure of closure along the complete length of the spine, resulting in parallel rows of echocenters on longitudinal scan but abnormal distance between the two columns (Figure 6-25), as well as absence of a cranium. Iniencephaly results in

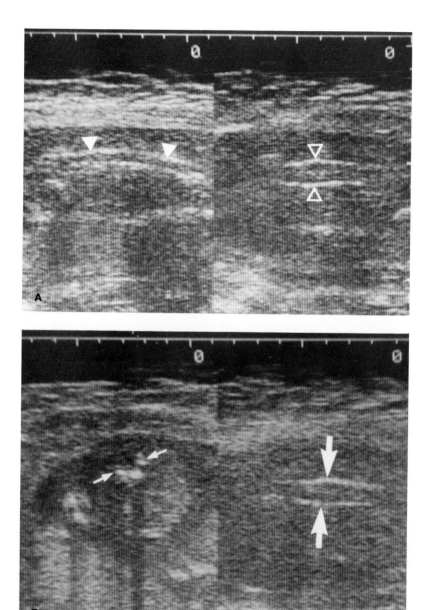

Figure 6-19 A, The oblique longitudinal view (solid triangles) of this fetal spine on the left gives no clue as to the dysraphic lesion (open triangles) seen on the coronal view of the same fetus shown on the right. **B,** To complete the examination of the fetal spine shown in A, here is shown the transverse view in the area of the defect. The separation of the dorsal paramedian echocenters is clearly visible (small arrows) on the left. **C,** This is the fetus shown in A and B. *Source:* Reprinted from *Practical Obstetrical Ultrasound* by JW Seeds and RC Cefalo, Aspen Publishers Inc, © 1986.

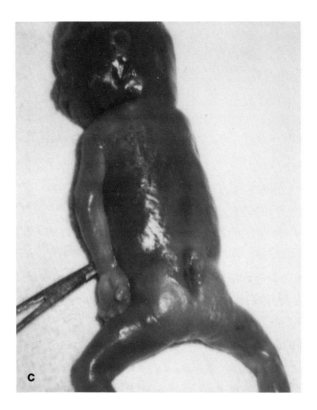

c

extreme dorsiflexion of the cranium on the neck, with fusion of the occiput to the dysraphic cervical spinal segments (Figure 6-26).

Biochemical or Visual Confirmation

Amniocentesis may be performed with analysis for both amniotic fluid alpha-fetoprotein, which will be increased in the presence of an ONTD and also a ventral wall defect, and for acetylcholinesterase, which is more specific for ONTD. The need for this additional testing depends on the clarity of the ultrasound images and the confidence of the diagnosis of a defect. Further confirmation may be derived from fetoscopy, which would allow direct visualization of the defect and some measure of its size, but this is rarely done.

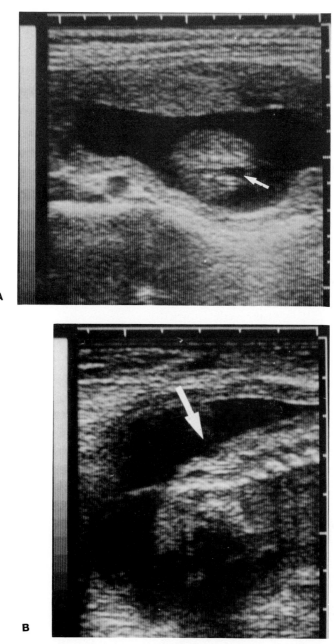

Figure 6-20 A, A very superficial coronal scanplane of the lumbosacral spine of a fetus with a small neural tube defect shows the echo-free area of the defect (arrow), filled with amniotic fluid. **B,** A sagittal midline view of the defect shown in A also shows the defect (arrow).

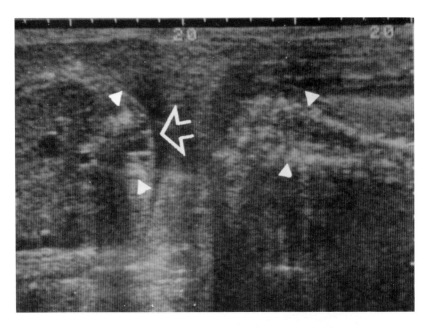

Figure 6-21 Spina bifida later in gestation may be more visibly disruptive to normal spinal anatomy. On the left is a transverse view of the dysraphic lesion (triangles), and on the right is a longitudinal view. *Source*: Reprinted from *Practical Obstetrical Ultrasound* (p 101) by JW Seeds and RC Cefalo, Aspen Publishers Inc, © 1986.

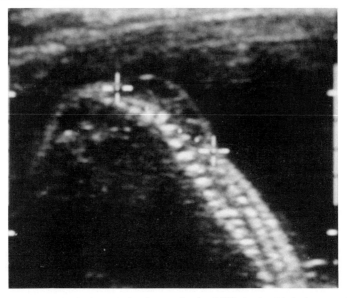

Figure 6-22 This sagittal view of a lumbosacral spina bifida in the third trimester shows the meningocele sac rising from the dorsal midline.

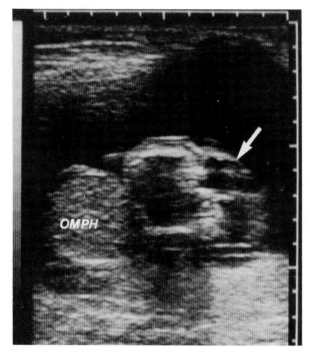

Figure 6-23 Both a meningocele (arrow) and an omphalocele (OMPH) were detected in this 19-week fetus being examined because of elevated MSAFP.

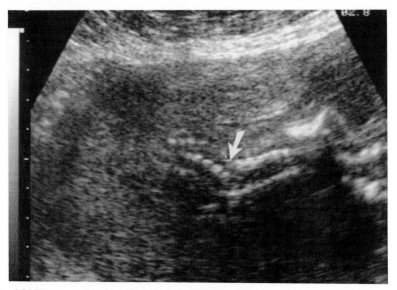

Figure 6-24 The arrow here identifies a point of extreme scoliosis on this coronal view of a fetal spine. Scoliosis is sometimes associated with spina bifida.

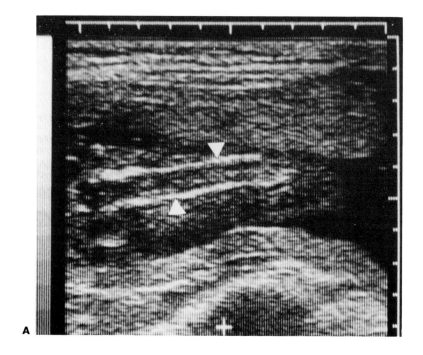

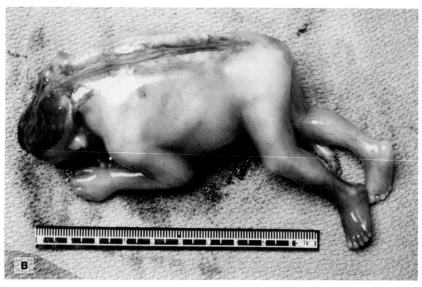

Figure 6-25 A, This coronal view of the spine of a fetus with craniospinal rachischisis illustrates the fact that the two rows of echocenters (triangles) are parallel but widely separated. **B,** Fetus depicted in A. *Source*: Reprinted from *Practical Obstetrical Ultrasound* (p 104) by JW Seeds and RC Cefalo, Aspen Publishers Inc, © 1986.

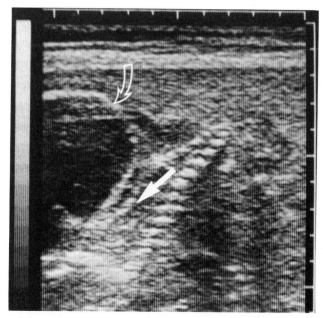

Figure 6-26 Iniencephaly, with the cranium (open curved arrow) in extreme dorsiflexion on the dysraphic cervical spine (solid straight arrow), is illustrated in this nearly sagittal scan of a 20-week fetus.

COUNSELING AND CARE AFTER THE DIAGNOSIS

Detection of the presence of an ONTD should include some estimate of the size and location of the defect. The rough relationship among size, location, and functional prognosis should be shared with the parents and specialized consultation with neurosurgery or pediatric consultants provided if desired. Prior to viability, pregnancy termination is an option for the parents to consider, but the decision is both unique to each family and very private. The patient should be convinced that full support of the counseling and health care team will be given to whatever decision is made regarding continuation or termination of the pregnancy.

If the pregnancy is continued, special arrangements should be made for prenatal care. In the case of anencephaly, special attention should be paid to the growth of the uterine fundus as a measure of amniotic fluid volume. Dangerous overexpansion of the uterus should be avoided. Usually, when faced with a complication of pregnancy that may threaten the mother's health, induction of labor is indicated and accepted.

Considerable controversy surrounds the best choice of method of birth in the case of spina bifida. Although it seems reasonable to assume that there is a considerable risk of sac rupture and bacterial contamination with vaginal birth, no clear clinical evidence supports the benefits of arbitrary abdominal delivery. If hydrocephalus complicates the case and fetal biparietal diameter exceeds normal limits, then cesarean delivery is indicated to avoid trauma to the fetal head. If the fetus presents in breech position with spina bifida and hydrocephalus, then abdominal delivery seems clearly superior. But in the absence of an enlarged head and malpresentation, the evidence is unclear regarding the benefits to the infant of abdominal delivery. Regardless of birth method, it is generally agreed that management for best outcome includes delivery at a center prepared for the special needs of these infants and the prompt repair of the defect.

SPINA BIFIDA: NEONATAL CARE

Since the postnatal survival of the anencephalic infant beyond a few days is not expected, we focus on the condition and management of the infant with spinal dysraphism and various cephaloceles. As stated above, spinal dysraphism (spina bifida) can occur anywhere along the spine or include the entirety of the spine (rachischisis). Survival with craniospinal rachischisis, as with anencephaly alone, is not possible.

In infants with spinal dysraphism, both a myelomeningocele and a meningocele are seen as a posterior midline cystic mass covered by thin, friable integument or full-thickness skin. The spinal membranes (meninges) protrude through a posterior vertebral bony defect and form the inner lining of the sac. These membranes are usually fused with the apical epithelial covering of the lesion (Figure 6-27). The most obvious common clinical difference between myelomeningocele and meningocele is the degree of neurological deficit observed. Infants with meningocele generally have much less severe neurological deficits, and when significant deficits occur, these can be attributed to other lesions within the craniospinal axis. At least 25% of children with meningocele have hydrocephalus.

The neonate with myelomeningocele usually shows significantly diminished motor and sensory functions, the severity of which will depend on the level of involvement of the spinal cord. Flaccid paralysis, absent reflexes, and amyotrophy commonly occur in the case of lumbosacral myelomeningocele. Thoracocervical or high lumbar lesions are most often associated with spastic paraplegia. Sensory deficits may also be apparent from absent or limited discrimination to pinpricks. Disordered rectal sphincter function is readily recognizable in severe forms. The loss of urethral and bladder sphincter tone, although difficult to detect in the neonate, complicates virtually all cases of spina bifida and will be significant later in childhood as the child bears the consequences of a neurogenic bladder.

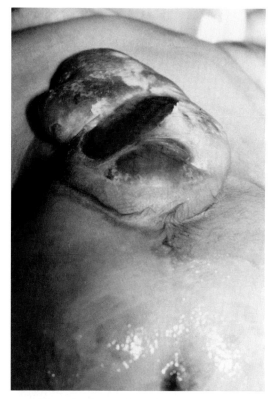

Figure 6-27 Neonate with large lumbar myelomeningocele. *Source*: Photograph courtesy of Thomas Lawrence, M.D.

In about 85% of children with spina bifida, the defects are located in the lumbosacral region. Rarely (less than 1%), the meningocele protrudes ventrally, producing an internal mass in the thorax, abdomen, or pelvis. Ventral meningoceles are found most commonly in the thoracic and sacral regions. Curiously, ventral sacral meningoceles are more commonly found in girls than in boys. At least 15% to 25% of the fetuses with spinal dysraphism are not detected antenatally because they have a very small bony defect covered by skin. Therefore, MSAFP is not elevated, and infants with these anomalies seldom come to a high-detail or level II ultrasound. These infants have what is termed spina bifida occulta and may be totally asymptomatic. A few will be seen with an area of hypertrichosis, a lipoma (see discussion of lipomyelomeningocele in Chapter 7), pigmented skin, or a dermal sinus overlying the spina bifida. Although obvious neurological deficits are absent at birth, a few of these patients have a tethered spinal cord that may become symptomatic and manifest as distal spinal cord or cauda equina–related neurological dysfunction as the child grows.

Associated Defects

Over 75%, and perhaps closer to 100%, of the infants born with myelomeningocele have or develop hydrocephalus, and virtually all such infants have type II Arnold-Chiari malformation of the brainstem and posterior fossa. The Arnold-Chiari malformation consists of an abnormal extension of cerebellar tissue, which is adherent to the underlying brainstem and protrudes into the spinal canal to the level of the second or third cervical vertebra. The medulla and the fourth ventricle are displaced caudally in the spinal canal. It is this posterior fossa deformity that is associated with the cerebellar compression and loss of cisterna magna noted in the review of ultrasound findings above. Reversal of the angles of the upper cervical nerve roots leaving the cord, cervical hydromelia, and a tethered cord often accompany this malformation. Although hydrocephalus in these patients can usually be attributed to the Arnold-Chiari malformation, up to one third will also have an aqueductal stenosis.

Other congenital anomalies are often found with major spinal dysraphic malformations and are listed in Table 6-5. The high incidence of clubfoot in association with overt and occult forms of spina bifida strongly implies a specific relationship. Local neurological deficits may or may not be demonstrable in the affected extremity.

Early Postnatal Management

Following delivery the infant with spina bifida should be placed in a prone position and the myelomeningocele or meningocele sac protected from desiccation, contamination, and trauma. Sterile saline-moistened gauze should be layered over the lesion, and the gauze should then be covered by clean plastic wrap to further retard drying. Protection is particularly important for the myelomeningocele patient, in whom the skin may be especially deficient. The meningeal layer may also be deficient, and in these infants the neural elements are exposed. Meningitis becomes an ever-present threat and

---

Table 6-5 Congenital Anomalies Associated with Spinal Dysraphism

Hydrocephalus
Vertebral-sacral anomalies
Clubfoot
Hip dislocation
Absent ribs
Bladder exstrophy
Genitourinary abnormalities
Cardiac anomalies
Klippel-Feil anomalies

a serious complication for these infants. Parenteral antibiotics and continued protection of the sac are warranted until the earliest possible surgical repair can be safely accomplished. Baseline measurements of the head circumference should be performed, along with evaluation of the fontanelles for evidence of increased intracranial pressure. The preoperative differentiation of myelomeningocele and meningocele is not based on the size of the lesion or the character of its covering. Appropriate diagnosis is supported by the presence or absence and degree of overt neurological deficit. Some recovery of neurological dysfunction may occur after repair if any part of the deficit is related to contusion of the neural elements during delivery. Furthermore, if a neurological deficit is associated with a simple meningocele, it points to neural dysplasia elsewhere in the craniospinal axis.

Surgical repair is accomplished by imbricating the lumbodorsal fascia and closing the skin without tension. The latter may be difficult in the face of a large skin defect. In some cases local undermining of skin may suffice; however, in large defects a rotation flap or extensive undermining with releasing incisions and lateral skin grafts may be required (Figure 6-28). Some infants with significant hydrocephalus will require ventriculoperitoneal shunting prior to or soon after repair of the spina bifida. Not infrequently, hydrocephalus that was not apparent before repair appears after excision of the meningocele sac. Prior to repair, the sac may serve in utero and after birth as a vent for cerebrospinal fluid (CSF) loss, allowing the ventricular system to remain relatively undilated. Following closure, postoperative inflammation or blood in the CSF may overwhelm the mechanisms for CSF resorption. A sudden decrease in the spinal CSF may further augment herniation of the cerebellar protrusion of an Arnold-Chiari malformation. This event could tamponade the foramen magnum and significantly increase the hydrocephalus.

Postoperative Care

The child should be maintained in a prone position. Daily evaluation of the wound to detect and deal with any infection or fluid collections is important. Daily measurements of head circumference and evaluation for increased intracranial pressure should be performed, especially for those infants who are not initially shunted. The widespread use of newer imaging techniques such as the CT scan and MRI have significantly improved our ability to evaluate and care for these infants.

Neonatal Outcome

Both the likelihood of survival and the degree of permanent disability as a result of spina bifida are roughly dependent on the level of neurological

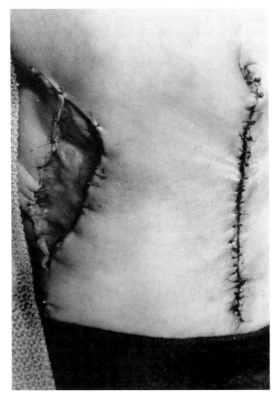

Figure 6-28 Same infant immediately following myelomeningocele repair. Extensive mobilization of skin flaps and lateral releasing incisions were required for closure of this defect. *Source:* Photograph courtesy of Thomas Lawrence, M.D.

deficit and the size of the defect. Survival is far less probable with large thoracic or cervical lesions than it is with small sacral defects. The majority of cases, however, involve lumbosacral defects (85%) that are most often survivable, but with significant permanent disabilities such as motor paralysis and mental retardation. In the absence of other central nervous system malformations and meningitis and if prompt neonatal closure and ventriculoperitoneal shunting are accomplished, 80% of these infants will demonstrate intelligence in the normal range. Often, as noted previously, the child with a successfully closed lumbosacral spina bifida can learn to ambulate with the assistance of braces as a child but by early adulthood becomes confined to a wheelchair. On the other hand, in the case of small sacral lesions, survival is expected, and the preservation of sufficient motor control to allow unassisted ambulation is the rule, although even here loss of some bowel or bladder control is expected.

Severe hydrocephalus is clearly associated with a poor prognosis in these patients. However, with appropriate neurosurgical intervention and decompression of the hydrocephalus if needed, many of these infants with lumbosacral and lower spina bifida can have a good functional outcome. Early postnatal shunting is also associated with optimal intellectual development. It is, of course, impossible to know if these individuals would have enjoyed a higher level of function in the absence of the malformation. In one recent study children who were shunted had a mean IQ of 91, whereas those not requiring a shunt had a mean IQ of 104. When complications such as ventriculitis arose, however, the mean IQ of those infants shunted fell to 70.

Surviving infants will often face many problems as they grow older. Not the least of these is the possible need for multiple neurosurgical shunt procedures. Significant musculoskeletal abnormalities, such as clubfeet, neurogenic dislocation of the hips, and paraplegia, pose tremendous obstacles for ambulation. Incomplete bladder emptying and urinary stasis with subsequent atony of the upper genitourinary tracts predispose these children to repeated and chronic urosepsis and the possibility of renal failure. Therefore, a dedicated myelodysplasia team of neurosurgical, orthopedic, urological, and pediatric physicians and a host of allied health personnel including nursing specialists and physical and occupational therapists are invaluable, providing the highest level of medical care and optimizing the chances for any individual child to achieve a reasonable physical status and lead a productive life.

CEPHALOCELE

Cephalocele is defined as a protrusion of the intracranial contents through a bony defect in the skull. Cephaloceles may present in a variety of configurations, as a cranial meningocele (sac of fluid) or as an encephalocele (sac containing neural elements). Cephaloceles most often are located in the cranial occiput but also rarely occur in the frontal, parietal, or basal region of the skull. Prognosis is tied to the amount of neural tissue within the sac and to the effect on brain growth. In the case of a sac filled with neural tissue and/ or associated with microcephaly, the prognosis is very poor. If the cephalocele is fluid filled and the cranium is of appropriate size, the prognosis can be good for repair and survival, although significant neurosurgical intervention may be required.

Sonographic verification of the cephalocele includes the visualization of a paracranial mass, usually in the midline, combined with a skull defect. The latter finding may be difficult to see since the bony defect is often much smaller than the herniated intracranial contents. More than two thirds of all occipital cephaloceles are associated with hydrocephalus. In contrast only 15% of the frontal cephaloceles are associated with significant ventriculomegaly. Large paracervical teratomas and cystic hygromas may be confused for a cephalocele. However, their paracervical location, the presence of multiple loculated cysts, and the absence of a cranial defect allow the sonographer to distinguish these lesions from cephaloceles. Other neural tube defects can be found in siblings, implying a genetic predisposition. Cephaloceles are a recognized component of a number of genetic (Meckel's syndrome, Chemke's syndrome, cryptophthalmos syndrome) and nongenetic (amniotic band syndrome, Wolfram's syndrome, nonfamilial frontonasal dysplasia) syndromes. The distinction of one of these syndromes is of importance in family counseling in order to provide accurate recurrence risk information.

Neonatal Care and Prognosis

Following delivery and initial stabilization, a thorough neurological evaluation of the infant should be performed (Figure 6-29). Postnatal ultrasound is useful in delineating the basic anatomy of the intra- and extracranial structures, particularly in unstable infants who cannot safely leave the neonatal intensive care unit (Figure 6-30). A CT or magnetic resonance

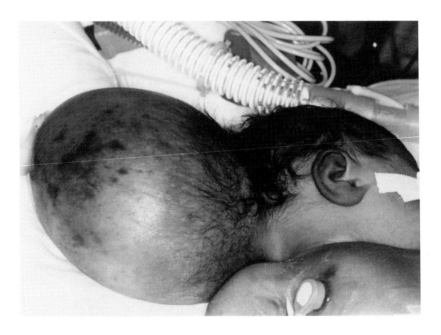

Figure 6-29 Neonate with a large occipital encephalocele. *Source*: Photograph courtesy of Dennis Vollmer, M.D.

image scan can provide further information as to the extent and involvement of the lesion (Figure 6-31). A careful search for other anomalies in these patients is warranted. In the case of the occipital encephalocele, between 65% and 85% will have associated hydrocephalus.

The protruding cephalocele should be carefully protected from direct trauma. Open lesions tend to be more complex anomalies and are usually associated with a much more dismal prognosis. Prognosis is adversely influenced by several factors, including the presence of brain tissue in the herniated sac, significant hydrocephalus, and microcephaly. Mortality has been reported as high as 40% with encephaloceles and as low as 5% with cranial meningoceles.

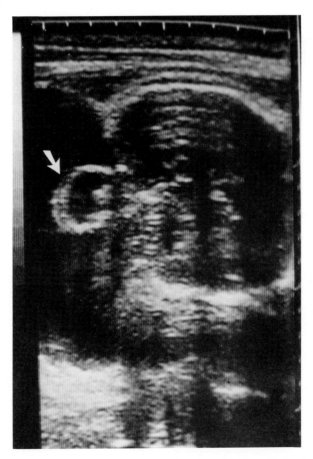

Figure 6-30 Antenatal ultrasound of same fetus with large occipital encephalocele demonstrates small amount of neural tissue (arrow) herniated into sac.

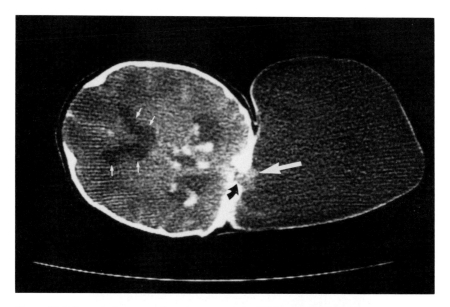

Figure 6-31 Computed tomography prior to repair establishes that this infant has hydrocephalus (small white arrows). The small occipital bony defect (black arrow) and the herniated brain tissue (large white arrow) are readily visible.

Surgical repair of the cranial meningocele includes removal of the sac, closure of the dural opening, and provision of a watertight soft tissue cover over the dural repair. Repair of the encephalocele is much more complex and may require resection of herniated brain tissue. If there is associated hydrocephalus, ventriculoperitoneal shunting should be performed with the repair of the encephalocele (Figure 6-32).

Intellectual development in children with occipital meningoceles has been reported as normal in up to 60% of the affected infants, whereas only 9% of infants with occipital encephaloceles have normal intellectual development. Significant ventriculomegaly or microcephaly in these patients was associated with profound intellectual impairment.

FURTHER READING

Burton BK, Sowers SG, Nelson LH. Maternal serum α-fetoprotein screening in North Carolina: Experience with more than twelve thousand pregnancies. *Am J Obstet Gynecol.* 1983; 146:439.

Campbell S, Thomas A. The use of ultrasound in the antenatal diagnosis of neural tube defects. *Birth Defects.* 1977; 13:209.

Drugan A, Zador IE, Syner FN, et al. A normal ultrasound does not obviate the need for amniocentesis in patients with elevated serum alpha-fetoprotein. *Obstet Gynecol* 1988; 72:627.

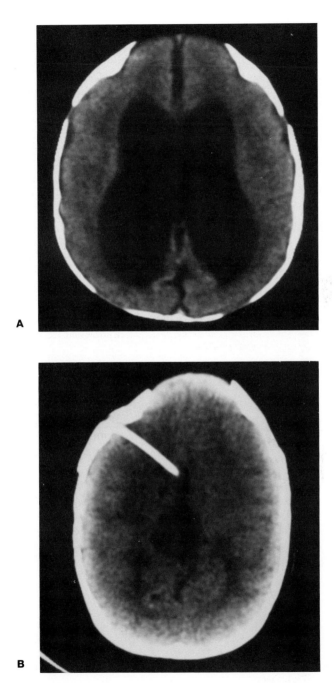

Figure 6-32 A, The marked hydrocephalus is easily seen in this infant following resection of an occipital encephalocele. **B,** The same infant following ventriculoperitoneal shunting, demonstrating marked improvement in ventriculomegaly. The intracranial portion of the shunt is seen.

Fiske CE, Filly RA. Ultrasound evaluation of the normal and abnormal fetal neural axis. *Rad Clin North Am*. 1982; 20:285.

Freeman JM, ed. *Practical Management of Meningomyelocele*. Baltimore: University Park Press; 1974.

Greenberg F, James LM, Oakley GP. Estimates of birth prevalence rates of spina bifida in the United States from computer-generated maps. *Am J Obstet Gynecol*. 1983; 145:570.

Haddow JE, Kloza EM, Smith DE, et al. Data from an alpha-fetoprotein pilot screening program in Maine. *Obstet Gynecol*. 1983; 62:556.

Leonard CO, Freeman JM. Spina bifida: A new disease. *Pediatrics*. 1981; 68:136.

Mapstone TB, Rekate HL, Nulsen FE, et al. Relationship of CSF shunting and IQ in children with myelomeningocele. A retrospective analysis. *Child's Brain*. 1984; 11:112.

Matson DD. *Neurosurgery of Infancy and Childhood*. 2nd ed. Springfield, Ill: Charles C Thomas, 1969.

Mealey J, Dzenitis AJ, Hockey AA. Prognosis of encephaloceles. *J Neurosurg*. 1970; 32:209–218.

Milunsky A, Alpert E. Results and benefits of a maternal serum α-fetoprotein screening program. *JAMA*. 1984; 252:1438.

Nager GT. Cephaloceles. *Laryngoscope*. 1987; 97:77–84.

The NICHD National Registry for Anmiocentesis Study Group. Midtrimester amniocentesis for prenatal diagnosis: Safety and accuracy. *JAMA*. 1976; 236:1471.

Nicolaides KH, Campbell S, Gabbe SG, et al. Ultrasound screening for spina bifida: Cranial and cerebellar signs. *Lancet*. 1986; 2:72.

Persson PH, Kullander S, Gennser G, et al. Screening for fetal malformations using ultrasound and measurements of α-fetoprotein in maternal serum. *Br Med J*. 1983; 286:747.

Roberts CJ, Hibbard BM, Roberts EE, et al. Diagnostic effectiveness of ultrasound in detection of neural tube defect. *Lancet*. 1983; 2:1068.

Wald NJ, Cuckle HS. Estimating an individual's risk of having a fetus with open spina bifida and the value of repeat alpha-fetoprotein testing. *J Epidemiol Community Health*. 1982; 36:87.

Chapter 7

Non-Neural Tube Malformations of the Head, Neck, and Neural Axis

The ability of high-resolution real-time ultrasound to provide good-quality images of the anatomy of the central nervous system of the fetus is well illustrated in the previous chapter. However, the visualization of certain malformations does not imply certain knowledge of prognosis and therefore places a special burden on those who would counsel pregnancy management on the basis of such visualization.

The organ system that is the second most frequently affected by serious malformation is the neural axis. In addition to malformations of the neural axis itself, by virtue of their anatomic proximity a variety of other malformations of the head and neck are also discussed in this chapter, including a variety of types of hydrocephalus, teratomas, and facial clefting.

The normal sonographic anatomy of the fetal neural axis is well described in the previous chapter, and the reader is referred to that description if a review is needed.

HYDROCEPHALUS WITHOUT SPINA BIFIDA

Isolated hydrocephalus is diagnosed when dilatation of the lateral ventricles without other associated intracranial or spinal abnormality is detected. Normal lateral ventricles show little growth, measuring an average of 7.5 mm at 15 weeks and 12 mm at term, so their normal early appearance is relatively large, and the brain and cranium grow around them. The upper limit of normal is 10 mm prior to 22 weeks, and up to 19 mm at term. The lateral ventricles may be measured at the frontal horns only if both are seen, in order to be sure that a correct scanplane, exactly perpendicular to the midline, has been derived. However, hydrocephalus appears first and is typically most severe at the level of the choroid plexus (Figure 7-1). Therefore, the most sensitive measurements of the ventricles for the purpose of early and sensitive diagnosis of hydrocephalus are made here. If the ventricular measurements exceed the limits of normal, hydrocephalus should be suspected. The diagno-

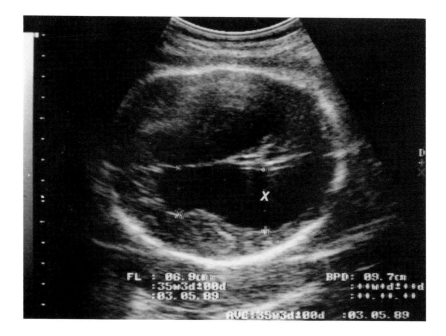

Figure 7-1 It is clear from an inspection of these moderately dilated lateral ventricles that the posterior portion of the ventricle is most severely affected. The width marked X is the most sensitive area to measure.

---

sis may be further supported by a comparison of the ventricular width to the hemispheric diameter in the same sonogram. Prior to 17 weeks this ratio may be as high as 0.50, but after 17 weeks it normally drops to under 0.33. This is simply another example of the phenomenon of the brain and cranium growing at a much more rapid rate than the ventricles.

Commonly, in the case of hydrocephalus, the choroid plexuses will be seen to droop dependently away from the transducer, and the midline membranes will be seen to waver flaccidly with uterine motion (Figure 7-2). Typically, there is a discontinuity of the midline membranes over the thalami in the case of severe hydrocephalus (Figure 7-3).

A sequential anatomic evaluation of the ventricular system may help identify the location of the obstruction. The third ventricle is located between the thalami and is not normally seen. If dilated, it would suggest that the site of obstruction is more distal, perhaps in the aqueduct of Sylvius (Figure 7-4). The fourth ventricle is located between and below the cerebellar hemispheres and, again, is not normally seen. If the third ventricle is dilated and the fourth is not, then the aqueduct is the likely location of obstruction. If the fourth ventricle is dilated, separating the cerebellar hemispheres, it indicates ob-

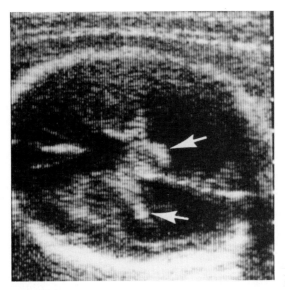

Figure 7-2 This sonogram of moderate hydrocephalus illustrates the dependent nature of the choroid plexuses (arrows), as they are here noted to droop dependently within the dilated ventricles. *Source*: Reprinted from *Practical Obstetrical Ultrasound* (p 109) by JW Seeds and RC Cefalo, Aspen Publishers Inc, © 1986.

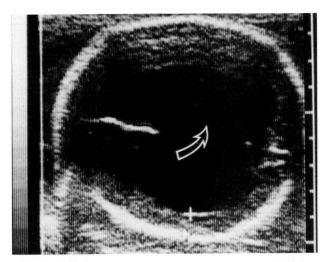

Figure 7-3 In the case of severe hydrocephalus, as shown here, the midline membranes are often seen to be discontinuous in the area of the midbrain (open arrow), as well as to undulate with motion. The thickness of the cortical mantle in the midparietal area is no longer thought to have prognostic value, as once was believed. *Source*: Adapted from *Practical Obstetrical Ultrasound* (p 110) by JW Seeds and RC Cefalo, Aspen Publishers Inc, © 1986.

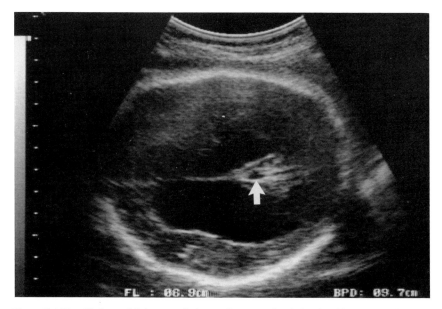

Figure 7-4 The third ventricle is normally located between the thalami and is not normally seen. In the case of aqueductal stenosis or atresia, dilatation of the third ventricle is expected, as seen here (arrow).

struction below that level, usually at the foramina of Luschka and Magendie, constituting a diagnosis of Dandy-Walker malformation.

The sonographic discovery of hydrocephalus should prompt an immediate examination of the posterior fossa and the spine, since up to one third of cases of congenital hydrocephalus are associated with spina bifida. A common error of the examiner after the discovery of any malformation is to concentrate on that anatomy and fail to adequately examine the remainder of the fetus. This is particularly unfortunate in the case of hydrocephalus associated with spina bifida since the final functional prognosis for the two conditions is significantly different.

Isolated hydrocephalus may occur as the result of multifactorial genetic factors, in utero infection with agents such as toxoplasmosis, in utero intraventricular hemorrhage, or less commonly as the result of a genetic syndrome such as a rare sex-linked recessive hydrocephalus or fetal aneuploidy. Therefore, consideration of fetal blood sampling or amniocentesis for fetal karyotype is appropriate. The majority of cases of symmetrical, isolated hydrocephalus result from multifactorial factors and therefore demonstrate a relatively low rate of recurrence, 2% to 4%. If the hydrocephalus is associated with infection, the risk of recurrence is typically much lower because the greatest risk of the fetus's being affected in most cases is only during the primary infection. If the hydrocephalus is part of a more general genetic syndrome or aneuploidy, the risk of recurrence is the risk associated with the specific syndrome diagnosed.

The prognosis for isolated fetal hydrocephalus can be good. Historical efforts to associate prognosis with the thickness of preserved cortical mantle have proven grossly inaccurate, however. In the case of isolated, symmetrical hydrocephalus that is the result of stenosis or atresia of the aqueduct of Sylvius and that receives appropriate neonatal neurosurgical intervention, the prognosis is good. Under these circumstances, normal intelligence and neurobehavioral function are expected in over 80% of cases. Even cases severe enough to make it difficult to visualize cortical mantle at all may achieve surprising functional recovery with proper treatment. It is necessary, however, to attempt to discriminate extreme hydrocephalus from other entities with differing prognoses, such as hydranencephaly or holoprosencephaly, which have a very poor prognosis regardless of care. Certainly, the majority of infants with hydrocephalus will require ventricular shunting, either to the cardiovascular system or the peritoneal cavity, and multiple procedures during childhood are the rule.

The functional prognosis for infants with hydrocephalus who are victims of in utero infection or genetic syndromes is poorer, and there are few therapeutic options. In the case of infection, other organ systems are often also affected, and the functional integrity of these other systems will often affect the final prognosis. It is also significant that several cases of apparently transient fetal ventriculomegaly have been reported, emphasizing the benefit of serial surveillance of the condition.

Obstetrical management may be altered by the presence of congenital hydrocephalus. If the condition is discovered prior to viability, the option of pregnancy termination should be considered. If the pregnancy continues or the condition is discovered after the point of viability, the influence of the diagnosis on pregnancy management depends on the size of the fetal head. If the biparietal diameter (BPD) exceeds 100 mm, then the absolute outside diameter of the fetal head generally exceeds 105 mm, and consideration of cesarean delivery is appropriate. Furthermore, it is common in cases of a BPD this large for the fetus to be in breech position, prompting consideration of cesarean.

The first example of the in utero treatment of fetal hydrocephalus was reported in 1981 using serial cephalocentesis. In 1982 the placement of an indwelling ventriculoamniotic diversion catheter was reported, and during the next 5 years, over 30 cases of such therapy were recorded by the International Registry of Fetal Surgery, maintained at the University of Toronto, Canada. The rationale for performing such intervention was based on the traditional information at the time that suggested a very poor prognosis for infants with congenital hydrocephalus, overt at birth, and also on the standard neurosurgical axiom that in the care of hydrocephalus, the earlier the decompression is accomplished, the better.

Such in utero therapy was considered in cases of isolated, progressive, symmetrical hydrocephalus. The intervention involved percutaneous placement of a thin-walled cannula through the occipital cranium into the dilated ventricle. A Silastic catheter was then advanced into the ventricle and the cannula removed, leaving the catheter to permit communication between the ventricle and the amniotic cavity (Figure 7-5). Although the technical feasibility of this treatment was established, three factors have led to general abandonment of the approach. First, with traditional treatment the outcome for isolated, symmetrical hydrocephalus has been shown to be much better than previously believed, making it very difficult to show significant benefit from fetal treatment. Second, at least six fetal deaths were apparently associated with the intervention, clearly emphasizing the possible dangers of such treatment. Third, in the majority of cases recorded by the International Registry, the condition was not isolated hydrocephalus. In these infants a

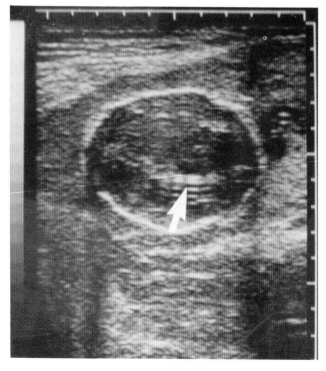

Figure 7-5 Following the placement of a ventriculoamniotic shunt, the internal terminus of the shunt can be seen within the cranium (arrow).

wide variety of associated significant malformations were overlooked, or the hydrocephalus was part of a broader syndrome with a prognosis not influenced by any therapy. Fetal therapy of isolated congenital hydrocephalus, therefore, is now not considered necessary or helpful.

HYDRANENCEPHALY

Hydranencephaly is characterized by an absence of cerebral cortical tissue within an intact cranium. It may be difficult to distinguish from extreme hydrocephalus using sonography alone, and therefore other imaging modalities such as CT or MRI may be used to confirm the diagnosis. Reported antenatal diagnoses have involved late gestations; therefore the appearance of this condition in early pregnancy is not known. Typically, by late in the third trimester, the cranium of a fetus with hydranencephaly is quite large, with a completely anechoic (echo-free or black) interior (Figure 7-6). Although there may be midline membranes, these are often absent. There is no cortex or peripheral soft tissue substance at all. Facial features are typically normal, and fetal movement is typically normal. This is characteristically an isolated defect and not associated with aneuploidy or genetic syndromes. The recurrence risk is very low.

The etiology of hydranencephaly is thought to be an early embryonic vascular accident or failure of the internal carotid arteries, with either resorption or failure of formation of cerebral cortical tissues. Neonatal survival for variable periods up to and possibly exceeding a year is possible, but neurobehavioral development is not possible, and eventually the infant's growth and development fail.

The early diagnosis of hydranencephaly must be based on very clear sonograms or the alternative imaging techniques mentioned above. If this diagnosis is confidently made early in gestation, termination of pregnancy should be considered. If the diagnosis is made later, obstetrical management may be based on consideration of maternal welfare. If the cranium at the time of delivery has achieved great size, transabdominal or transcervical cephalocentesis may increase the probability of vaginal delivery. However, even with cephalocentesis, vaginal delivery is not guaranteed. Furthermore, although cephalocentesis often leads to the intrapartum or neonatal death of the infant, this also is not guaranteed. Therefore, it is possible that despite cephalocentesis, cesarean delivery may be required anyway and produce a surviving but disabled infant with no chance of functional long-term survival.

The confident diagnosis of hydranencephaly should lead to prompt consideration of induction of labor and delivery to prevent further growth of the head and to optimize the probability of vaginal delivery of this infant with no chance of long-term survival.

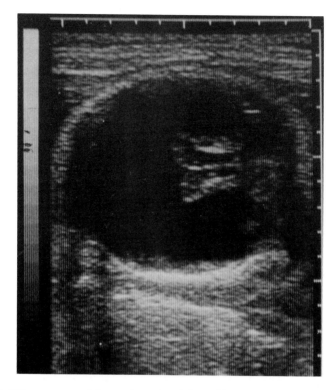

Figure 7-6 This sonogram of the cranium of an infant with hydranencephaly illustrates the absence of cortical matter. The cranium is filled with fluid only.

HOLOPROSENCEPHALY

Holoprosencephaly describes a family of cortical anomalies that result from a failure of the prosencephalon to divide in the 8th embryonic week to form bilateral cerebral hemispheres. The resulting single cortical structure may demonstrate no tendency toward bilaterality, constituting a subtype of holoprosencephaly known as alobar holoprosencephaly; there may be a slight tendency toward bilaterality, constituting semilobar holoprosenceph-aly, or there may be considerable evidence of bilaterality, called lobar holoprosencephaly.

The sonographic image of holoprosencephaly seen on the occipitofrontal scanplane is one of a single central anechoic ventricle surrounded by a cortex of variable thickness (Figure 7-7). This appearance may vary, however, and often complex malformations of the brain alter the appearance (Figure 7-8).

Ultrasound may not always be of sufficient clarity to allow a confident diagnosis because of artifact or fetal position. In those cases alternative imaging techniques may be helpful. Figure 7-9 illustrates a case of holoprosencephaly with inadequate ultrasound images. Magnetic resonance imaging was utilized to eliminate acoustic artifact and provided a definitive diagnosis (Figure 7-10).

Holoprosencephaly is often associated with facial deformities such as hypotelorism, anophthalmia, and absence or deformities of the nose, ears, and mouth. These malformations result from abnormal development of the relevant cranial nerves, which is related to the abnormal brain development. There is a vague correlation between the severity of holoprosencephaly and the presence of facial deformities.

In general, functional disabilities increase with decreased structural bilaterality, and prognosis for survival increases with increased structural bilaterality. There are reports of otherwise functionally normal patients identified to have a form of holoprosencephaly diagnosed incidentally. However, the alobar and semilobar forms of the disorder are not generally associated with functional survival.

Holoprosencephaly may occur as an isolated multifactorial central nervous system malformation, or it may be associated with genetic syndromes or

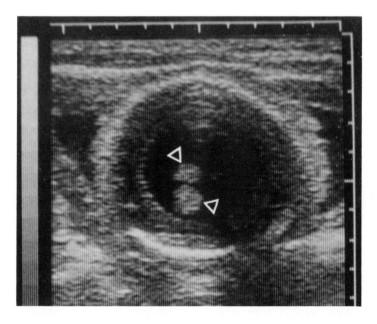

Figure 7-7 The paired choroid plexuses (triangles) float within the single ventricle of alobar holoprosencephaly pictured here. *Source*: Reprinted from *Practical Obstetrical Ultrasound* (p 114) by JW Seeds and RC Cefalo, Aspen Publishers Inc, © 1986.

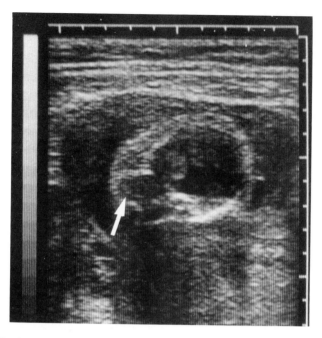

Figure 7-8 Similar in nature to the case illustrated in Figure 7-7, this sonogram is of an infant even more severely affected with holoprosencephaly. The single ventricle was associated with severe microcephaly. Only the single orbit (arrow) was present, and the fetus lacked a face altogether at birth.

aneuploidy. Triploidy and tetraploidy particularly have been seen in association with holoprosencephaly. The recurrence risk is low.

If the diagnosis is made in early pregnancy, the option of pregnancy interruption should be considered. Depending on the gestational age, either fetal blood sampling or amniocentesis should be considered to establish fetal karyotype. If the diagnosis is made in later gestation, the precise subtype of the condition can be important in assessing the potential viability of the fetus. A careful examination of the fetal face, including interorbital distances, is recommended as a correlate to the functional development of the central nervous system. Alternative imaging techniques such as CT or MRI can be important in discriminating lobar from semilobar or alobar holoprosencephaly.

If facial anatomy appears normal and the diagnosis is lobar or semilobar in nature, fetal survival is more likely. However, functional integrity cannot be accurately predicted. In the case of alobar holoprosencephaly with or without facial deformities, management for maternal welfare is appropriate. If there is semilobar or lobar holoprosencephaly, without more complex brain de-

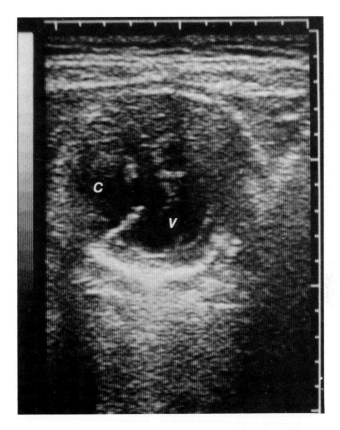

Figure 7-9 This sonogram appears to show a single ventricle (V) and possibly a posterior fossa cyst (C), but acoustic artifact significantly degrades the image. *Source*: Reprinted with permission from *American Journal of Perinatology* (1989;6:418–420), Copyright © 1989, Thieme Medical Publishers Inc.

formities and without significant facial deformities, then management for best fetal outcome is more appropriate. However, as mentioned above, final functional outcome cannot be predicted and is often imperfect.

DANDY-WALKER MALFORMATION

Obstruction of the foramina of Luschka or Magendie results in dilatation of the fourth ventricle and secondary supratentorial hydrocephalus, also known as the Dandy-Walker syndrome. The obstruction may result from failure to canalize the above-named foramina during development or secondary obstruction associated with intrauterine hemorrhage or infection.

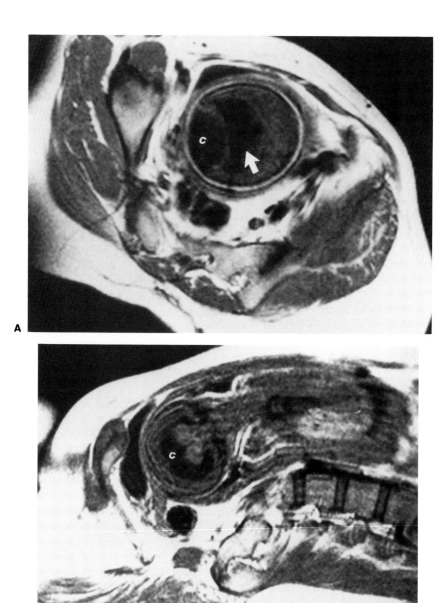

Figure 7-10 A, Magnetic resonance imaging of the fetus in Figure 7-9 eliminates the acoustic artifact and in this confirms a case of holoprosencephaly with a single ventricle (arrow) and a posterior fossa cyst (c). **B,** A longitudinal view of the MRI study of the infant shown in A shows the horseshoe-shaped ventricle (c) over the paired but fused thalami. *Source:* Reprinted with permission from *American Journal of Perinatology* (1989;6:418–420), Copyright © 1989, Thieme Medical Publishers Inc.

The sonographic appearance is one of hydrocephalus with dilatation of the lateral, third, and fourth ventricles (Figure 7-11). The roof of the fourth ventricle may be elevated to obliterate the cisterna magna, and the cerebellar hemispheres are separated by the dilated fourth ventricle.

The result varies from modest dilatation (Figure 7-12) to severe dilatation, with complete obliteration of visible soft tissue in the posterior fossa (Figure 7-13). The hydrocephalus can be severe.

The prognosis is poorer for hydrocephalus associated with Dandy-Walker malformation than it is for hydrocephalus associated with aqueductal stenosis or atresia. The neonatal therapy is more complex, because sudden decompression of the supratentorial pressure can result in upward herniation of posterior fossa tissues.

Although aneuploidy with Dandy-Walker malformation is rare, the diagnosis of hydrocephalus with Dandy-Walker malformation in early gestation should result in consideration of amniocentesis or fetal blood sampling for fetal karyotype. Obstetrical management is not necessarily altered for this diagnosis, and management for best fetal outcome is appropriate. If the fetal

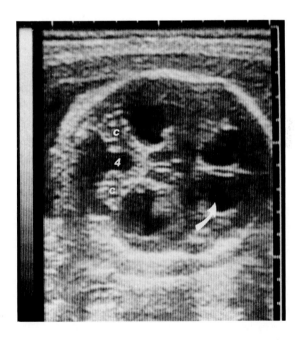

Figure 7-11 This posterior fossa scanplane of the fetal cranium (plane B of Figure 6-2) of a fetus with Dandy-Walker malformation shows the cerebellar hemispheres (c) separated by a dilated fourth ventricle (4) and the supratentorial hydrocephalus (arrow).

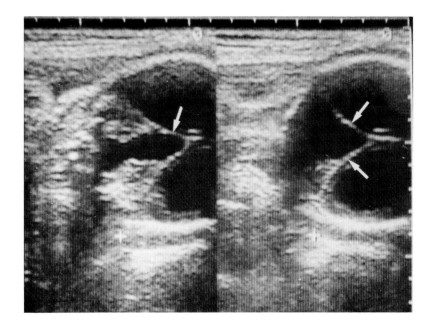

Figure 7-12 These views of the posterior fossa of a fetus with moderate to severe Dandy-Walker malformation shows the expansion of the fourth ventricle to fill and elevate the tentorium (arrows).

cranium grows to excessive proportions late in gestation, then cesarean delivery offers the best results. Malpresentation is common in these cases.

ARACHNOID CYST

Arachnoid cyst formation may occur in many locations and produce asymmetrical and confusing anatomic deformation. Whenever cystic mass abnormalities are found that do not appear to coincide with anatomic structures, arachnoid cyst formation should be suspected (Figure 7-14).

Arachnoid cysts appear to be sporadic malformations that have a low association with other anomalies and a low probability of aneuploidy. The recurrence risk is very low.

Prognosis varies from very good to poor and cannot be precisely assessed antenatally. However, the prognosis is often much better than would be expected from the degree of malformation.

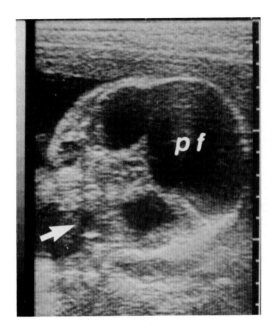

Figure 7-13 An extreme example of Dandy-Walker malformation is illustrated here, with a hugely dilated posterior fossa (pf). An orbit is indicated by the arrow for orientation. *Source*: Reprinted from *Practical Obstetrical Ultrasound* (p 113) by JW Seeds and RC Cefalo, Aspen Publishers Inc, © 1986.

TERATOMAS

Teratomas are germ cell tumors that may arise anywhere, including the sacrum, the cauda equina, the soft tissue of the neck, or even the fetal lip.

Sacrococcygeal Teratoma

A sacrococcygeal teratoma (SCT) may be internal or external, cystic or solid (or both). It may be resected with no residual disability, or with disability depending on size and location. If the tumor is mainly internal and remains undiagnosed in early infancy, SCTs do show a malignant potential of up to 10%.

Sacrococcygeal teratomas may be diagnosed in early or late gestation and may appear to grow quite rapidly. A large sacrococcygeal teratoma has been seen only 10 weeks after a normal sonogram. The early diagnosis of such a tumor should, as with other malformations, lead to the careful search for other anomalies and to discussion of management options, including possibly

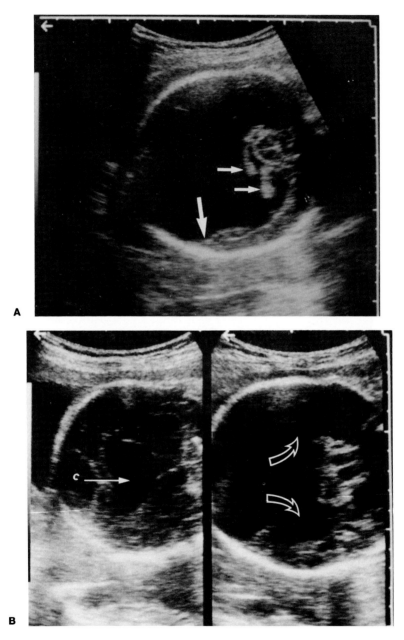

Figure 7-14 A, An arachnoid cyst has grown between the hemispheres and into the ventricular system to create unusual anatomy. The cortex very atypically stops at a midparietal point (large arrow). The choroids (small arrows) are seen drooping from the thalami (t). **B,** Similar views to A but sequenced from anterior to posterior; the arachnoid cyst (c) can be seen arising from above the cortex frontally, then extending down (arrows) between the hemispheres.

interruption. However, careful observation and atraumatic delivery with neonatal resection offer a very good prognosis for normal functional outcome.

At the time of antenatal ultrasound, the SCT appears to be a solid soft tissue mass arising from the sacral area of the fetus (Figure 7-15). The texture is typically mixed, with both solid and cystic areas. There are often dense areas with shadowing, indicating calcification. There is little or no organizational structure within the typical SCT. Occasionally the SCT appears to be purely cystic or fluid filled and may achieve great size.

Obstetrical management may be altered either by the fetal malpresentation that is common in these cases or by the size of the mass, which may result in soft tissue dystocia. A potential for difficult soft tissue manipulation should prompt consideration of cesarean delivery since vascular structures within these tumors are not well supported and internal hemorrhage with life-threatening potential can occur rapidly.

Nuchal Teratoma

Cervical teratomas also present a mixed internal sonographic appearance, most often mixed cystic and solid (Figure 7-16). The nuchal teratoma may

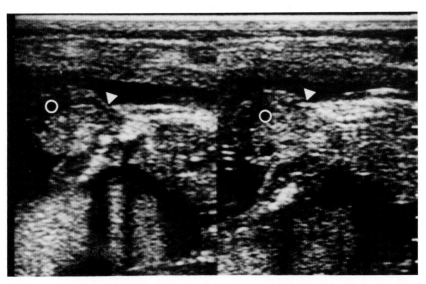

Figure 7-15 A sacrococcygeal teratoma arises from the caudal aspect of the fetus, may be cystic or solid, and most often presents a mixed pattern, as seen on this sagittal scan showing the teratoma (o) arising at the sacrum (triangle). *Source:* Reprinted from *Practical Obstetrical Ultrasound* (p 120) by JW Seeds and RC Cefalo, Aspen Publishers Inc, © 1986.

arise from the soft tissue surrounding the trachea or from the base of the tongue or hypopharyngeal tissues (Figure 7-17). These teratomas have also been seen to arise from the fetal lip. Frequently the fetal head is seen to be forced into extreme dorsiflexion suggesting the need for cesarean delivery because of the extremely unfavorable fetal posture. These tumors may also result in immediate neonatal ventilatory difficulty and are resectable only with difficulty, but are most often survivable. Delivery should occur in a center prepared for the immediate special needs of such an infant, including possible emergency tracheotomy.

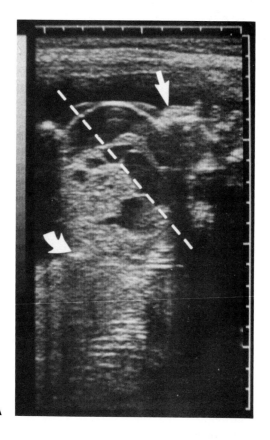

A

Figure 7-16 A, This sagittal scan of the neck of this fetus shows the fetal chin (straight arrow) dorsiflexed by a large cystic/solid mass arising from the ventral neck. *Source*: Reprinted from *Practical Obstetrical Ultrasound* (p 118) by JW Seeds and RC Cefalo, Aspen Publishers Inc, © 1986. **B**, A transverse view at the level of the dashed line on A confirms the disorganized cystic/solid and even calcified architecture typical of teratomas.

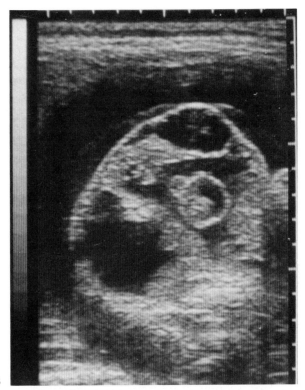

B

Lipomyelomeningocele

A fatty teratoma of the cauda equina that protrudes through an occult spina bifida and is associated with a subcutaneous infiltrative lipomatous tumor is called a lipomyelomeningocele. Most often the infant is neurologically normal at birth, with a soft subcutaneous mass overlying the lumbosacral spine. The mass may be easily ignored if not recognized for what it is. Resection of these tumors is necessary to prevent ascending neuropathy due to tethering of the cord as the child grows. Recurrence is possible, but only one case of recurrence within a sibship has been reported.

The sonographic appearance is that of a vaguely outlined echogenic mass of the lumbosacral midline extending into the spinal canal (Figure 7-18). There may or may not be a cystic component essentially constituting a meningocele sac. The mass is of variable size (Figure 7-19).

Although technically a defect of the neural tube, the neural tube defect itself appears to be secondary to the protrusion of the teratoma and not a primary closure failure of the neural tube.

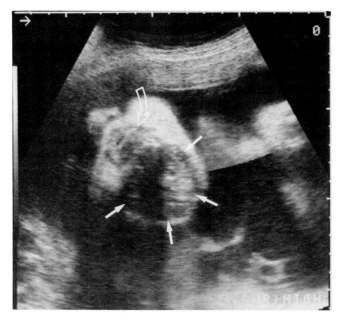

Figure 7-17 Teratomas may also arise from the base of the tongue, as seen here. The teratoma (arrows) is seen on this frontal facial view just below the fetal lips (open arrow).

There appears to be no clear association with other major malformations or aneuploidy, and no clear basis for alteration of obstetrical management based on this diagnosis. The early diagnosis of this tumor has been reported. The prognosis for successful resection and normal neurobehavioral development is very good.

INTRACRANIAL TUMORS

Glioblastomas, teratomas, and craniopharyngiomas have been diagnosed antenatally and may carry a poor but not absolute prognosis that depends on the malignant potential of the tumor in question, its size, and its surgical resectability.

The sonographic appearance of such tumors is variable. Most create a disorganized disruption of the normal intracranial anatomy. As the tumor grows, the midline is shifted by a soft tissue mass of variable echogenicity and lacking in internal architectural organization.

Diagnosis in early pregnancy is not expected and has not been reported. If found later in gestation, delivery as soon as fetal lung maturity is documented is recommended to allow the earliest possible resection. Delivery before 38 weeks often involves a cesarean delivery due to noncompliance of the

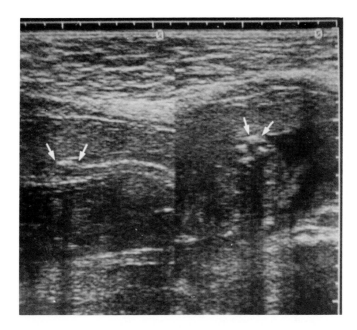

Figure 7-18 The sagittal view on the left and the transverse view on the right show the appearance in early gestation of the fatty subcutaneous tumor of the lipomyelomeningocele (arrows). *Source*: Reprinted with permission from The American College of Obstetricians and Gynecologists from *Obstetrics and Gynecology* (1988; 72:469–471), Copyright © 1988, Elsevier Science Publishing Company Inc.

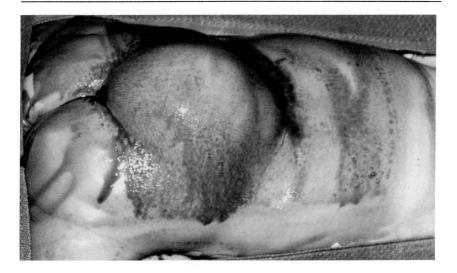

Figure 7-19 The lipomyelomeningocele is variable in final size but may be quite large, as illustrated here in the case of a 3-month-old infant prepared for surgical resection.

undilated cervix. Delivery is best performed in a center where appropriate neurosurgical services are available.

PORENCEPHALIC CYST

Often the result of vascular accident with subsequent soft tissue resorption, the porencephalic cyst can present considerable diagnostic difficulty because normal anatomic structures are often lost. The finding of a large, discretely outlined but irregularly shaped cystic (anechoic) mass within the cranium should suggest this possibility (Figure 7-20).

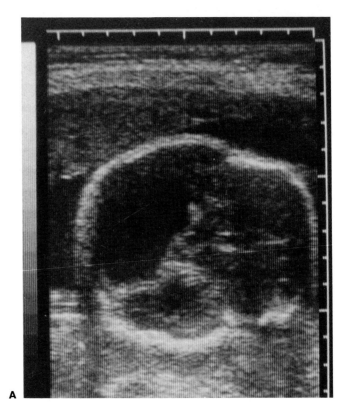

A

Figure 7-20 A, The irregular outline of the cystic mass of the porencephalic cyst is typical. **B,** The porencephalic cyst may grow with advancing gestation, as illustrated here. *Source*: Reprinted from *Practical Obstetrical Ultrasound* (p 111) by JW Seeds and RC Cefalo, Aspen Publishers Inc, © 1986.

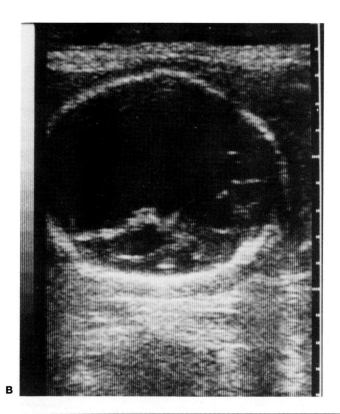

B

AMNIOTIC BAND SYNDROME

The entanglement of various fetal parts in fibrous bands thought to arise when the amnion breaks but the chorion remains intact in early gestation results in amputations, constriction rings, nonembryonic facial and trunk clefting, and rarely a kind of pseudoanencephaly. When the fetal cranium becomes entangled in such fibrous bands, no calcification occurs above the level of constriction, creating an image possibly consistent with encephalocele but often irregular in outline. The development of brain and scalp may closely simulate normal, but no cranium is formed (Figure 7-21). The detection of echogenic strands crossing the amniotic cavity, attached to the fetus, along with an associated fetal malformation indicates the diagnosis of amniotic band syndrome (Figure 7-22).

CHOROID PLEXUS CYSTS

Cystic defects in one or both choroid plexuses are seen in about 5% of infants. These vary in size from very small (Figure 7-23) to up to 1 to 2 cm in

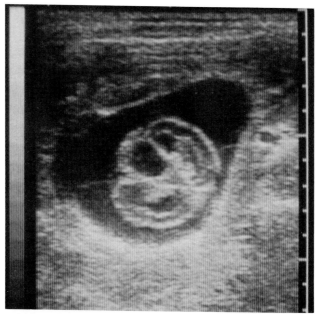

Figure 7-21 This sonogram is at the approximate level of the thalami and posterior fossa, showing remarkable brain development but no cranium.

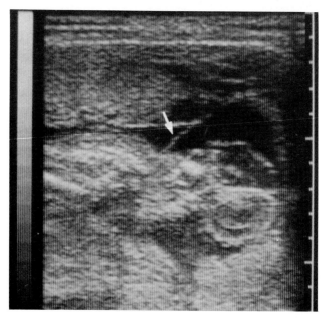

Figure 7-22 A longitudinal view of the fetus shown in Figure 7-21 reveals one of many transamniotic bands (arrow) eventually found to be responsible for the malformation.

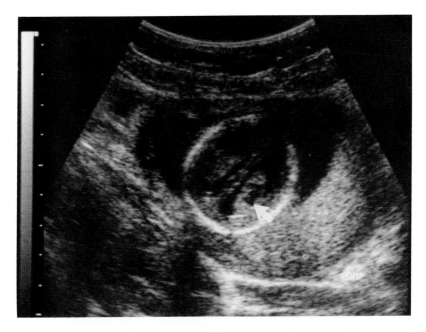

Figure 7-23 Choroid plexus cysts may be small (arrow), and most resolve spontaneously with advancing gestation.

diameter (Figure 7-24). The majority of these cystic areas spontaneously resolve as pregnancy progresses, but if the cysts are 2 cm in size or greater, or fail to disappear before 22 weeks' gestation, there is an increased risk of fetal aneuploidy—as high as 10%. If choroid plexus cysts are noted at scan and measure over 1 cm at or near midgestation, amniocentesis or fetal blood sampling should be considered.

FACIAL CLEFTING

Cleft lip and palate are the most common facial malformations. Cleft lip may be associated with a wide variety of genetic syndromes, is likely with certain types of aneuploidy such as trisomies 13 and 18, and may result from teratogenic exposure. However, over 90% of cases of cleft lip or cleft palate occur as isolated multifactorial malformations.

The incidence varies from 0.4 to 1.7 per 1000 live births, with a slight male predominance. About four out of five cases are unilateral. The risk of other associated anomalies is greater if the cleft involves both lip and palate. The recurrence risk is about 4% after the birth of an affected child, double that if there have been two previous children with clefts, and double that again if there is an affected parent and a previous child.

Cleft lip and palate have been successfully diagnosed in early pregnancy; facial anatomy may be examined with ultrasound in two planes, either a frontal or a coronal plane (Figures 7-25 and 7-26). A bilateral cleft lip and

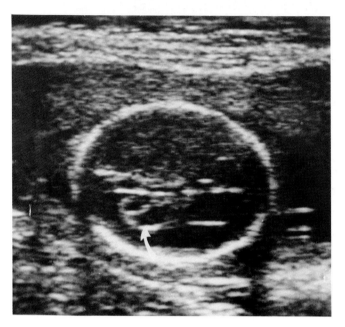

Figure 7-24 If choroid plexus cysts are large (curved arrow) or persistent, consideration of fetal karyotype should follow.

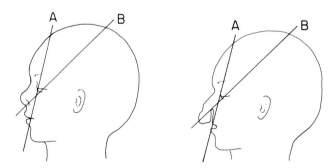

Figure 7-25 Scanplane A in this drawing in the normal case will show frontal fetal anatomy similar to that found in Figure 7-26. A slightly more coronal view may also be helpful in detecting facial clefting, as seen in Figure 7-27. *Source*: Reprinted with permission from The American College of Obstetricians and Gynecologists from *Obstetrics and Gynecology* (1983; 62:2S–7S), Copyright © 1983; Elsevier Science Publishing Company Inc.

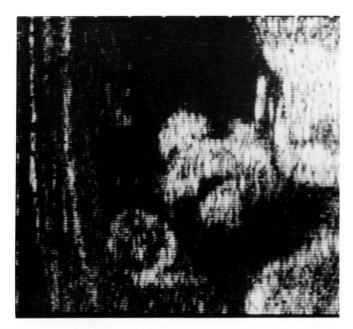

Figure 7-26 A frontal view of a normal fetal mouth. The intact lips and both nostrils are clearly seen, which excludes clefting of the lips but not necessarily of the palate. *Source*: Reprinted with permission from The American College of Obstetricians and Gynecologists from *Obstetrics and Gynecology* (1983; 62:2S–7S), Copyright © 1983, Elsevier Science Publishing Company Inc.

palate leave a bulbous premaxillary process that commonly protrudes from the facial midline (Figure 7-27); a wide separation of the sphenoid bones in the frontal scanplane (Figure 7-28) makes antenatal diagnosis possible (Figure 7-29). Unilateral clefting results in disruption of the normally intact upper lip on the superficial coronal scanplane. Typically both fetal nares can be imaged and the upper lip seen just below. With a cleft, the disruption produced relative to the nostril on the affected side is apparent.

The diagnosis of facial clefting should prompt a diligent search for associated anomalies and consideration of amniocentesis or fetal blood sampling to establish fetal karyotype. The diagnosis of a fetal cleft lip or cleft lip and palate does not alter obstetrical management. The prognosis for survival for an isolated cleft lip is not different, in the absence of genetic syndromes or aneuploidy, from that without the anomaly.

Isolated cleft palate is a much more difficult malformation to detect antenatally due to the absence of surface disruption. In a frontal scanplane behind the face, the tongue is normally noted to remain in the mouth, at the level of the mandible. In the case of cleft palate, the tongue is seen to migrate upward to the level of the sphenoid bones. The presence of isolated cleft palate cannot be confidently excluded by early ultrasound examination.

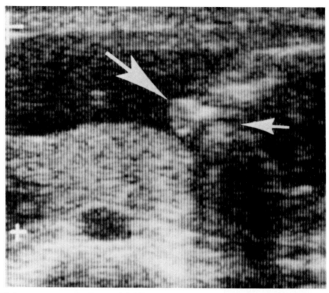

Figure 7-27 A sonogram of a fetus with bilateral cleft lip and palate, made in plane B of Figure 7-25. Note the prominent premaxillary process (large arrow). *Source*: Reprinted with permission from The American College of Obstetricians and Gynecologists from *Obstetrics and Gynecology* (1983; 62:2S–7S), Copyright © 1983, Elsevier Science Publishing Company Inc.

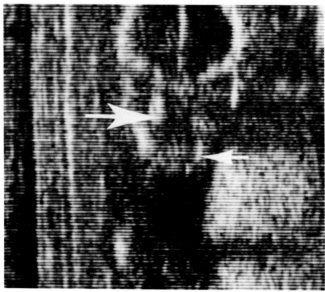

Figure 7-28 The same fetus illustrated in Figure 7-27, but seen in plane A. Note the wide separation of the sphenoid bones (large arrow). *Source*: Reprinted with permission from The American College of Obstetricians and Gynecologists from *Obstetrics and Gynecology* (1983; 62:2S–7S), Copyright © 1983, Elsevier Science Publishing Company Inc.

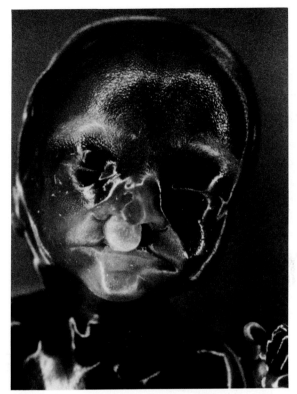

Figure 7-29 The fetus whose sonograms are shown above, demonstrating the antenatal diagnosis of bilateral cleft lip and palate. *Source*: Reprinted with permission from The American College of Obstetricians and Gynecologists from *Obstetrics and Gynecology* (1983; 62:2S–7S), Copyright © 1983, Elsevier Science Publishing Company Inc.

NEONATAL CONSIDERATIONS

Hydrocephalus

As noted above, hydrocephalus is frequently diagnosed in utero, but the majority of infants with hydrocephalus come to medical attention some time well after birth. In infancy the most common presentation of hydrocephalus is an enlarging head that increases in size beyond the normal growth curves. Serial examination and cephalic measurements are crucial in establishing the diagnosis in infants with this more insidious form of hydrocephalus. The fetus with aqueductal stenosis, which accounts for nearly half of the congenital hydrocephalus, may present with a very large head that results in dystocia and requires cesarean delivery (Figure 7-30). In suspected hydrocephalus in the neonate, CT is now the major diagnostic procedure performed postnatally

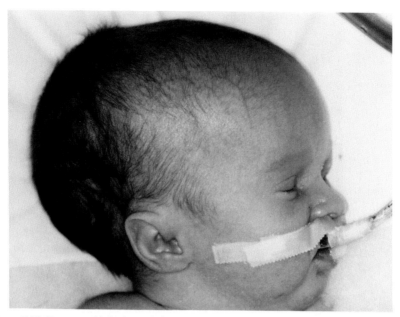

Figure 7-30 Neonate with hydrocephalus secondary to aqueductal stenosis.

not only to determine the diagnosis but also to rule out intracranial anomalies, tumors, and other fluid collections such as posterior fossa cyst. A CT scan may be sufficient to establish the diagnosis of aqueductal stenosis, communicating hydrocephalus, or Dandy-Walker malformation. However, in some complex cases the CT scan does not clearly demonstrate communications between ventricles and cysts; therefore, other diagnostic studies including ventriculocephalography and more recently MRI may provide additional information.

Operative Treatment

Infants with congenital hydrocephalus usually require ventriculoperitoneal shunting. At the time of insertion an extra coil of catheter is placed within the abdomen to accommodate the expected growth of the infant. Shunt dysfunction with either obstruction or infection is a not infrequent occurrence and may necessitate shunt revision or replacement. Alternatively, ventriculoatrial shunts or other shunting options may be necessary as a child ages. The shunt catheters are constructed of Silastic. A slit valve at the end of the catheter opens at a predetermined pressure, thus protecting the end of the catheter from being obstructed by tissue. The catheter is then connected to a one-way pump mounted on the skull, which is then connected to Silastic tubing placed within the ventricular system (Figure 7-31). Although complication rates are

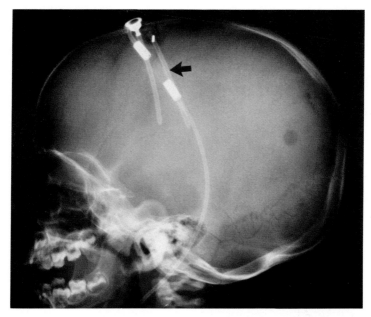

Figure 7-31 A retained segment of catheter from a previous nonfunctioning shunt may be seen (black arrow) in this radiograph of a child following placement of a ventriculoperitoneal shunt.

low, ventriculoperitoneal shunts are more likely to be obstructed but less likely to become infected than ventriculoatrial shunts. In young infants ventriculoperitoneal shunting is the procedure of choice.

Prognosis

Intellectual development is often normal in treated surviving infants. However, a significant number of infants have been reported to die in utero or in the early postnatal period and are not always included in long-term follow-up studies. The information available indicates that the mortality rate for aqueductal stenosis is between 10% and 20%. The infant with successfully treated hydrocephalus has a good outlook for relatively normal intellectual development (Figure 7-32). The prognosis depends on the extent of functional brain tissue that remains. As mentioned earlier, the amount of cortical mantle prior to treatment does not necessarily correlate with normality of intellectual development later in childhood. Aggressive early neurosurgical treatment is associated with improved prognosis for intellectual development, with average IQs of over 80 in the majority of patients. Communicating hydrocephalus without other associated defects appears to have a better prognosis for intellectual development than aqueductal stenosis. If the communicating hydrocephalus is associated with a neural tube defect, then prognosis may be adversely altered (see Chapter 6). Infants with intracranial malformations and hydrocephalus such as that associated with Dandy-Walker malformation or holoprosencephaly are more likely to have a poor prognosis, with diminished survival and severe intellectual impairment.

Dandy-Walker Malformation

Dandy-Walker malformation is characterized by a retrocerebellar cyst, a defect in the cerebellar vermis, and hydrocephalus. The hydrocephalus may occur prenatally but is more likely to be recognized after birth. Postnatal management includes shunting of the posterior fossa cyst. Reported mortality is between 12% and 25%. The prognosis for normal intellectual development is in the range of 40% to 60%.

Sacrococcygeal Teratoma

Postnatal Management

A teratoma arising from the presacral region is the most common extragonadal site for teratomas in childhood, which are usually diagnosed in the neonatal period. Large teratomas protrude posteriorly and extend between the coccyx and rectum (Figure 7-33). Ten percent of these tumors extend intra-abdominally. Large exophytic tumors and intra-abdominal tumors can become necrotic due to compromised blood supply. Life-threatening hemorrhage, although rare, may occur in these patients. Infants with SCTs require careful evaluation to establish the presence or absence of intra-abdominal tumor prior to surgical excision. In this regard abdominal ultrasound and CT are useful preoperative imaging techniques.

Complete surgical excision is the primary therapy for all patients with SCT (Figure 7-34). The coccyx must be removed in continuity with the tumor. A combined transabdominal and trans-sacral approach may be required for those tumors with a large intra-abdominal component or when excessive spontaneous hemorrhage has occurred in an exophytic tumor. In these patients the middle sacral artery must be ligated to secure the bleeding. Since the incidence of malignancy is 10% with the neonatally excised tumors, all children require close postoperative follow-up (3- to 6-month evaluations), including serial physical examinations, alpha-fetoprotein levels, and imaging studies. If no problems have been identified by age 3, yearly follow-up until adulthood is advised. Following resection, long-term functional and cosmetic results are usually excellent in children with a benign SCT (Figure 7-35). The incidence of malignancy in untreated teratomas increases with the age of the child. Nearly 40% to 50% of children with untreated teratomas have malignant tumors by the time the child is 6 months to a year of age. The prognosis of children with malignant SCT is poor despite aggressive chemotherapy and surgical excision.

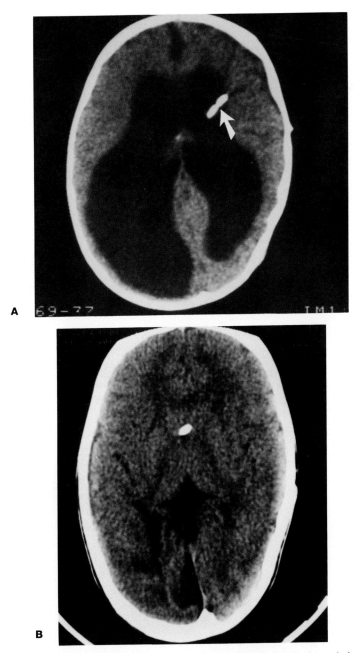

Figure 7-32 A, This is a cranial computed tomogram of an infant with hydrocephalus immediately following placement of a ventriculoperitoneal shunt (arrow). **B,** A CT study of the same infant 6 years later shows the hydrocephalus well controlled and considerable brain development since shunting.

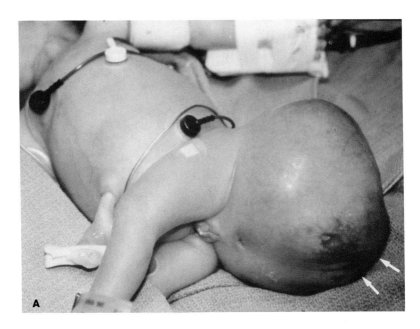

Figure 7-33 A, This large sacrococcygeal teratoma was prenatally diagnosed. The tumor was necrotic in some areas (white arrows), making planned surgical excision more urgent. The infant is now healthy at 5 years of age. **B,** A fetal sonogram at 28 weeks' gestation showing the complex solid and cystic mass (arrows) at the caudal end of the spine. The fetal head (asterisk) is seen. **C,** A lateral radiograph of the same infant after birth, demonstrating calcifications (arrow) within the teratoma.

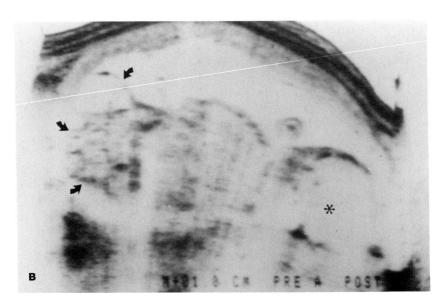

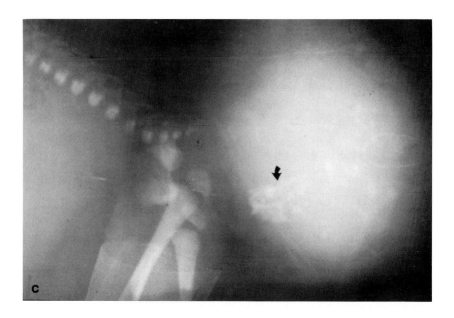

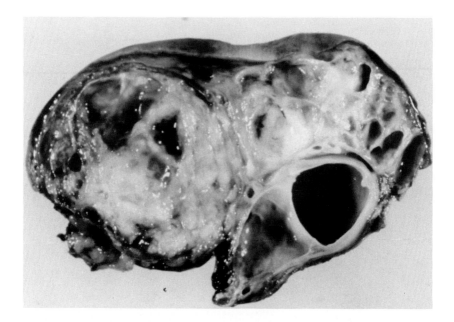

Figure 7-34 This cross-section of an excised sacrococcygeal teratoma shows the complex solid and cystic nature typical of these tumors.

Nuchal Teratomas

Nuchal teratomas are associated with high mortality (80% when untreated). Respiratory obstruction in the delivery room or in the early neonatal period is the most frequent cause of death (Figure 7-36). In these patients intubation may not be feasible without specialized approaches, including fiberoptic bronchoscopy or emergency tracheotomy in the delivery room. Prognosis following surgical resection is very good (Figure 7-37). Malignancy is exceedingly rare in these patients.

Amniotic Band Syndrome

Amniotic band syndrome is a wide spectrum of anomalies that are associated with craniofacial defects, limb anomalies, and abdominal wall defects. Prognosis depends on the severity of the anomalies. Multiple severe anomalies are incompatible with life, but infants born with isolated extremity bands may be normal except for the limb anomalies. Postnatal surgical treatment may improve functional outcome in selected patients.

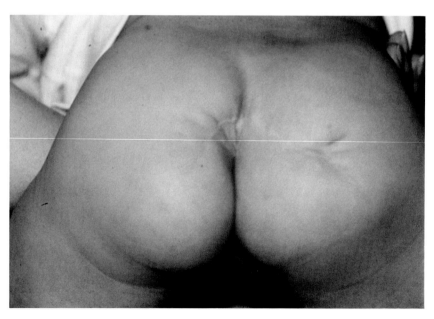

Figure 7-35 Nine months following resection of the sacrococcygeal teratoma, the infant has an excellent result.

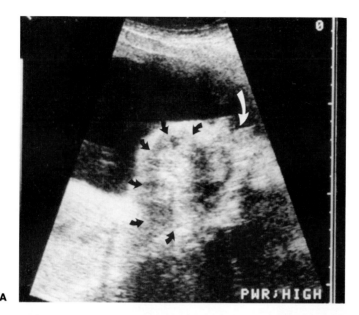

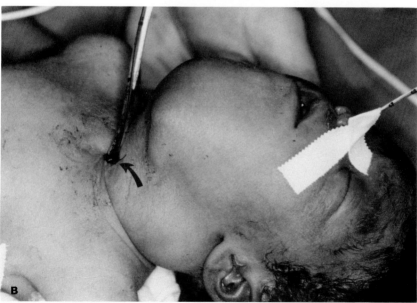

Figure 7-36 **A**, On this antenatal sonogram of a fetal neck and face at 32 weeks' gestation, the large nuchal teratoma is well outlined (black arrows). The open fetal mouth is identified with a curved white arrow. **B**, At delivery, this infant had complete airway obstruction secondary to laryngeal and tracheal compression. Emergency tracheostomy (arrow) was required to secure the airway. Orotracheal intubation was not feasible because of severely distorted oropharyngeal anatomy.

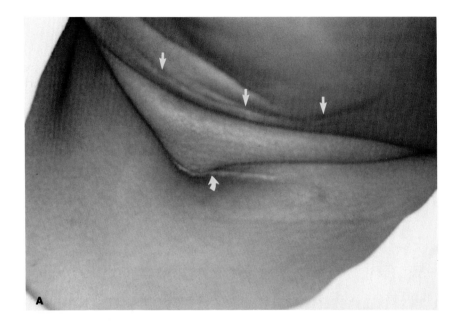

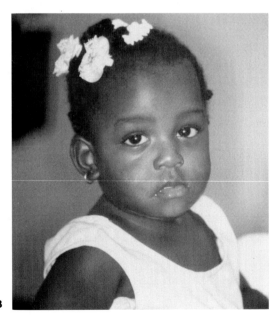

Figure 7-37 A, The teratoma seen here was identified antenatally, and, with some difficulty, orotracheal intubation was accomplished at birth. Resection of these tumors requires extreme care in dissection to avoid damage to critical nerve tracts. **B,** The same infant 2 years after resection, demonstrating the positive outcome possible.

Cystic Hygroma

Cystic hygroma is a form of cystic lymphangioma found primarily in the occipital cervical region of the fetus. These lymphatic anomalies are frequently found in association with chromosomal abnormalities, particularly Turner's syndrome. Cystic hygroma has also been recognized with significant frequency in patients with trisomies 21, 18, and 13 as well as in genetic and noninherited syndromes such as Noonan's syndrome or fetal alcohol syndrome. Cystic hygromas seen in the fetus with Turner's syndrome are bilateral posterior cervical lesions frequently associated with severe nonimmune hydrops, progressive peripheral lymphedemal and fetal demise (Figure 7-38).

Pathoembryology

Improper development of the jugular lymphatic sacs and failure of the joining of the cervical lymphatic structures to the venous system are thought to be the etiology of the obstruction and subsequent dilatation of the lymphatic system. The resultant cystic structures, lined by endothelium, range widely in size and extent within the cervicomediastinal region. Some patients may have a small circumscribed lesion, while others may have extensive infiltration of lymphangioma into the base of the tongue and all the soft tissues of the neck, including the supraglottic structures, cervical muscles, and salivary glands (Figure 7-39). These infants may have compression of their tracheas from mediastinal extension.

Diagnosis

Characteristic cystic structures in the posterior cervical region can be visualized by prenatal ultrasound (Figure 7-40). The diagnosis can be established as early as the first trimester. Differential diagnosis includes cephaloceles and nuchal teratoma. Cephalocele is associated with a bony defect in the skull; furthermore, hydrocephalus is more likely to occur in the fetus with a cephalocele. Nuchal teratomas have a more complex appearance sonographically. Commonly, cystic hygromas have a multiseptated appearance. Hydrops and generalized edema are also more common in infants with cystic hygroma.

Prognosis

The presence of hydrops in a fetus with cystic hygroma is associated with nearly 100% mortality. Spontaneous fetal death frequently occurs by the end of the second trimester. The fetus with isolated cystic hygroma without fetal hydrops is likely to survive to term. At least 25% of delivered infants develop airway obstruction in the early neonatal period. Some may require emergency intubation in the delivery room.

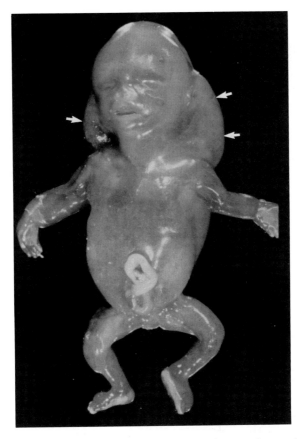

Figure 7-38 Spontaneously aborted fetus with Turner's syndrome and severe hydrops fetalis. Bilateral cervical cystic hygromas (arrows) are present.

Obstetrical Management

Determination of fetal karyotype is advised for all patients. The karyotype may provide important diagnostic information for the index pregnancy and is useful in counseling for occurrence risks for future pregnancies. Pregnancy termination before viability should be offered. Following viability the fetus with associated hydrops should be managed nonaggressively because of the extreme prognosis. Standard obstetrical management is recommended for patients with isolated cystic hygroma. Cesarean delivery may be indicated for extremely large lesions that preclude vaginal delivery. These infants should be delivered in a tertiary medical center because of significant risk of airway obstruction (Figure 7-41). We have used flexible bronchoscopy to guide tracheal intubation for the occasional infant in whom the laryngopharyngeal anatomy is distorted and intubation by traditional means was unsuccessful.

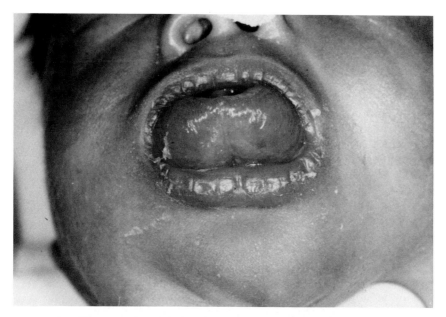

Figure 7-39 This neonate has an infiltrating cystic lymphangioma of the tongue and entire anterior lateral cervical region.

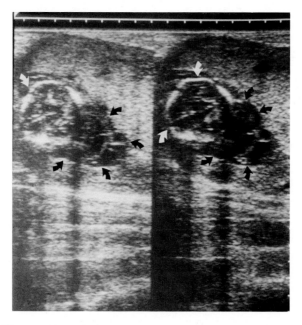

Figure 7-40 These two views of a fetus show a large, septate, cystic mass (black arrows) adjacent to the fetal calvarium (white arrows).

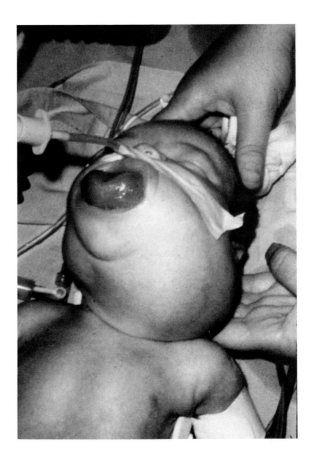

Figure 7-41 This term neonate has a large cervical cystic hygroma, resulting in life-threatening airway obstruction.

Postnatal Management and Prognosis

The results of surgical excision vary with the extent of involvement. Regionally circumscribed cystic lesions are often removed completely with little chance of recurrence and excellent cosmetic results. Lymphangiomas with infiltrating smaller cysts may be very extensive, involving the soft tissue of a wide region (Figure 7-42). Complete excision may be impossible because of the involvement of vital structures in the infiltrating process. Extensive lesions that involve the base of the tongue and pharynx may require tracheostomy and multiple surgical procedures to render satisfactory function and cosmetic appearance (Figure 7-43).

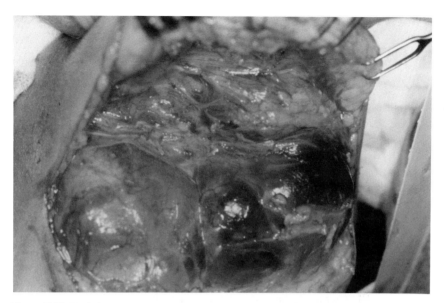

Figure 7-42 Both large and small cysts were found during the resection of this large cystic hygroma.

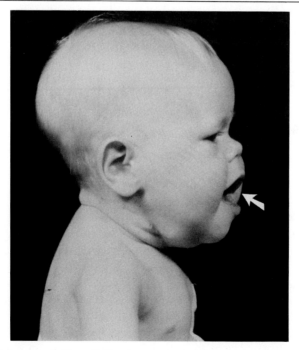

Figure 7-43 Infant seen in Figure 7-41 at 2 years of age, following several surgical procedures. Persistent swelling of the left cheek (arrow) remains.

Cleft Lip

Neonatal Management

After birth, infants with incomplete unilateral cleft lip can be bottle or breast fed. Infants with more severe clefting and those with a cleft palate have feeding difficulties and require other methods of feeding (such as use of the Brecht feeder).

It is helpful for the surgeon and multidisciplinary orofacial team to evaluate the child in the neonatal period and outline for the parents the expected course of treatment and results. As long as the infant is otherwise healthy, operative correction of the cleft lip can be performed in the first 6 to 12 weeks. A number of operative procedures have been successfully applied to the repair of cleft lips. Prognosis depends on the extent of clefting and whether other facial anomalies are present. Infants with isolated unilateral cleft lips have excellent cosmetic appearance (Figure 7-44). Bilateral cleft lip may require single or multistaged procedures. Cases with complete bilateral cleft lip and severe premaxillary projection often require neonatal maxillary orthopedics before soft tissue repair. Almost all patients require special orthodonture once eruption of secondary teeth has occurred. This improves the dental, alveolar, and maxillary abnormalities associated with cleft lip. Lengthening of the nasal columella, scar revision, and procedures to improve nasal blunting may be performed later in childhood to improve the child's cosmetic appearance.

Cleft Palate

Surgical closure of the palate is performed early in childhood before the child has significantly developed speech patterns and habits. Very successful palatoplasty techniques are available. Early functional results are generally good, but nearly all children require speech therapy and orthodonture.

SUMMARY

The very different prognoses and obstetrical implications of these malformations and fetal conditions underscore the need for accurate diagnostic information. Both obstetrical management and future family planning can be inappropriately altered by an inaccurate diagnosis. It is important to consider a second opinion prior to management counseling in order to minimize the possibility of misinformation. It is also important for the patient to understand the limits of ultrasound and the possibility that the diagnosis might be changed after birth. Access to further diagnostic testing, such as karyotype, CT, or MRI, may be helpful in providing optimal antenatal diagnostic

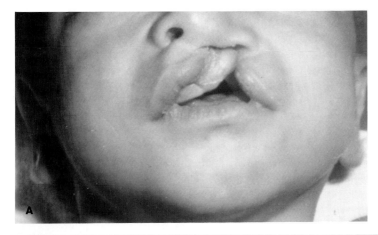

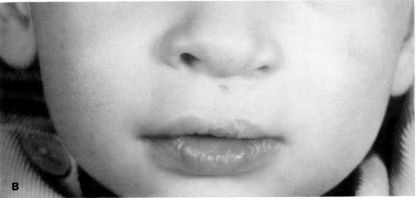

Figure 7-44 A, Term neonate with unilateral cleft lip. **B,** The same infant following repair shows an excellent functional and cosmetic result 9 months later. *Source:* Photograph courtesy of A. Griswald Bevin, M.D.

information. Once optimal antenatal diagnostic information is accumulated, specialized counseling should provide the most accurate prognostic information, including the potential range of prognosis and the possible alternative conditions and their prognoses.

The patient should understand that pregnancy interruption in most cases is not clinically necessary, although if the gestational age is under 24 weeks it is usually available. Optimally, she should understand that the health care provider is willing to support her in her pregnancy regardless of the decision and the prognosis for a specific diagnosis. It is critical that an accurate confirmation of diagnosis be obtained after birth in order to provide the most accurate recurrence risk counseling.

Perinatal management and counseling are predicated on a careful evaluation of the following:
1. Accuracy of diagnosis
   * What is the quality of images and interpretation?
2. Accuracy and precision of prognosis
   * Do we really know the full meaning of what we see?
3. Quality of management counseling
   * Are we really letting the patient decide?
   * What should the patient's input be?
4. Adequacy of follow-up
   * Are we facilitating or disabling grieving?
   * Does the husband grieve?
   * Does the couple understand recurrence risk?
   * Is the couple aware of early diagnosis?

FURTHER READING

Burton BK. Recurrent risks for congenital hydrocephalus. *Clin Genet.* 1979; 16:47.

Callen PW, Hashimoto BE, Newton TH. Sonographic evaluation of cerebral cortical mantle thickness in the fetus and neonate with hydrocephalus. *J Ultrasound Med.* 1986; 5:251.

Chervenak FA, Berkowitz RL, Tortora M, Hobbins JC. The management of fetal hydrocephalus. *Am J Obstet Gynecol.* 1985; 151:933.

Chervenak FA, Goldberg JD, Chin TH, Gilbert F, Berkowitz RL. The importance of karyotype determination in a fetus with ventriculomegaly and spina bifida discovered during the third trimester. *J Ultrasound Med.* 1986; 5:405.

Chervenak FA, Hobbins JC, Wertheimer I, O'Neal JP, Mahoney M. The natural history of ventriculomegaly in a fetus without obstructive hydrocephalus. *Am J Obstet Gynecol.* 1985; 152:574.

Chervenak FA, Isaacson G, Blakemore KJ, et al. Fetal cystic hygroma, cause and natural history. *N Engl J Med.* 1983; 309:822.

Chervenak FA, Isaacson G, Hobbins JC, Chitkara U, Tortoro M, Berkowitz RL, et al. Diagnosis and management of fetal holoprosencephaly. *Obstet Gynecol.* 1985; 66:322.

Chervenak FA, Isaacson G, Mahoney MJ. Advances in the diagnosis of fetal defects. *New Engl J Med.* 1986; 315:305.

Chervenak FA, Isaacson G, Tortora M. A sonographic study of fetal cystic hygroma. *J Clin Ultrasound.* 1985; 13:311.

Chervenak FA, Jeanty P, Cantraine F, et al. The diagnosis of fetal microcephaly. *Am J Obstet Gynecol.* 1984; 149:512.

Clewell WH, Meier PR, Manchester DK, Manco-Johnson ML, Pretorius DH, Hendee RW. Ventriculomegaly: Evaluation and management. *Semin Perinatol.* 1985; 9:98

Cochrane DD, Myles T. Management of intrauterine hydrocephalus. *J Neurosurg.* 1982; 57:590.

Donnellan WA, Swenson O. Benign and malignant sacrococcygeal teratomas. *Surgery* 1968; 64:834.

Garden AS, Benzie RJ, Miskin M, et al. Fetal cystic hygroma colli: Antenatal diagnosis, significance and management. *Am J Obstet Gynecol.* 1986; 154:221.

Greene MF, Benacerrof B, Crawford JM. Hydranencephaly: US appearance during in utero evolution. *Radiology.* 1985; 156:779.

Grosfeld JL, Cooney DR, Smith J, et al. Intraabdominal complications following ventriculoperitoneal shunt procedures. *Pediatrics.* 1974; 54:791–796.

Gundry SR, Wesley JR, Klein MD, et al. Cervical teratomas in the newborn. *J Pediatr Surg.* 1983; 18:382.

Guthkelch AN, Riley NA. Influence of aetiology on prognosis in surgically treated infantile hydrocephalus. *Arch Dis Child.* 1969; 44:29

Hirsch JF, Pierre-Kahn A, Renier D, et al. The Dandy-Walker malformation. *J Neurosurg.* 1984; 61:515.

Holzgreve W, Mahony BS, Glick PL, et al. Sonographic demonstration of fetal sacrococcygeal teratoma. *Prenatal Diagn.* 1985; 5:245.

Jackson IJ, Snodgrass SR. Peritoneal shunts in the treatment of hydrocephalus and increased intracranial pressure: A 4-year survey of 62 patients. *J Neurosurg.* 1955; 12:216–222.

Johnson ML, Dunne MG, Mack LA, Rashbaum CL. Evaluation of fetal intracranial anatomy by static and realtime ultrasound. *J Clin Ultrasound.* 1980; 8:311.

Kagan AR, Steckel RJ. Cervical mass in a fetus associated with maternal hydramnios. *AJR.* 1983; 140:507.

Lipman SP, Pretorius DH, Rumack CM, Manco-Johnson ML, et al. Fetal intracranial teratoma: US diagnosis of three cases and a review of the literature. *Radiology.* 1985; 157:491.

Mahoor GH, Woolley MM, Trivedi SN, et al. Teratomas in infancy and childhood: Experience with 81 cases. *Surgery.* 1974; 76:309.

Matson DD. *Neurosurgery of Infancy and Childhood.* 2nd ed. Springfield, Ill: Charles C Thomas, 1969.

McCullogh DC, Balzer-Martin LA. Current prognosis in overt neonatal hydrocephalus. *J Neurosurg.* 1982; 57:378.

Pretorius D, Davis K, Manco-Johnson ML, et al. Clinical course of fetal hydrocephalus: 40 cases. *AJR.* 1985; 144:827.

Raimondi AJ, Samuelson G, Yarzagaray L, et al. Atresia of foramina of Luschka and Magendie: The Dandy-Walker cyst. *J Neurosurg.* 1969; 31:202.

Riboni G, Simoni MD, Leopardi O, Molla R. Ultrasound appearance of a glioblastoma in a 33-week fetus in utero. *J Clin Ultrasound.* 1985; 13:345.

Sawaya R, McLaurin RL. Dandy-Walker syndrome. *J Neurosurg.* 1981; 55:89.

Seashore JN, Gardiner LJ, Ariyan S. Management of giant cystic hygromas in infants. *Am J Surg.* 1985; 149:459.

Seeds JW, Mittelstaedt CA, Cefalo RC, Parker TF. Prenatal diagnosis of sacrococcygeal teratoma: An anechoic caudal mass. *J Clin Ultrasound.* 1982; 10:193.

Snyder JR, Lustig-Gillman I, Milio L, Morris M, Pardes JG, Young BK. Antenatal ultrasound diagnosis of an intracranial neoplasm (craniopharyngioma). *J Clin Ultrasound.* 1986; 14:304.

Strauss S, Bouzouki M, Goldfarb H, Uppal V, Costales F. Antenatal ultrasound diagnosis of an unusual case of hydranencephaly. *J Clin Ultrasound.* 1984; 12:420.

Sutton LN, Bruce DA, Schut L. Hydranencephaly versus maximal hydrocephalus: An important clinical distinction. *J Neurosurg.* 1980; 6:35.

Vassilouthis J. The syndrome of normal-pressure hydrocephalus. *J Neurosurg.* 1984; 61:501.

Chapter 8

Skeletal Dysplasias

There are over 55 distinct varieties of congenital long bone dysplasias. Some types are mild and associated with minimal disability, while others are severely disabling if not lethal. All categories of genetic inheritance may be identified in the study of congenital dwarfism, including autosomal dominant, autosomal recessive, polygenic/multifactorial, and acute mutations. The prenatal diagnosis of these conditions can be important for planning appropriate obstetrical management, and an accurate diagnosis forms the basis for appropriate reproductive counseling of the parents of such an infant.

Although it may be difficult to discriminate specific varieties of long bone dysplasia antenatally, it is usually possible to make a categorical diagnosis and estimate a reasonably accurate prognosis, deferring the definitive diagnostic evaluation until after delivery. It is possible, therefore, to answer in most cases the most frequently asked questions from the parents of a fetus with a bone dysplasia: "Will my baby look abnormal?" and, "Will my baby live?"

We review the normal sonographic anatomy of fetal long bones, examine established normal growth relationships, outline the general and specific techniques for risk identification and detection of fetal dwarfism, and, finally, survey a selected group of congenital long bone conditions that have been successfully diagnosed antenatally.

NORMAL ANATOMY

All fetal long bones may be seen with real-time ultrasound and measured from 12 weeks to term. The femur is perhaps the easiest to image and measure due to its more limited range of motion at the hip, and it is therefore the long bone most often measured during basic screening ultrasound examinations (Figure 8-1). All of the long bones, however, including the humerus, tibia and fibula, radius and ulna, and even the clavicles, demonstrate equally precise growth characteristics as a function of gestational age. Growth of the femur and the other long bones has been reported to be nearly linear through early pregnancy, with a slight negative slope later.

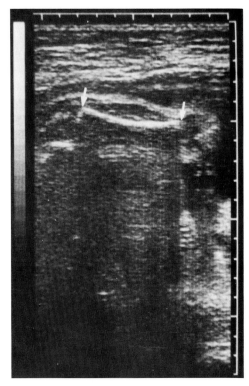

Figure 8-1   This sonogram of a fetal femur illustrates the typical shaft, with often a shallow curve, blunt metaphyseal ends (arrows), and the expected acoustical shadowing. *Source*: Reprinted from *Practical Obstetrical Ultrasound* (p 62) by JW Seeds and RC Cefalo, Aspen Publishers Inc, © 1986.

In general, once the transducer is located in the general area of the desired long bone (Figure 8-2), rotation will bring the entire length of the bone into view (Figure 8-3). The femur is found arising from the caudal aspect of the fetal trunk, and the upper segment of the lower limb is discriminated from the lower by the fact that the solitary femur is found within it, compared to the tibia and fibula within the lower segment. The humerus is found arising from the upper trunk near the heart and, again, is differentiated from the distal segment of the upper limb because there is a single bone in the upper segment. Special care is necessary to ensure that the entire length of any bone has been captured on the sonogram. Unclear endpoints without good landmarks suggest the possibility that the scanplane does not include the entire bone and that any measurement, therefore, would underestimate the true bone length. The acoustical shadowing characteristic of the bone shaft can help in truly

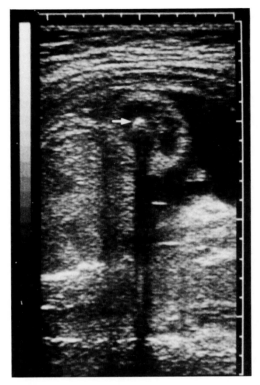

Figure 8-2 One popular method of imaging the femur, aligning the transducer across the trunk and sliding caudally, finds this femur (arrow), within the thigh, casting the expected shadow. *Source*: Reprinted from *Practical Obstetrical Ultrasound* (p 59) by JW Seeds and RC Cefalo, Aspen Publishers Inc, © 1986.

defining the endpoint for measurement. Waterbath studies have shown that the sonographic image does not include the relatively echolucent epiphyseal areas and therefore underestimates the palpable length of the bone by 8% to 17%, depending on gestational age. This undermeasurement is not clinically relevant, however, since individual measurements are empirically compared to a normal reference database imaged and measured in a comparable manner. The bone is measured parallel to its shaft, from metaphyseal plate to metaphyseal plate. Shadows should be dense and sharply defined. Endpoints should be clear and blunt. It is recommended that an attempt be made to align the shaft of the bone as parallel to the transducer surface as possible and perpendicular to the direction of propagation of the sound pulses, to avoid any image or measurement error due to differential sound speed through tissues.

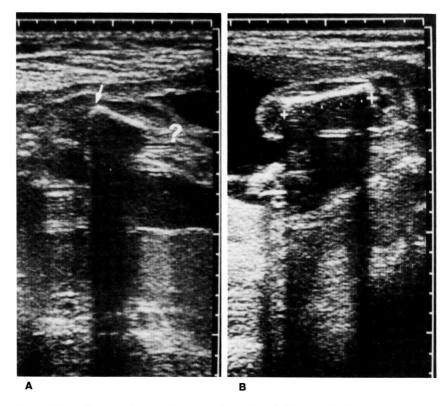

A   **B**

Figure 8-3 A, Rotating the transducer from its position in Figure 8-2 will capture a greater length of the femur in the scanplane, but if not perfectly aligned with the shaft, one end will terminate with poor definition as seen here. The arrow indicates one metaphyseal terminus of the femur. Further rotation is necessary. *Source*: Reprinted from *Practical Obstetrical Ultrasound* (p 61) by JW Seeds and RC Cefalo, Aspen Publishers Inc, © 1986. **B**, Further rotation of the transducer will successfully image the entire length of the femur and satisfy minimum criteria for measurement, including sharply defined landmarks and shadowing.

GROWTH RELATIONSHIPS

Gestational Age

There are many different long bone/gestational age reference charts available, and none are identical. All charts appeared correct to the reporting author. It is for individual practitioners to validate a particular chart with their own sonographic and clinical data or construct their own. Most investigators have found the relationship early in gestation to be nearly linear, with a slight negative slope later on. For most cases of antenatal diagnosis, growth

Table 8-1 Long Bone Dimensions (mm) in Early Gestation

Gestational Age (Wks)	Femur	Humerus	Tibia and Fibula	Radius and Ulna
14	14	15	2	12
16	20	20	16	17
18	26	25	22	21
20	32	31	27	26
22	38	36	32	30

characteristics before 22 weeks are most important since diagnostic information at that time is most useful for early management considerations.

From 14 to 25 weeks, in the case of our own scanning laboratory, femur length (FL) as a function of gestational age (GA) age was found to be

$$FL = -29.49 + 3.09(GA) \ (\pm 4.3 \text{ mm, } 95\% \text{ confidence interval})$$

(See Table 8-1.)

Biparietal Diameter

Most investigators have found that the relationship between fetal long bones and BPD is linear throughout gestation. This allows the observer to index a given measurement of a long bone to an internal measure of the fetus itself, and not to a clinical gestational age that might be in error.

$$BPD = -9.79 + 0.864(FL) \ (\pm 5.3 \ 95\% \text{ CI})$$
$$BPD = -4.94 + 0.73 \ (Humerus) \ (\pm 5.7 \ 95\% \text{ CI})$$

Tibia and fibula (T/F) and radius and ulna (R/U) complexes bear a relatively linear relationship to the femur and humerus in early pregnancy that may be easily used to assess the symmetry of long bone development:

$$T/F = 0.80 \ FL \pm 0.06$$
$$R/U = 0.83 \ Hu \pm 0.05$$

The primary characteristic of bone growth that enables the detection of a defect in bone growth is the measurement of length and the observation of abnormally small dimensions. As we will soon see, the detection of other collateral abnormalities of the fetus, such as diminished chest size and cranial development, can enhance the confidence of the diagnosis and contribute to discriminating certain types of dysplasia, but it is the bone length that forms

Table 8-2 Clinical Indications for Screening

Previously affected child
Affected parent
Polyhydramnios: Short limbs noted at ultrasound done for other purposes

the basis for diagnosis. The femur, for example, demonstrates a very tight relationship with gestational age in early pregnancy. The 95% confidence levels for femur length under 20 weeks' gestation are ± 1 week. It would be inappropriate to diagnose or suspect a bone dysplasia, however, unless there was a discrepancy between femur length and both clinical gestational age and other dimensions of the fetus, such as BPD of over 2 weeks.

LONG BONE DYSPLASIAS

An examination for the prenatal diagnosis of a congenital bone dysplasia is based on a clinical assessment of the risk of occurrence, the severity of the condition in question, and the risks of the diagnostic process.

Indications for prenatal diagnosis include both clinical and screening information (Table 8-2). Polyhydramnios in particular has been associated with severe long bone dysplasias that have thoracodystrophy as a part of the syndrome (Table 8-3).

DIAGNOSTIC TECHNIQUES

Ultrasound is capable of evaluating the length of bones, their shape, fetal trunk proportions, and, in the extreme, their density. Radiography is capable of assessing bone shape, rough size, and density but is of limited value prior

Table 8-3 Dwarf Conditions Associated with Polyhydramnios

Camptomelic dysplasia
Thanatophoric dysplasia
Achondroplasia
Asphyxiating thoracodystrophy
Hypophosphatasia
Achondrogenesis

to 19 weeks' gestation and carries a small but real risk of the induction of childhood cancer or leukemia in the child examined. Amniography involves the injection of radiographic contrast medium into the amniotic cavity. The technique allows the visualization and assessment of fetal surface soft tissue but also involves the use of radiation, with its inherent dangers, and offers little additional information over that available from ultrasound.

SELECTED SPECIFIC CONDITIONS

Achondroplasia

The most common type of unexpected congenital dwarfism is achondroplasia, which is inherited as an autosomal dominant trait but is the result of an acute mutation in up to 80% of cases. Achondroplasia is most often mild in its expression, and prenatal diagnosis in early gestation is difficult. Confident exclusion in early gestation is not possible. Successful antenatal diagnosis using ultrasound has been accomplished at 22 weeks, but normal bone lengths were recorded earlier. A significant clue to the presence of a growth disorder in the preceding case was that bone measurements crossed percentiles with advancing gestation, so serial observation is suggested in the diagnostic approach. Achondroplasia demonstrates an autosomal dominant pattern of inheritance, so there is a 50% risk that children of an affected parent will be affected also. Since the majority of cases occur as acute mutations, if such a child is born to normal parents, there is only slightly increased risk of recurrence.

Achondrogenesis

Achondrogenesis is a severe, lethal dysplasia with markedly short long bones, often cloverleaf skull deformity (Figure 8-4), polyhydramnios, and a 25% risk of recurrence. Another sonographic characteristic is the soft tissue echotexture of the bones (Figure 8-5).

Asphyxiating Thoracodystrophy

This condition produces markedly short bones (Figure 8-6), an extremely small funnel-shaped chest (Figure 8-7), polyhydramnios, and neonatal death due to pulmonary hypoplasia.

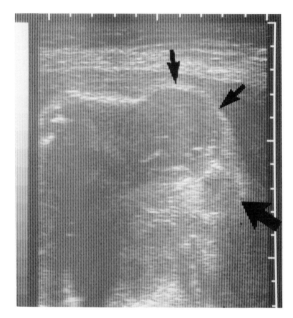

Figure 8-4 This sonogram of the cranium of a fetus with achondrogenesis at the level of the orbit demonstrates the bulbous cloverleaf skull deformity associated with this bone dysplasia. The arrows indicate the abnormal retro-orbital bulging of the cranium.

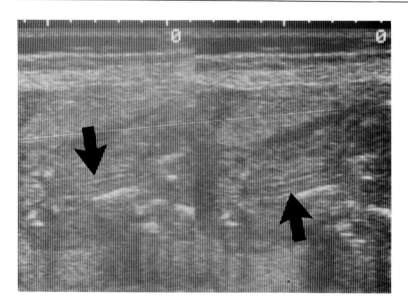

Figure 8-5 These longitudinal views of the spine of a fetus with achondrogenesis demonstrate the unusual echolucency of all fetal bones typical of this condition. Note that no bony elements are seen, including spinal segments. The arrows indicate the neural canal.

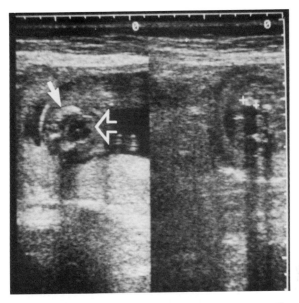

Figure 8-6 On the left is a four-chamber heart view showing the severe disproportion of the heart (open arrow) to the chest (small arrow). This is the typical appearance of severe thoracodystrophy seen with lethal dwarf conditions. The femur on the right measures 10 mm at 20 weeks' gestation (expected, 32 mm). *Source*: Reprinted from *Practical Obstetrical Ultrasound* (p 156) by JW Seeds and RC Cefalo, Aspen Publishers Inc, © 1986.

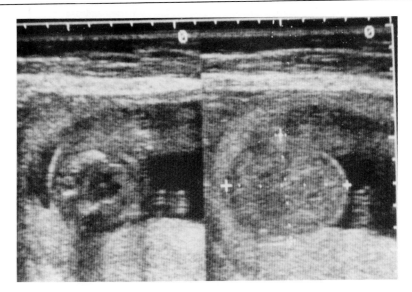

Figure 8-7 In addition to the disproportion of the heart to the chest, here is apparent the disproportion of the chest girth to the abdominal girth in the same fetus. The abdominal circumference was appropriate for gestational age.

Camptomelic Dysplasia

This rare disorder produces markedly short, bowed long bones (Figure 8-8). The lower limbs are more severely affected, and polyhydramnios is common. Survival is possible.

Chondroectodermal Dysplasia

This condition demonstrates short limbs, polydactyly, and a low recurrence risk.

Diastrophic Dwarfism

Diastrophic dwarfism is characterized by short limbs, spinal deformities, normal intelligence, and a good probability of survival. Diastrophic dwarfism is inherited as an autosomal recessive trait.

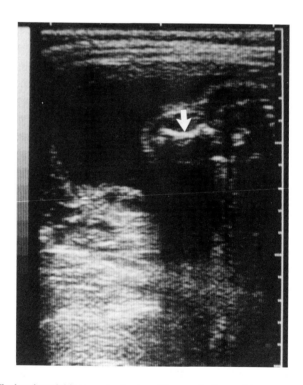

Figure 8-8   The bowing of this severely shortened femur of a fetus with camptomelic dysplasia is apparent. Note that the metaphyseal plates are nearly coplanar with the shaft of the bone.

Osteogenesis Imperfecta

Osteogenesis imperfecta probably occurs in over a dozen discrete genetic forms but for clinical simplicity has been described as four types with somewhat different clinical and genetic characteristics. Brittle bones, short limbs, and fractures to a variable extent characterize all of these types.

1. Type I: mild, survivable, and inherited as an autosomal dominant trait
2. Type II: severe, lethal, marked long bone shortening with multiple fractures, and inherited as an autosomal recessive trait
3. Type III: severe, marked long bone shortening, fractures, survivable for variable time, inherited as an autosomal recessive trait with a 25% risk of recurrence (Figure 8-9)
4. Type IV: milder, survivable, an autosomal dominant trait with early antenatal diagnosis unlikely

Thanatophoric Dysplasia

This is the commonest form of lethal dwarfism. There is marked shortening of bowed long bones and a small chest (Figures 8-10 and 8-11). It is lethal due to pulmonary hypoplasia. Inheritance is non-Mendelian, with low recurrence.

Robert's Syndrome

This lethal condition causes short limbs, renal dysplasia, tetraphocomelia, oligohydramnios, and no bladder filling. Death is due to pulmonary hypoplasia. The recurrence rate is 25%.

Hypophosphatasia

This disorder is characterized by nonmineralization of the entire skeleton, which is not visualized on ultrasound or radiography. Hypophosphatasia causes markedly short limbs, a small chest, and echolucent bones, including the spine, and is lethal.

POTENTIAL SOURCES OF ERROR IN ANTENATAL DIAGNOSIS

An important potential source of inaccurate negative diagnostic results is that the dwarf condition in question is not yet manifest at time of examination. This is particularly true in the case of mild achondroplasia. Bone length early

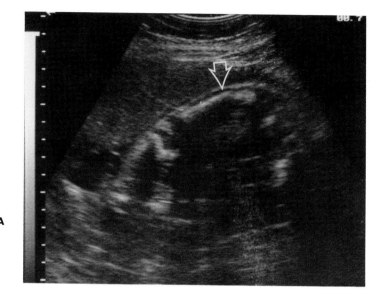

A

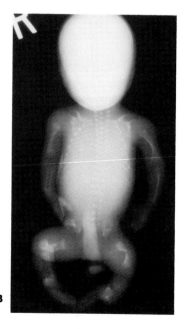

B

Figure 8-9 A, Fractures, in addition to short dimensions, are the hallmark of osteogenesis imperfecta. Note here the angulation (arrow) characteristic of in utero fractures. **B,** This radiograph of an infant with one of the severe forms of osteogenesis imperfecta clearly demonstrates the multiple fractures and the severely attenuated long bones.

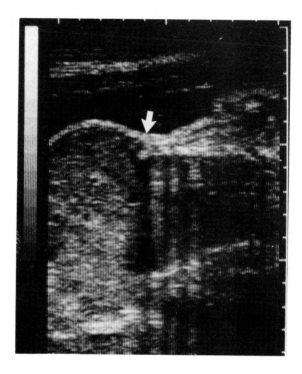

Figure 8-10   Thoracodystrophy is characteristic of thanatophoric dysplasia and is seen here in early pregnancy compared to the same infant's abdomen. It is important when comparing chest girth to abdominal girth not to include the skin edema that might be present.

in gestation is often normal, but the later growth rate is not normal. Therefore, serial examination is recommended to document normal interval growth.

A common basis for inaccurate positive diagnoses is familial short stature. Using 95% confidence intervals as a diagnostic discriminator could lead to false-positive diagnosis of short limbs in 1 out of every 20 patients, since 5% of the normal population lies outside these limits. It is suggested that the diagnosis not be suspected unless the growth rate over an interval is clearly abnormal, or the length is more than 3 standard deviations (SD) below the average for the gestational age (i.e., 10 mm at 20 weeks). Furthermore, in the majority of severe forms of dysplasia, there are other sonographically detectable abnormalities, such as skull deformities or thoracodystrophy, that should be sought. In later pregnancy, as the growth curve flattens, a mild discrepancy in bone growth in millimeters can translate into a much larger apparent discrepancy if expressed in terms of weeks of gestation, and it is very important, therefore, to adhere to a dimensional criterion for suspecting dysplasia to avoid producing unnecessary anxiety.

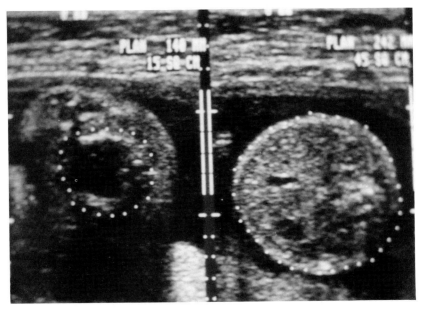

Figure 8-11 Thanatophoric dysplasia later in pregnancy, with the narrow chest seen as the abdominal contour bulges out from the base of the chest (arrow).

GENERAL CONSIDERATIONS

Once a deviation from normal long bone growth is identified, the examiner must address the two primary questions mentioned above. In general, the fetus with sonographically short limbs falls into two distinct categories. Most often, a discrepancy is noted that may appear to be significant in terms of time length of gestation, such as 2 or 3 or even 4 weeks shorter than expected for gestational age or BPD, as noted above. If the pregnancy is in the third trimester, however, even a 4-week discrepancy amounts to less than a centimeter between what is observed and what was expected. At birth, the parents are not going to notice a discrepancy of a centimeter and might feel misled if it has been overly emphasized as pathological. Furthermore, in the absence of associated abnormalities of the chest or shape of bones that would indicate a significant or disabling dysplasia, such a discrepancy most likely represents familial or constitutional variation. The identification of a mild bone length discrepancy should not, however, be completely ignored. A careful examination of the fetus should be performed, and any associated abnormality should lead to consideration of performing fetal blood sampling or amniocentesis for karyotype. Mild long bone shortening is one recognized characteristic of Down's syndrome.

The other category of bone length abnormality that will be encountered much less frequently is the severe discrepancy. When the long bone length demonstrates a severe deviation from the expected, the sonographer should examine the shape of the bones and pay particular attention to the shape of the skull and the shape and size of the chest. The proportion of the heart to the chest measurements should be assessed in an attempt to diagnose or exclude the most frequent basis for lethality in dwarf conditions, which is pulmonary hypoplasia. A comparison of the chest circumference to abdominal circumference will be helpful in this regard. If there is a significant reduction in chest size, with a disproportionately large heart within the chest, then one of several lethal short limb dysplasias may be diagnosed. It may not be possible antenatally to make the precise diagnosis, but that is not clinically essential to forming an appropriate obstetrical management plan. If the diagnosis of a lethal dwarf condition is made, obstetrical management may then focus on maternal welfare. Radiographic evaluation of bone density, connective tissue biopsies, and gross and microscopic examinations of the infant may be performed postnatally to establish with precision the exact diagnosis for purposes of accurate family planning.

If the diagnosis of a severe long bone dysplasia is made in early gestation, management options include termination of pregnancy. Later, if a lethal dysplasia is diagnosed, at least unproductive surgical interventions for fetal indications might be avoided.

FURTHER READING

Aylsworth AS, Seeds JW, Guilford WB, et al. Prenatal diagnosis of a severe deforming type of osteogenesis imperfecta. *Am J Med Genet.* 1984; 19:707.

Golbus MS, Hall BD, Filly RA, Poskanzer LB. Prenatal diagnosis of achondrogenesis. *J Pediatr.* 1977; 91:464.

Hobbins JC, Bracken MB, Mahoney MJ. Diagnosis of fetal skeletal dysplasias with ultrasound. *Am J Obstet Gynecol.* 1982; 142:306.

Kaitila I, Ammala P, Karjalainen O, et al. Early prenatal detection of diastrophic dysplasia. *Prenatal Diagn.* 1983; 3:237.

Kurtz AB, Wapner RJ. Ultrasonographic diagnosis of second trimester skeletal dysplasias: A prospective analysis in a high risk population. *J Ultrasound Med.* 1983; 2:99.

Mahoney BS, Filly RA. High resolution sonographic assessment of the fetal extremities. *J Ultrasound Med.* 1984; 3:489.

Nimrod C, Davies D, Iwanicki S, et al. Ultrasound prediction of pulmonary hypoplasia. *Obstet Gynecol.* 1986; 68:495.

Seeds JW, Cefalo RC. Relationship of fetal limb lengths to both biparietal diameter and gestational age. *Obstet Gynecol.* 1982; 60:680.

Shaff MI, Fleischer AC, Battino R, et al. Antenatal sonographic diagnosis of thanatophoric dysplasia. *J Clin Ultrasound.* 1980; 8:363.

Skiptunas SM, Weiner S. Early prenatal diagnosis of asphyxiating thoracic dystrophy (Jeune's syndrome). *J Ultrasound Med.* 1987; 6:41.

Wong WS, Filly RA. Polyhydramnios associated with fetal limb abnormalities. *AJR.* 1983; 140:1001.

Chapter 9

Congenital Heart Disease

The heart is the most common site of congenital malformation. The general incidence of congenital heart disease is 0.1% to 0.8%, or 10 to 80 per 1000 live births, compared to the 1 to 2 per 1000 incidence of neural tube defects, the next most frequent type of congenital malformation. Although in the majority of cases of a liveborn with congenital heart disease the lesion is not associated with a genetic syndrome or aneuploidy, evidence suggests that a substantial proportion of cases of congenital heart disease discovered in early or midpregnancy are associated with aneuploidy. This apparent inconsistency may be due to a substantial number of midtrimester fetal deaths that do not come to autopsy or karyotyping. It is perhaps due to the complexity of cardiac embryogenesis that congenital heart defects occur with greater frequency than any other single organ system defect.

Antenatal diagnosis of congenital heart disease is based on familiar principles of early prenatal risk assessment and careful sonographic evaluation. Historical and clinical factors that suggest an increased risk of congenital heart disease are listed in Table 9-1. The expected recurrence risks of common congenital heart lesions are listed in Table 9-2. Routine screening of cardiac anatomy whenever ultrasound is performed is another important method of making the antenatal diagnosis of congenital heart disease, since up to 90% of cases occur without previous history. Doppler velocimetry and color flow Doppler imaging add exciting new sources of data to the evaluation of fetal cardiac structure and function.

Table 9-1 Congenital Heart Disease Clinical and Historical Risk Factors

Previous child with congenital heart disease
Parent with congenital heart disease
Maternal diabetes
Maternal autoimmune disease
Maternal teratogen exposure
Fetal aneuploidy
Intrauterine growth retardation
Excess or deficiency of amniotic fluid
Fetal cardiac dysrhythmia
Fetal dysmorphology of other organ systems

Table 9-2 Congenital Heart Disease Recurrence Risk

Malformation	Recurrence in Sibling
Ventricular septal defect	3%–4.5%
Tetralogy of Fallot	2.5%
Transposition of arteries	1.5%–1.9%
Atrioventricular septal defect	2%–2.6%
Ebstein's anomaly	1%
Truncus arteriosus	1.2%
Hypoplastic left or right heart	2%

CARDIAC EMBRYOLOGY

The development of the fetal cardiovascular system begins early in the 3rd week after conception. The aggregation of mesenchymal angioblasts into blood islands occurs within both the embryo and the yolk sac. Cavities develop within these islands, and then the cavities fuse to form primitive networks of blood vessels. Formation of the heart begins by the end of the 3rd week with the fusion of paired heart tubes in the chest area. By the end of the 3rd week circulation of blood begins with the beating of this primitive heart. A functional level of development is reached by the heart before any other system.

Initially the atrium of the primitive heart tube is at the caudal end of the tube structure, the single contractile ventricle in the middle, and the bulbus cordis at the top. The bulbus cordis represents the common root of the two main outflow tracts of the early heart. During the 4th week, longitudinal growth of the heart tube at a greater rate than that of the thoracic cavity requires a convolution of the tube, bringing the ventricle both ventral and caudal relative to the atrium, which at the same time rises in a cephalic direction and moves to a more dorsal position in the chest. The bulbus cordis rotates to the right of the ventricle. During the 4th and 5th weeks, the heart tube is divided into the familiar four chambers by the growth of septa sometimes known as endocardial cushions, which appear first in the atrioventricular area and grow toward each other and toward the developing interventricular septum, which grows inward from the apex of the ventricle.

In the 5th week the aortopulmonary septum begins to develop, dividing the previously single outflow tract (truncus arteriosus) into the aorta and the pulmonary artery. By the end of the 7th week, the interventricular septum is completed with the closure of the membranous portion.

The bulk of the eventual left ventricle originates from the middle portion of the original primitive heart tube, while the right ventricle has its origins in the initially more cephalic bulbus cordis of the original heart tube. The original atrium is divided first by the growth of the septum primum. As the septum primum fuses caudally with the endocardial cushion to close the foramen primum, it breaks down superiorly to result in the foramen secundum. The septum secundum forms to the right of this secondary foramen, and a valve effect is produced, with the septum primum preventing left-to-right flow but allowing flow from right to left across the foramen secundum.

The most common congenital cardiac defect is the interventricular septal defect. The majority of these occur in the membranous portion, and many are not clinically significant. The most severe variety of septal defect is the endocardial cushion defect, also known as atrioventricular septal defect, which essentially results functionally in a single atrium–single ventricle complex with complete mixing of circulations. Errors in the formation of the aortopulmonary septum that normally divides the truncus arteriosus and bulbus cordis into the aorta, pulmonary artery, and right ventricle can result in malformations such as transposition of the great vessels, persistent truncus arteriosus, double outlet right ventricle, and tetralogy of Fallot. Hypoplastic left heart and hypoplastic right heart syndromes may result from abnormal development of the aortopulmonary septum, resulting in either aortic or pulmonary outflow obstruction very early in development.

CLINICAL SCREENING

Over 90% of congenital cardiac defects occur without previous history, and the majority of antenatal diagnoses will be made during sonographic examinations done for other indications. Although only 10% to 12% of liveborn fetuses with congenital cardiac disease are aneuploid, some observers report a risk of over 30% in the case of congenital lesions diagnosed antenatally. The discrepancy, as noted above, probably results from death of many affected fetuses in utero or in early neonatal life, without documentation of karyotype.

Certainly, the history of the previous birth of a child with congenital cardiac disease or the history of congenital cardiac disease in one of the parents justifies a careful fetal cardiac examination. Clinically, the identification of a significant abnormality of amniotic fluid volume justifies careful fetal cardiac examination. Both global cardiomegaly and, specifically, left atrial enlargement have been associated with polyhydramnios. Heart failure resulting from a variety of causes, including congenital malformation, has been associated with hydrops fetalis both with and without oligohydramnios. Finally, fetal heart dysrhythmias, particularly fixed bradydysrhythmias, have been associated with congenital malformations and justify careful fetal cardiac examination. A lower but still increased risk of malformation has also been seen with tachydysrhythmias. The prognosis for fetuses with fixed bradycardias even without malformation is poor, with a perinatal mortality of up to 50%.

Antenatal fetal pharmacologic cardioversion of tachydysrhythmias is now possible, however, improving the clinical prognosis for these fetuses.

FETAL ECHOCARDIOGRAPHY

Fetal echocardiography consists of two-dimensional imaging in each of several specific scanplanes, M-mode motion analysis, Doppler velocity determinations of blood flow across atrioventricular valves and in each outflow tract, and, if indicated, real-time Doppler color flow imaging of the fetal heart.

The most commonly performed screening examination of the fetal heart, and an important part of every complete antenatal ultrasound examination, is the four-chamber view. This image is seen on a nearly transverse scan of the fetal chest at about one third of the distance from the diaphragm to the clavicles (Figure 9-1). The fetal heart assumes a nearly horizontal orientation within the chest, rather than the more oblique position of the neonate or adult, because of the uninflated lungs and the relatively higher position of the fetal diaphragm. The scanplane most nearly coincident with the cardiac long axis parallels the fetal ribs.

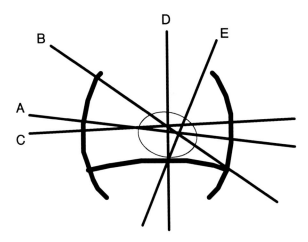

MAJOR FETAL CARDIAC SCANPLANES
FRONTAL PERSPECTIVE

Figure 9-1 This drawing illustrates the major scanplanes that are helpful for the antenatal examination of the fetal heart. Plane A is appropriate for the four-chamber view. Scanplane B will show the long-axis aortic outflow anatomy, while plane C is most appropriate for pulmonary outflow anatomy. Plane D is intended to show the aortic arch and descending aorta, and plane E is for the short-axis biventricular view.

The easiest sequence for the sonographer is to align the transducer with the fetal spine, rotate 90° transverse to the fetus in the region of the heart, and then make the small adjustments necessary to align the scanplane with a fetal rib. Slight movement of the scanplane either cephalically or caudally to an intercostal space will produce the clearest four-chamber cardiac view. The ideal four-chamber view, then, is not quite perfectly transverse to the fetal spine (Figure 9-2).

The chest outline seen with the cardiac four-chamber view is nearly circular. The heart occupies about one third of the area of the chest at this level, normally never over half, and is shaped vaguely like an arrowhead with the point directed toward the left. The anteroposterior midline passes through the left atrium, the base of the interventricular septum, and the right ventricle. The long axis of the heart intersects the anteroposterior midline at about 45° plus or minus 10° (Figure 9-3). The left ventricle is the more posterior of the two, is slightly longer, and comes to a sharper point. There is a prominent papillary muscle (moderator band), often seen to cross the cavity of the right ventricle (Figure 9-4). The ventricles are normally of equal width at their base and synchronous in their movement. Ventricular size has been measured throughout gestation, and normative charts have been constructed against which individuals can be compared. It may prove useful to compare the biventricular diameter to the biparietal diameter or the femur length in the

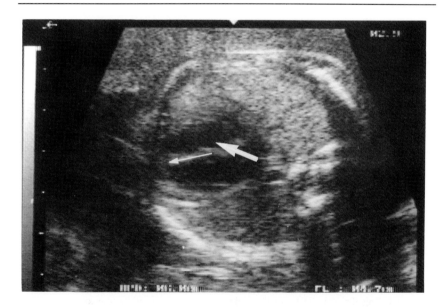

Figure 9-2   This four-chamber view illustrates the long axis of the heart (small arrow), inclined to the left of the anteroposterior axis of the chest (large arrow). The spine is to the right in this view. The left ventricle is the more posterior of the two. Compare to Figure 9-3.

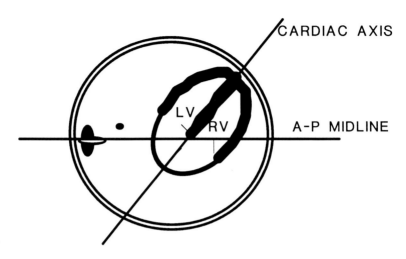

FOUR CHAMBER VIEW: FETAL HEART

Figure 9-3 The cardiac axis and the anteroposterior (A-P) midline are drawn here to illustrate the normal inclination and centering of the fetal heart. The anteroposterior midline should pass through the left atrium, the base of the septum, and the right ventricle. LV, left ventricle; RV, right ventricle.

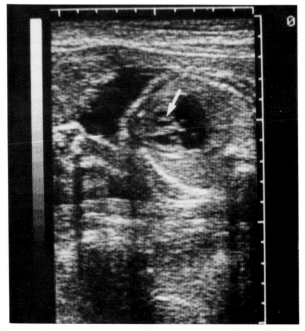

Figure 9-4 This four-chamber view again shows the correct centering and inclination of the fetal heart, and the prominent papillary muscle (moderator band) crossing the right ventricle (arrow).

case of a fetus with unsure gestational dates. In the normal fetus, the biventricular end-diastolic diameter–femur length ratio is 0.60 ± 0.10. End-diastolic dimensions are easily obtained from M-mode sonograms (see below). Significant asymmetry of the ventricular diameters at the base is very suggestive of significant pathology.

Left ventricular enlargement may result from relative or absolute obstruction of aortic outflow or coarctation of the aortic arch. Right ventricular enlargement can be seen with relative or absolute obstruction of outflow of the pulmonary valve or acute or chronic fetal distress.

Displacement of the heart to the right or the left, abnormality of the orientation of the long axis, and abnormality or asymmetry of the size of the ventricles or atria are observations that should suggest the presence of a major defect and lead to a more detailed examination or referral. Slight cephalic rotation of the scanplane from the standard four-chamber view should produce a long-axis, left ventricular outflow tract view (Figure 9-5). To achieve this view, note the position of the fetal back on the video monitor, then slide the transducer (scanplane) slightly toward the fetal head, angle the plane back toward the fetal abdomen, and rotate the end of the transducer nearest the fetal spine slightly cephalically. This will move the scanplane superiorly at the base of the ventricles but keep the apex in view, and the aortic root should be seen (Figure 9-6). The aortic valve will be seen to flicker in and out of view.

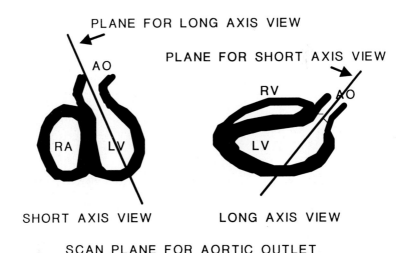

Figure 9-5   The short-axis view, to the left in this drawing, illustrates the approximate scanplane for the examination of the long-axis left ventricle and outflow tract shown to the right. AO, aortic outlet; RA, right atrium; RV, right ventricle; LV, left ventricle.

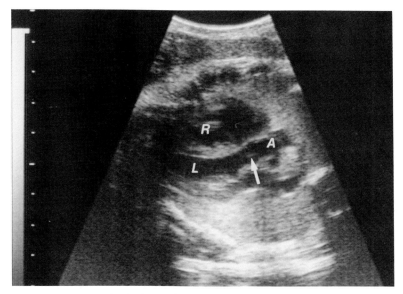

Figure 9-6   A sonogram in the long-axis, left ventricle orientation is shown here. The left ventricle (L), much of the right ventricle (R), and the aorta (A) are seen, along with a part of the aortic valve (arrow).

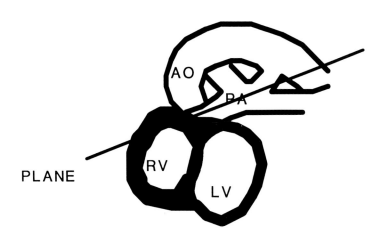

APICAL SHORT AXIS PERSPECTIVE

PULMONARY OUTFLOW SCANPLANE

Figure 9-7   This drawing in a short-axis orientation with the outflow tracts superimposed shows the approximate plane for imaging of the pulmonary outflow. PA, pulmonary artery; other abbreviations explained in legend for Figure 9-5.

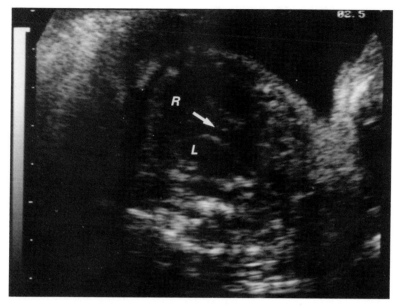

Figure 9-8   The right ventricular outflow is shown here (arrow) with a small portion of right ventricle (R) and a minor portion of the left (L).

A slight sliding motion of the transducer in a caudal direction with an angle a bit more transverse to the chest will lead to visualization of the pulmonary outflow tract crossing over the aortic root, with pulmonary valve action being apparent (Figure 9-7). The infundibulum leading into the pulmonary artery is seen to be slightly broader than the aortic root (Figure 9-8).

Rotation of the transducer 90° to the long axis of the heart will show the short-axis view of both ventricles (Figure 9-9), and sliding toward the atria will show the short-axis view of the pulmonary outflow (Figure 9-10).

Rotation of the transducer from the transverse to the oblique sagittal left paraspinal area of the fetus will usually capture the entire aortic arch (Figure 9-11). A sagittal plane just to the right of the fetal spine should allow viewing of both superior and inferior venae cavae.

M-Mode Echocardiography

M-mode (motion-mode) echocardiography, sometimes also known as T-M-mode (time-motion-mode) echocardiography, identifies a technique that uses the graphic display over time of the echoes along one scanline that may be positioned as desired throughout the field of view. The visual display over

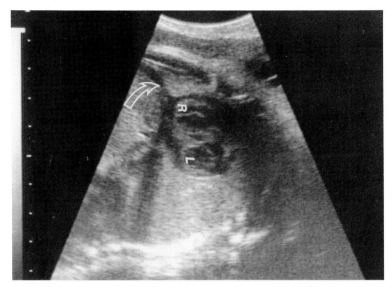

Figure 9-9 The left (L) and right (R) ventricles are nicely shown on this short-axis sonogram of a normal fetal heart. The diaphragm is also seen below the heart (arrow).

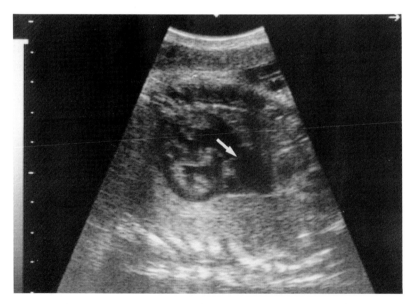

Figure 9-10 This short-axis view of the fetal heart is close to the base of the heart and shows the pulmonary outflow from the right ventricle (arrow).

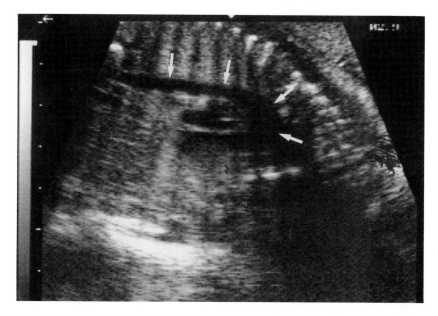

Figure 9-11 A slightly oblique sagittal scan of the fetal chest from right anterior to left posterior should allow the imaging of the descending aorta and the aortic arch (arrows), as illustrated here.

a finite time period of the movements of the echoes located along that scanline allows the viewer to compare the characteristics of movement of related structures along that scanline. For instance, if the M-mode cursor tracks through the two ventricles at a right angle to the interventricular septum, then the movements of the two ventricular walls will be seen on the M-mode display together (Figure 9-12). The rate of excursion, the synchrony of movement, and a variety of other measurements may be made from such a tracing; these are not available either from two-dimensional images or freeze frame imaging. The diameter of either or both ventricles at end diastole and end systole may be derived from such an M-mode display, as well as the movement and thickness of the interventricular septum. Positioning the M-mode cursor over one ventricle and an atrium allows the comparison of mechanical activity as an analogue of electrical activity (Figure 9-13). Atrial contraction should occur just slightly before ventricular contraction. Many dysrhythmias that result in the partial or complete disassociation of atrial and ventricular activity can be examined using this tool. The positioning of the cursor parallel to the interventricular septum over a valve leaflet of the mitral or tricuspid valve should document valvular excursion.

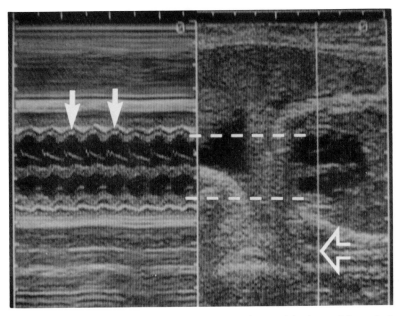

Figure 9-12 Passing the M-mode cursor (large open arrow) through both ventricles at the base shows the systolic excursion and allows the measurement of end-diastolic diameters. The wavering images on the left (arrows) correspond to the ventricular walls, as indicated by the dashed lines. *Source:* Reprinted from *Practical Obstetrical Ultrasound* (p 94) by JW Seeds and RC Cefalo, Aspen Publishers Inc, © 1986.

Doppler Flow Techniques

Sound reflected from a moving object is altered in frequency and wavelength in relation to the direction of movement of the object and in proportion to the velocity of the object (see Chapter 3). Sound reflected from an object moving away from the sound source has a lower frequency (negative frequency shift) and a longer wavelength than the original, while sound reflected from an object moving toward the source has a higher frequency (positive frequency shift) and a shorter wavelength than the original. The degree of frequency shift, positive or negative, is proportional to the velocity of the object and to the cosine of the angle of insonation. This means that the frequency shift is greatest when the angle is zero or the object is moving directly away from or toward the sound source, and the frequency shift is zero if the object is moving in a path at 90° to the direction of the sound.

The Doppler effect may be applied to medical purposes by using it to measure the velocity of blood flow in a noninvasive manner. Ultrasound pulses generated at the skin surface and directed at a vessel of interest are used as the source, and the frequency shift detected in reflected echoes is then

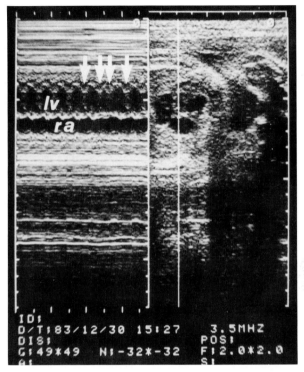

Figure 9-13 This M-mode echocardiogram has the M-mode cursor passing through one ventricle and an atrium. The arrows indicate regular rhythm except for one premature beat. The blood in the left ventricle (lv) and in the right atrium (ra) appears continuous on the left. *Source*: Reprinted from *Practical Obstetrical Ultrasound* (p 127) by JW Seeds and RC Cefalo, Aspen Publishers Inc, © 1986.

used to calculate blood flow velocity. Difficulty arises from imprecision in the measurement of the angle of insonation, however, and imprecision in the measurement of the diameter of the vessel interrogated makes it impossible to precisely estimate volume flow. However, the graphic display of the maximum frequency shift associated with arterial pulsatile flow allows some significant qualitative conclusions regarding the hemodynamic characteristics of the vascular system being studied. Furthermore, if the angle of insonation can be measured with reasonable accuracy, as it can be on most contemporary pulse duplex systems, velocity may be accurately estimated even if volume flow cannot.

The typical maximum frequency shift profile seen from the insonation of a fetal umbilical artery demonstrates a systolic peak followed by a diastolic minimum. Analysis of this waveform may be accomplished by a variety of methods. This waveform appears to change with changes in the vascular resistance of the vascular bed distal to the point of interrogation.

The simplest method is the ratio of the systolic peak frequency shift to the diastolic minimum, the S/D ratio. In a normal fetus this ratio falls slightly with advancing gestation, from a mean of 3.4 at 20 weeks to a mean of 2.4 at term, reflecting a slow drop in placental vascular resistance. Elevated S/D ratios are seen in cases of intrauterine growth retardation, fetal malformation, and aneuploidy. The use of Doppler velocity studies for the monitoring of fetal well-being in high-risk pregnancies is under investigation. Pulsed Doppler may be used to evaluate the velocity of blood flow in the pulmonary and aortic outflow tracts and to establish competence of cardiac valves by placing the interrogation sample cursor on either side of a cardiac valve.

Color flow Doppler technology provides color-coded visual representation of the direction of blood flow within a two-dimensional real-time image. The color (blue or red) indicates whether the blood is flowing toward (red) or away (blue) from the transducer. Such information can, in addition to the anatomic information, provide the basis for a more specific diagnosis than might otherwise be available. For instance, color flow studies can actually document right-to-left shunting across an apparent interventricular septal defect that might otherwise be unclear. Availability of color flow Doppler studies is limited, due to the very high expense of the equipment and the limited number of individuals with experience in its use. The actual number of cases in which color flow information is of critical clinical management value also appears to be limited, but the technique offers significant investigational potential.

DIAGNOSIS OF CARDIAC MALFORMATIONS

The antenatal diagnosis of cardiac malformations generally involves the detection of an abnormality of overall cardiac size, heart rate, size or shape of one or both ventricles or atria, mechanical activity of one or both ventricles or atria, cardiac axis, or outflow tracts.

Ventricular Malformations

Enlargement of one or both ventricles may be diagnosed by comparison of one to the other in the case of asymmetry, or by comparison of the biventricular end-diastolic diameter to either biparietal diameter or femur length, as mentioned above. Enlargement of the left ventricle may be seen in cases of aortic valvular stenosis or atresia or proximal coarctation of the aorta, while enlargement of the right ventricle is seen in cases of acute fetal distress, Ebstein's anomaly, and pulmonary stenosis or atresia.

Hypoplastic right or left heart may be seen in cases of aortic or pulmonary outflow obstruction, leading to hypoplastic development of the related ventricle.

Dilatation of both ventricles may be seen in cases of fetal cardiomyopathy of a variety of etiologies, endocardial fibroelastosis, end-stage erythroblastosis fetalis, and large capillary chorioangiomas.

Interventricular septal defects may be relatively limited or may involve the entire septum and the atrial septum as well, creating functionally a single atrium–single ventricle complex.

Outflow tract anomalies that may be detectable prenatally include transposition of the great vessels, tetralogy of Fallot, double outlet right ventricle, and possibly coarctation of the aorta.

General Prognosis and Management Considerations

In general, a cardiac malformation that is detected antenatally will not cause a fetal emergency prior to labor and delivery. However, with the birth of the infant the necessity for perfusion of the lungs and separation of the systemic and pulmonary circulations often results in critical and life-threatening circumstances if these functions are not properly performed.

Monitoring and Delivery

Referral and delivery in a tertiary center prepared for the birth of an infant with potentially life-threatening cardiac disease is recommended for optimal outcome in the case of the antenatal diagnosis of a congenital lesion. Ideally, pediatric cardiologists can be involved antenatally and given the opportunity to counsel the parents on issues such as neonatal care and possible therapies and therapeutic interventions that might be appropriate.

In many cases, depending on the nature of the defect, no immediate neonatal emergency is likely. Often neonatal echocardiography combined with cardiac catheterization is recommended for complete characterization of the malformation and its effect on neonatal cardiovascular function. However, some malformations carry a strong possibility of neonatal compromise because of variable perfusion of pulmonary or systemic circulation. Neonatal survival, for instance, in cases of pulmonary stenosis or atresia may be dependent on continued patency of the ductus arteriosus, because that is the only route of pulmonary perfusion. If the ductus closes, pulmonary perfusion will be impossible. In cases of atrioventricular septal defects with essentially complete mixing of the right and left circulations, the degree to which the neonate can oxygenate blood depends on the relative distribution of ventricular output between the systemic and pulmonary circulations, and this cannot be predicted antenatally.

In most cases of congenital cardiac disease, normal labor and vaginal delivery are possible. Continuous electronic fetal heart rate monitoring is indicated, and prompt response to any sign of fetal distress is important in achieving an optimal outcome. Fetal scalp blood pH evaluation may be helpful in evaluation of heart rate changes. In cases of fixed fetal bradycardias, fetal heart rate monitoring does not offer complete reassurance that the fetus is tolerating labor well. Since the baseline is generally 60 to 70 beats per minute, it is not clear that transient fetal hypoxemia would cause periodic decelerations from this baseline with a similar sensitivity to that seen with a normal baseline. Many practitioners therefore choose to deliver fetuses with fixed bradycardia by cesarean.

Recognition of specific cardiac anatomical defects in utero sets the stage for appropriate and early postnatal evaluation and management. Following birth, the diagnosis and the degree of severity of the cardiac anomalies should be confirmed. In addition, other major cardiac or noncardiac anomalies should be excluded. For a simple lesion such as a ventricular septal defect, echocardiography may provide crucial information regarding the size and location of the septal defect, as well as evidence of shunting. More complex cardiac lesions may require much more detailed anatomic and physiological investigations, including the use of cardiac catheterization and biplanar angiocardiography. The recent addition of color flow Doppler imaging combined with Doppler velocitometry may noninvasively provide crucial physiological information.

Appropriate medical or surgical therapy should be carried out once the diagnosis of specific cardiac lesions is confirmed. Therapy is based on the pathophysiology and cardiac anatomy of the patient. For example, infants with small asymptomatic ventricular septal defects require no specific therapy in the early postnatal period. However, neonates with more complex anomalies, and especially those with unstable cardiorespiratory physiology, may require emergency palliative or corrective surgery. The management of an infant with transposition of the great arteries illustrates this point. The pulmonary and systemic vascular circulations function independently and do not mix in these infants, who may rapidly deteriorate and die soon after birth. Immediate balloon atrial septostomy and creation of an interatrial communication at the time of initial diagnostic cardiac catheterization may be lifesaving. The procedure permits significant mixing of systemic and pulmonary circulations at the atrial level. Although this procedure is palliative, it has successfully been applied to tricuspid and pulmonary atresias as well as to anomalous pulmonary venous return. Recently balloon atrial septostomy has been guided using echocardiographic visualization. Following balloon atrial septostomy and initial stabilization, these patients usually require additional surgical treatment for physiologic correction (discussed below).

Some of the most critically ill infants following birth are those with duct-dependent lesions such as hypoplastic left heart syndrome or interrupted aortic arch. Blood flow to the distal aorta is dependent on patency of the ductus arteriosus and right-to-left shunting. To maintain oxygen saturation in these patients, prostaglandin E_1 infusions are used to prevent early ductal closure. Infants with isolated interrupted aortic arch may survive after neonatal repair of the aortic arch, but unfortunately, those with hypoplastic left ventricle have a dismal prognosis.

Operative intervention in the neonatal period is now performed with increasing success and safety. For many years palliative systemic-to-pulmonary shunts such as the Blalock-Taussig procedure (subclavian to pulmonary artery) have been used successfully for conditions such as tetralogy of Fallot. As experience and successes have increased, total correction of many defects is preferred and can be performed safely in infants. The combined use of cardiopulmonary bypass and deep hypothermia with circulatory arrest has been particularly useful for children with complex congenital heart disease.

ANTENATAL DIAGNOSIS OF SPECIFIC DEFECTS

Atrial Septal Defects

As noted above, the atrial septum develops as the result, first, of the growth of the septum primum, completed by the end of the 5th week, then of the septum secundum to the right side of the initial septum. The foramen ovale is an opening in the septum secundum, valved by the septum primum, allowing flow from right to left but not from left to right. Defects of the atrial septum may be located superiorly near the superior vena cava and are frequently associated with anomalies of pulmonary venous return. Alternatively, failure of the septum primum valve closure may occur more centrally, and finally, incomplete closure of the foramen primum by the septum primum may occur, leading to an atrial septal defect (ASD) located near the outlet portion of the atria.

An ASD is physiologic in utero. Therefore, it would not be expected to lead to any particular abnormality of flow or function. After birth, however, if ASD persists normal alterations in vascular resistance that accompany birth will lead to a significant left-to-right shunt and eventual right ventricular overload and possibly pulmonary vascular hypertension over the course of several years.

Because ASDs do not characteristically lead to chamber enlargement or physiologic abnormalities in utero, it is difficult to confidently diagnose or exclude their presence in utero. The atrial septum is difficult to image in early pregnancy due to its thin structure and rapid flapping movement in response to flow.

Although obstetrical management would not necessarily be altered by the antenatal diagnosis of an ASD, such a diagnosis, as with the diagnosis of any fetal anomaly, should lead to a careful search for other malformations that might be present.

Neonatal Care

Atrial septal defects, otherwise known as septum secundum defects, account for approximately 10% of the congenital heart lesions. Defects of the septum secundum can be placed into three categories based on the anatomic location of the septal defect. These defects include a patent foramen ovale (the most commonly encountered septum secundum defect), an ostium secundum defect, and a sinus venosus defect. The ostium secundum defect is the most common type of ASD recognized preoperatively and involves the area of the septum lateral and inferior to the foramen ovale. The sinus venosus defect occurs in the most superior portion of the atrial septum, immediately adjacent to the superior vena cava. This rare defect is often associated with anomalous drainage of the right pulmonary veins into the right atrium or the superior vena cava. Although ASDs may occur as isolated defects, they are frequently found in association with other complex congenital cardiac anomalies. The majority of infants presenting with secundum-type ASDs remain entirely asymptomatic. The diagnosis can be confirmed by both echocardiography and cardiac catheterization. In rare instances ASDs can cause significant congestive heart failure in infants. For the most part, however, the left-to-right shunting at the atrial level is remarkably well tolerated by most children. This altered physiology is tolerated until such patients reach the 3rd to 4th decades, when they may become symptomatic due to an increase in pulmonary vascular resistance secondary to chronic changes in the pulmonary vascular bed. The presence of a significant shunt at the atrial level is an adequate indication for surgical repair in childhood. Surgical repair of the ASD is associated with an extremely low mortality, less than 1% in asymptomatic patients. The sinus venosus defect presents a more significant challenge for operative repair since anomalously draining pulmonary veins would have to be appropriately dealt with in many of these patients.

Ventricular Septal Defect

Ventricular septal defects (VSDs) represent the most common cardiac defect, accounting for up to one third of all cardiac anomalies. They are also components of other more complex defects, such as double outlet right ventricle, tetralogy of Fallot, and transposition of the outflow tracts. Ventricular septal defects are also the most common cardiac anomaly resulting from diabetic embryopathy.

The ventricular septum results from the fusion by the 7th week of the endocardial cushions with the muscular septum originating from the apex of the ventricle. The majority of VSDs involve the membranous portion of the septum. Since the combined ventricular output of the fetus essentially provides flow through the aorta and systemic systems, with mixing in the aortic arch, even a large VSD would not be expected to produce significant abnormalities of cardiovascular function in utero. However, after birth increased pressures developed on the left side of the system will be transmitted to the right side and to the pulmonary vasculature. The majority of VSDs are small and close spontaneously in early childhood.

The antenatal diagnosis of a VSD is based on the visualization of discontinuity of the septum (Figure 9-14). However, confident diagnosis or exclusion in early gestation is very difficult due to the nature of the septum and the location of many membranous defects above the usual level of the four-chamber view. Furthermore, an apical four-chamber view, with the septum aligned in the direction of propagation of the sound waves (vertical orientation on the viewscreen) will often render the septum sufficiently echolucent to suggest the possibility of a defect. The ideal orientation of the septum in the scanplane is horizontal, resulting in maximum echo intensity from the tissue. Color flow imaging may be very helpful in the diagnosis of a VSD by color coding the blood flow in the area of the defect. Again, if the septum is oriented horizontally in the scanplane, blood flowing into or out of the horizontal ventricles will not produce a Doppler shift because the ultrasound pulses encounter the moving blood at a right angle to the direction of movement. However, blood shunting either right to left or left to right will produce a blue color if moving away from the transducer and red if moving toward the transducer. Such studies can be very helpful in diagnosing VSDs.

Obstetrical management in the case of VSDs is not altered, and the general prognosis for the majority of cases is very good if the defect is isolated. As with all other sonographic dysmorphology, the identification of a VSD should prompt the careful search for another defect and the consideration of fetal karyotype to exclude associated aneuploidy.

Neonatal Care

Ventricular septal defects occur in nearly one half of all children with complex congenital heart disease. The severity of the VSD lesion depends on the degree of left-to-right shunting and the sequelae of increased pulmonary blood flow and corresponding changes in pulmonary vascular resistance. The spontaneous closure of small VSDs less than 0.5 cm in diameter may occur in up to 50% of children before age 5. Ventricular septal defects between 0.5 and 2 cm in diameter are often associated with moderately severe left-to-right

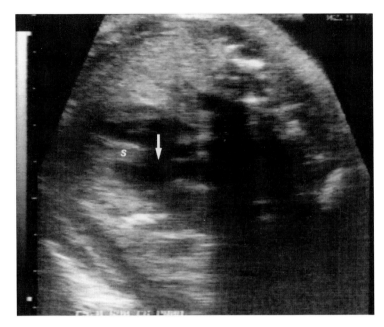

Figure 9-14 A large ventricular septal defect is seen here as a discontinuity (arrow) of the septum (s). Color Doppler examination would be confirmatory by showing the directional flow across the defect.

shunting with a pulmonary systemic blood flow ratio of greater than 1.5 to 1. Most of these patients remain asymptomatic in infancy, but as the pulmonary vascular resistance decreases, some children may present with congestive heart failure or failure to thrive. Less than 5% of these lesions will spontaneously close. A general rule is that if the child is older than age 2 and has persistently high pulmonary artery flow (greater than two times systemic blood flow) and increased pulmonary artery pressure, then the child has a significant chance of developing pulmonary vascular disease. Children with normal pulmonary artery pressure and pulmonary blood flow (less than two times systemic vascular flow) seldom develop pulmonary vascular disease. Ventricular septal defects greater than 2 cm are usually associated with failure of involution of the pulmonary vascular bed and commonly develop severe congestive heart failure and failure to thrive. Pulmonary vascular disease may occur despite aggressive medical and surgical therapy.

Echocardiographic studies are useful in the postnatal evaluation and management of these infants. Anatomic defects can be readily defined and the presence of a shunt detected. Angiocardiography and cardiac catheterization are useful to further define the anatomy and assess the size of ventricular cavities and the state of the atrioventricular valves.

Surgical closure of the VSD is recommended for all infants with significant anatomic or hemodynamic abnormalities. Large left-to-right shunts associated with increased cardiac size, a pulmonary-to-systemic flow ratio greater than 2:1, increased pulmonary artery pressure or slightly increased pulmonary vascular resistance, and supracristal or infracristal defects associated with aortic valvular insufficiency or a sinus of Valsalva fistula are all indications for repair of the VSD. In early infancy if the pulmonary-to-systemic blood flow ratio is less than 2:1 and the infant is asymptomatic, immediate surgical intervention is not required. Pulmonary artery banding, developed by Muller in 1952, was designed to reduce blood flow into the pulmonary vascular circuit. Currently this palliative operation has only selected use and has been replaced with intracardiac repairs even in early infancy. Intracardiac repairs using a synthetic patch material can be accomplished safely with cardiopulmonary bypass, deep hypothermia, and circulatory arrest. Associated lesions such as ASDs and incompetent atrioventricular valves should be repaired concomitantly. Operative mortality is now reported to be between 5% and 10%, even for infants with large symptomatic VSDs. These defects can be safely closed in the smallest children with an acceptable operative risk, with the ultimate result depending upon the degree of pulmonary vascular disease prior to repair. A small percentage of children may require pacemakers for third-degree heart block following repair of VSDs, particularly atrioventricular septal defects.

Atrioventricular Septal Defects

Atrioventricular septal defects (AVSDs) are often known as endocardial cushion defects and result, to a variable extent, in the failure of division of both the atria and the ventricles. Anomalies of the atrioventricular valves are also seen.

As noted above, the endocardial cushion grows to divide the primitive atrioventricular canal into two canals by the 6th week, then grows to fuse with the interventricular septum and the atrial septum to complete division of the right and left heart. Failure of the growth and development of the endocardial cushion results in some form of a single atrium–single ventricle complex with various forms of an abnormal valvular structure.

The functional result is complete mixing of venous and arterial blood, which in the fetus has limited impact. Often, however, the atrioventricular valve structure is incompetent, resulting in reduced effective output and also venous hypertension, with consequences that include hydrops fetalis. Furthermore, AVSDs are often associated with other significant cardiac defects, including most forms of truncal malformation. Persistent fetal bradycardia may be associated with a persistent atrioventricular canal and may be the key to antenatal diagnosis of this lesion. As with most other examples of fetal

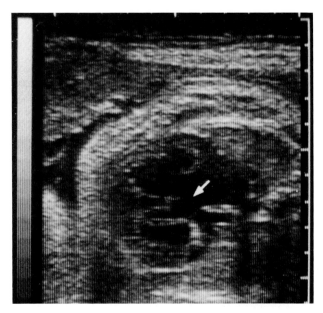

Figure 9-15 This sonogram shows an endocardial cushion defect (atrioventricular septal defect). Note the continuity between the right atrium and both ventricles (arrow). *Source*: Reprinted from *Practical Obstetrical Ultrasound* (p 122) by JW Seeds and RC Cefalo, Aspen Publishers Inc, © 1986.

dysmorphology, there appears to be a significant increase in the incidence of Down syndrome in the case of AVSD, indicating the need for consideration of fetal karyotype determination.

The diagnosis of AVSD may be made from the four-chamber view by demonstration of a defect in both the ventricular and atrial septa, resulting in confluence of the atria and the ventricles (Figure 9-15). There may be a single atrioventricular valve noted (Figure 9-16). Incomplete forms of the anomaly, however, may be difficult to detect. The demonstration of valvular incompetence using Doppler techniques may be valuable in estimating prognosis, as there is a lower probability of survival in the case of the infant with valvular incompetence and AVSD.

The survival of infants with AVSD without surgery is reported to be less than 5% beyond 5 years of age. Pulmonary artery banding to protect the pulmonary circulation from systemic pressures represents one surgical approach to this defect, but more recently, intracardiac repair of the abnormality has been attempted with good results.

Diagnosis of an AVSD should not necessarily alter obstetrical management. Amniocentesis or fetal blood sampling to perform fetal karyotype should be considered. Fetal heart rate monitoring may be difficult if a fetal bradydysrhythmia is present. If hydrops is present, the long-term prognosis

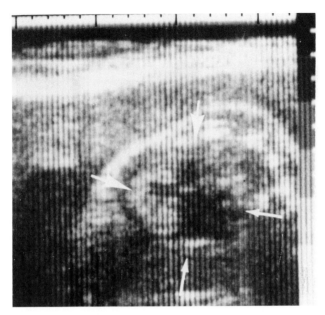

Figure 9-16 A severe atrioventricular septal defect results in a functional single atrium–single ventricle heart, as seen here. Arrows outline cardiac ventricle and atrium. *Source*: Reprinted from *Practical Obstetrical Ultrasound* (p 123) by JW Seeds and RC Cefalo, Aspen Publishers Inc, © 1986.

for the fetus is sufficiently grave, because of the valvular incompetence, that generally the detection of hydrops suggests that management for maternal welfare alone may well be appropriate.

Neonatal Care

The degree of atrioventricular valvular insufficiency and the extent of left-to-right shunting at the atrioventricular levels account for the severity of the symptoms the infant may exhibit after birth. Echocardiography is extremely useful for accurate diagnosis of atrioventricular defects. A deficiency in the muscular ventricular septum along with an abnormal attachment of the atrioventricular valve, specifically the mitral valve, can be typically seen both with echocardiography and angiocardiograms.

Pulmonary artery banding, once advocated to protect the pulmonary circulation from systemic pressures, is now rarely used, as the majority of these patients now have superior results with total correction of AVSDs. Operation is advised before the onset of severe pulmonary vascular disease. Furthermore, operation is indicated at any age when cardiac failure is not readily manageable, but more patients will do well with elective repair performed before the age of 2 or 3 years. Repair of AVSDs includes prosthetic closure of the defect and repair of the mitral valve. Survival following correction even in infants approaches 95%. However, heart block may occur postoperatively, which requires a pacemaker insertion. Nearly 5% of the patients will eventually require mitral valve replacement when their valves become or remain incompetent.

Ebstein's Anomaly

This rare congenital cardiac malformation is characterized by apical displacement of the tricuspid valve. The valve is often incompetent, and the resulting regurgitation causes cardiomegaly, right atrial enlargement, and often hydropic changes including fetal ascites. There are a variety of possible associated cardiac malformations, including septal and truncal malformations.

The diagnosis may be made visually by the detection of apical displacement of the tricuspid valve, with an enlarged right atrium (Figure 9-17). Doppler studies may be helpful in the identification of regurgitation of the tricuspid valve. Regurgitation is not only consistent with the diagnosis but also contributes to assessment of prognosis, which is much worse if valvular incompetence is documented. The natural history of this malformation includes up to a 50% mortality in early infancy, but recent advances in surgical intervention have led to a significant improvement in outcome.

Obstetrical management is not necessarily altered by this diagnosis. A careful search for associated anomalies and for signs of hydrops is indicated.

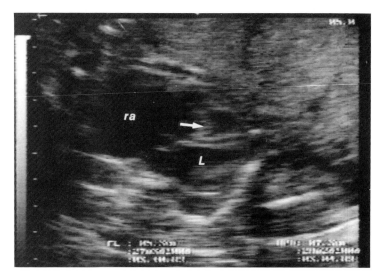

Figure 9-17 Ebstein's anomaly involves apical displacement of the tricuspid valve (arrow) and severe enlargement of the right atrium (ra), as seen here. The left ventricle (L) is below.

Fetal blood sampling or amniocentesis should be considered to diagnose or exclude aneuploidy in the case of this and any other fetal cardiac defect.

It should be noted that there is an unexpected disproportion of incidence of Ebstein's anomaly among babies of mothers treated continuously with lithium during pregnancy.

Neonatal Care

Ebstein's anomaly is seen neonatally about once in 100,000 live births. The characteristic downward displacement of the septal and posterior leaflets of the tricuspid valve along with apical displacement of the entire valve apparatus, as described above, is associated with both obstruction and insufficiency of the valve. Primary indications for surgical intervention are functional limitations from congestive heart failure and low cardiac output. Many of these patients require tricuspid valve replacement, closure of the ASD, and plication of the atrialized portion of the right ventricle. Because of the wide spectrum of anatomic and physiological severity, one cannot generalize about the long-term prognosis of the individual patient. However, even with surgical intervention many of these patients still have a significantly shortened life span. The average age of death is in the 3rd decade.

Hypoplastic Left Heart Syndrome

Hypoplastic left heart syndrome (HLHS) includes significant under-development of the left ventricle, aortic valvular atresia, and mitral valvular hypoplasia or atresia. It may be that the primary abnormality is aortic atresia. In the case of absolute obstruction of outflow, normal development of the left ventricle, atrium, and mitral valve would be impossible.

In the case of HLHS, the right ventricle is the primary pumping organ of the system. It supplies the pulmonary and systemic circulations. Descending aortic and coronary circulations are supplied in a retrograde fashion after blood is pumped through the ductus arteriosus. The right ventricle may be capable of supporting the entire circulation throughout gestation or may suffer failure due to overload. Regardless, usually shortly after birth, failure and death will occur. The long-term prognosis for survival of infants with HLHS is very poor.

The diagnosis may be made from the standard four-chamber view. Normally the cardiac ventricles are symmetrical in width at their base. In the case of HLHS, the left ventricle will be seen to be very small compared to the right, and also to any of the other fetal dimensions such as biparietal diameter or femur length (Figure 9-18). In some cases, the left side is sufficiently underdeveloped that the appearance of a single atrium–single ventricle complex is simulated. It is not clear that HLHS can be reliably excluded in early gestation.

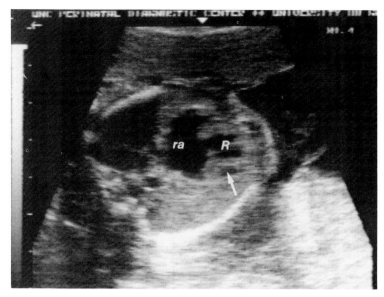

Figure 9-18 Hypoplastic left heart syndrome may result from aortic valvular atresia, as in this case. The left ventricle was hypoplastic and nonfunctional (arrow). The right ventricle (R) was the functional pump, and the right atrium (ra) was enlarged.

Early diagnosis of HLHS should result in a discussion of the option of pregnancy termination, a careful search for associated defects, and either fetal blood sampling or amniocentesis to establish fetal karyotype. The prognosis is sufficiently poor that obstetrical management will often focus on maternal welfare.

Neonatal Care

Surgical intervention for palliation or correction in this frequently lethal anomaly is experimental. Norwood and his colleagues have developed a complicated series of procedures in an attempt to physiologically repair infants with hypoplastic left heart. Long-term survival has been achieved in selected patients. Neonatal cardiac transplantation, another highly experimental procedure, is being pursued in a few centers worldwide.

Hypoplastic Right Ventricle

Hypoplastic right ventricle (HRV) is typically associated with pulmonary valvular obstruction and an intact interventricular septum. Atresia of the pulmonary valve is likely to be the primary malformation, with underdevelopment of the right ventricle simply resulting from the absolute obstruction of outflow. Some variability of appearance may be seen in the case of tricuspid incompetence, because that would allow greater right ventricular contractility, although the outflow is unproductive retrograde ejection.

In the fetus with HRV, right atrial blood is shunted through the foramen ovale to the left atrium and pumped by the left ventricle to the systemic circulation and by retrograde flow through the ductus arteriosus to the pulmonary circulation. Closure of the ductus arteriosus after birth produces, as expected, severe cyanotic heart disease, as pulmonary perfusion and oxygenation are blocked.

Antenatal diagnosis of HRV can be difficult. Although the ventricles are expected to be of equal diameter at the base, and the normal relationship of these diameters to biparietal diameter and femur length is known, the confident exclusion of HRV in early pregnancy is not always possible. If the right ventricle is clearly smaller than the left and Doppler investigation demonstrates little or no flow through the infundibulum of the right ventricle, the diagnosis may be considered (Figures 9-19 and 9-20). However, as noted above, with tricuspid incompetence, the right ventricle might be normal or even enlarged (Figure 9-21) in dimensions, making the diagnosis dependent upon demonstration of atresia of the pulmonary valve and retrograde flow through the tricuspid valve.

The prognosis for infants with HRV is very poor without palliative surgery. As many as one third of infants so affected may enjoy long-term survival with pulmonary valvulotomy combined with a **systemic-pulmonary artery shunt**. More recent experience suggests even further improvement in outcome using pharmacologic inhibition of closure of the ductus.

Obstetrical management of these patients is not necessarily altered by this diagnosis. However, once the diagnosis is made, a careful search for associated abnormalities, including any sign of hydrops fetalis, should be done. Fetal blood sampling or amniocentesis should be considered to exclude the possibility of aneuploidy. If the diagnosis is made in early gestation, the patient should be apprised of the option of pregnancy termination.

Neonatal Care

Right ventricular hypoplasia associated with pulmonary valvular atresia accounts for less than 1% of all congenital heart disease. In these patients the right ventricular myocardium is hypertrophied although the ventricular chamber is diminutive. The pulmonary circulation is maintained by flow through the patent ductus arteriosus. Death frequently coincides with closure of the ductus. Without palliative surgery death ensues rapidly. These patients are candidates for balloon atrial septostomy or other systemic-pulmonary shunts. Without treatment the prognosis is exceedingly poor; nearly 80% of the patients succumb within 6 months. The best hope for survival of

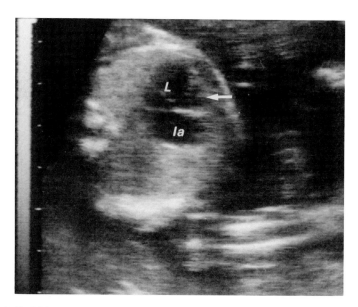

Figure 9-19   This example of hypoplastic right heart demonstrates the attenuated right side (arrow), the functional left side (L), and the enlarged left atrium (la).

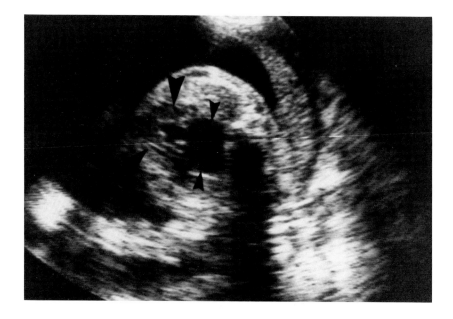

Figure 9-20   Again, in this example of a hypoplastic right heart, the attenuated right side is evident, with a dilated left atrium.

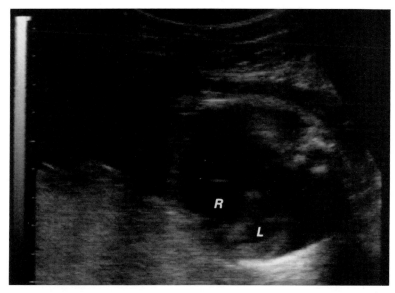

Figure 9-21 When there is incompetence of the tricuspid valve, the right ventricle can maintain mechanical activity despite pulmonary valvular atresia, and the right ventricle (R) may be seen to be enlarged, as in this case. The left ventricle (L) was normally functional.

the patient is a systemic-pulmonary shunt combined with pulmonary valvulotomy.

Tetralogy of Fallot

The classic tetralogy includes a VSD; displacement of the aortic root to the right, over-riding the interventricular septum; pulmonary artery stenosis; and hypertrophy of the right ventricle. The VSD usually involves the upper membranous part, and the degree of dextrodeviation of the aorta is variable.

Hemodynamic abnormalities in the fetus appear to be minimal, but after birth, the physiologic impact of the syndrome varies with the degree of pulmonary stenosis. The greater the degree of pulmonary perfusion, the less the immediate physiological detriment. There is a variable right-to-left shunt at the point of the VSD, and eventually right ventricular overload is to be expected due to the chronic exposure of the right ventricle to systemic pressures.

The diagnosis may be made from four-chamber images, showing a dilated aortic root over-riding the interventricular septum and receiving output from both ventricles (Figures 9-22 and 9-23). The pulmonary artery may be seen to be small or may be difficult to image at all with confidence. If the pulmonary artery cannot be identified at all and the single dilated outflow tract appears

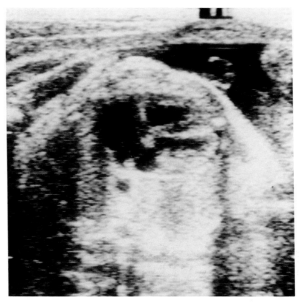

Figure 9-22 Tetralogy of Fallot need not alter the four-chamber view significantly, as illustrated here. The only abnormality evident on this scan was that the cardiac long axis intersected the midline at almost 90°.

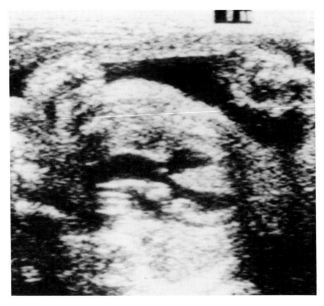

Figure 9-23 Moving the scanplane of Figure 9-22 slightly cephalically shows the single dilated ventricular outflow tract with inflow from both ventricles.

to serve as the origin for the pulmonary arteries, a diagnosis of truncus arteriosus should be considered.

The prognosis for infants with tetralogy of Fallot is variable, depending on the exact nature of the lesion, but has improved considerably with the evolution of surgical palliation followed by surgical correction of the abnormalities, with long-term survival exceeding 80%.

As with other malformations, diagnosis should lead to careful examination of the infant for associated malformations and also consideration of fetal blood sampling or amniocentesis to confirm fetal karyotype. There appears to be no benefit to alteration of obstetrical management, but as with most other significant intracardiac congenital defects, delivery in a tertiary center prepared for the special needs of such an infant is recommended.

Neonatal Care

The diagnosis of tetralogy of Fallot can be confirmed postnatally using echocardiography. Angiocardiography and cardiac catheterization provide the most precise information concerning the anatomy of the pulmonary arteries and the VSD and the physiology of the patient. The usual cause of death in children with tetralogy of Fallot is hypoxia. Without correction the prognosis is very poor, as hypoxia increases with age. During the past 30 years, operations for tetralogy of Fallot have evolved to include closure of the VSD and a patch enlargement of the pulmonary outflow tract. Complete intracardiac repair is now considered preferable to palliative systemic and pulmonary shunts. More than 85% of the patients have excellent long-term results with intracardiac repair. The mortality of patients older than 3 years of age with mild symptoms is less than 2% to 3%. Extremely small infants who initially require palliative systemic-pulmonary shunting may have long-term survival in the range of 95% after a period of appropriate growth and subsequent total correction. Infants less than 1 year of age undergoing a primary complete intracardiac repair have greater than an 85% survival, with excellent functional results.

Transposition of the Great Vessels

Transposition of the great vessels refers to a cardiac malformation involving the origin of the aorta from the right ventricle and the origin of the pulmonary artery from the left ventricle. This malformation may result from a failure of the aortopulmonary septum to develop along a spiral course within the primordial truncus. The resulting positions of the arteries may vary. Transposition is a common cardiac anomaly in the child of the diabetic.

Transposition may be associated with pulmonic stenosis with an intact septum, with a VSD, or with a VSD with pulmonic stenosis. In utero, transposition usually results in few pathophysiological changes. Output from both ventricles mixes normally in the ductus arteriosus anyway. However, after birth, if no pathway for significant mixing is present, survival is not possible.

The diagnosis rests with the detection of the absence of the normal diagonal relationship between the aorta and the pulmonary artery. The discrimination of transposition from other conotruncal malformations may be difficult, however, and it is always wise to include such diagnoses as double outlet right ventricle in the clinical discussion.

Prognosis is poor without surgical intervention, with mortality as high as 90% by 1 year of age. The creation of arteriovenous connections to promote mixing may be helpful.

Obstetrical management centers on a careful search for associated malformations, consideration of a fetal karyotype, and delivery at a tertiary center prepared for the special support of the fetus.

Neonatal Care

Transposition of the great vessels is seen in approximately 10% of all infants with congenital heart disease. These infants present with severe cyanosis from birth, and hypoxia threatens their survival. Since mixing of the pulmonary and systemic circulations is absent, many of these patients rapidly succumb in the neonatal period without the creation of a large opening between the pulmonary and systemic circulations. Although echocardiography can establish the diagnosis, angiocardiography should be performed to define the varied anatomical relationships with the cardiac chambers, structures, and great vessels prior to the planning and performing of major surgical procedures. The anatomy of the transposition of the great vessels is quite variable, which may affect the outcome of surgical repair. Although the balloon atrial septostomy is a useful initial palliative procedure in the neonatal period, additional palliative procedures such as the Blalock-Hanlon operation, which creates a large ASD, or other pulmonary-systemic shunts, including a Blalock-Taussig shunt (a subclavian-to-aortic shunt), may be required. Patients with transposition and VSDs often require operation prior to age 6 months because of severe progressive pulmonary vascular disease. The Mustard and Senning operations are the most commonly used intracardiac corrective procedures. These complex procedures correct the abnormal physiology by rearranging the atrial blood flow. Jatene and his colleagues have advocated a complete reversal of the great arteries, known as the "switch" operation. This procedure has been quite successful but is associated with a higher mortality than the intra-atrial corrective procedures. A few patients require valved external conduits to relieve left ventricular outflow obstruction (Rastelli procedure). The operation consists of placing a valve conduit from the left ventricle to the pulmonary artery. If a VSD is present, this is also repaired during the procedure. These operations are complex and difficult and are associated with significant complications in over half of the patients; mortality is as high as 20%.

Despite advances in cardiac surgical management, 20% of the initial transposition survivors develop grave complications and succumb in the first 10 years. Children with transposition often require reoperation for pulmonary venous or severe vena caval obstruction. In addition dysrhythmias, progressive pulmonary vascular obstructive disease, and chylothorax have been reported.

Double Outlet Right Ventricle

This condition is characterized by the origination of both great vessels from the right ventricle. Double outlet right ventricle (DORV) may be viewed as an extreme of tetralogy of Fallot, in which the aorta is sufficiently displaced to the right as to be originating from the right ventricle. Ventricular septal defects are commonly found, as are abnormal atrioventricular valves, anomalous pulmonary venous return, and coarctation of the aorta. There is a relatively high rate of associated extracardiac anomalies.

The fetal implications of DORV are variable. Often, no specific hemodynamic effect is seen. Typically, significant asymmetry of ventricular development is noted, but rarely signs of failure. After birth the right ventricle will often develop failure in response to its required workload, which includes both the systemic and pulmonary circulations.

The diagnosis is based on the visualization of the origin of both great vessels from the right ventricle, and supported by significant asymmetry of the ventricles. However, confusion with tetralogy of Fallot is common, as these are related anomalies and visually similar. Tracing the aortic arch with visible origins of the head and neck vessels to the right ventricle and identifying pulmonary origin from the right ventricle as well are compelling evidence for DORV.

The common recommendations include a search for associated anomalies, consideration of fetal karyotype, and delivery at a tertiary center. There is no basis, in the absence of hydrops or other evidence of failure, to alter obstetrical management.

Neonatal Care

Angiocardiography is crucial for accurate preoperative diagnosis and assessment of infants with DORV. Echocardiography is also useful in these patients, but there are a number of subtle variations of anatomy that may require different surgical procedures for correction. At least six different types of operative techniques have been developed to correct these variations. In some patients a patch graft reconstruction of the pulmonary outflow tract is required, whereas other patients require an extra cardiac conduit from the right ventricle to the pulmonary artery. Repair of the VSD and creation of intra-atrial transposition of venous return are useful in some patients. The risks of operation for these more complex repairs are significantly higher than for repair of simple VSDs or tetralogy of Fallot. Infants, despite aggressive medical management, may develop congestive heart failure due to increased pulmonary blood flow, progressive pulmonary vascular obstructive disease, and severe cyanosis. Palliative procedures such as systemic-to-pulmonary artery shunting can be very useful to salvage small infants who cannot tolerate intracardiac repair.

Truncus Arteriosus

Truncus arteriosus describes a single large outflow tract originating almost equally from both ventricles, with a single truncal valve that is commonly incompetent. The lesion results from defective conotruncal septation, and offers origin for pulmonary and systemic vessels.

In utero, hemodynamic aberrations are minimal, but after birth the dramatically lower resistance in the pulmonary vascular bed results in substantially higher-volume perfusion of the lungs and often congestive ventricular failure due to the volume overload. In time, damage to the pulmonary vessels results in pulmonary hypertension, with a very poor long-term prognosis. Most infants with truncus arteriosus demonstrate congestive failure shortly after birth, and the expectation of survival is poor.

The detection of a single large outflow tract over-riding the interventricular septum may be difficult to discriminate from tetralogy of Fallot. If a pulmonary outflow can be identified, tetralogy becomes the more likely diagnosis, but even in the absence of a visible separate pulmonary outflow, tetralogy with pulmonic stenosis or atresia may be present.

In the absence of fetal hydrops, there is no basis for altering obstetrical management. The fetus should be carefully examined to exclude other malformations, and a karyotype should be considered. If the diagnosis is made in early gestation, termination should be discussed.

Neonatal Care

Truncus arteriosus is a rare congenital cardiac malformation that accounts for approximately 1% to 2% of congenital cardiac defects. The congestive heart failure that is very common in infants born with truncus arteriosus manifests when pulmonary vascular resistance decreases and the pulmonary blood flow increases within the first few weeks after birth. The presence of truncal valvular insufficiency significantly aggravates the congestive heart failure. Infants with congestive heart failure often die within the 1st year of life. Echocardiography is diagnostic, but cardiac catheterization and angio-cardiography are required to provide precise anatomic information, such as the location of the pulmonary arteries and truncal valve function, prior to consideration for surgical correction. The steps at operative repair include separation of the pulmonary arteries from the truncus, closure of the truncal defect, closure of the VSD, and establishment of the continuity between right ventricle and the pulmonary artery using a Dacron conduit containing a heterograft valve. Many of these infants require palliative banding of a pulmonary artery trunk or separate bandings of the right and left pulmonary arteries. However, pulmonary artery banding increases the risk of definitive correction later. Salvage of many children by corrective operations has been possible, with excellent to good functional results present in most of the patients. The presence of truncus valve insufficiency diminishes the chances for successful outcome.

Cardiomyopathy

Fetal cardiac dysfunction may result from viral infection such as cytomega-lovirus or parvovirus, drug toxicity such as betamimetic drug therapy, or genetic myopathy such as endocardial fibroelastosis (Figure 9-24). In general, these conditions are characterized by cardiomegaly and often pericardial effusions, intrauterine growth retardation, and fetal hydrops.

Management includes efforts to diagnose the etiology of the failure, including consideration of fetal blood sampling for antibody identification. Supportive observation is in most cases the only appropriate management option. Prognosis is variable. In the case of endocardial fibroelastosis the prognosis is very poor, and no therapeutic intervention is likely to alter this. Viral cardiomyopathy may recover partially or totally, and toxic failure related to pharmacologic treatment may recover if the agent is discontinued.

Cardiac Dysrhythmias

The most common variety of fetal cardiac dysrhythmia is the isolated ectopic beat that may represent an atrial or ventricular premature contrac-tion. These produce an irregular heart rate of variable severity. Premature atrial or ventricular contractions are typically benign, are not associated with cardiac anomalies, are not associated with altered prognosis, and resolve with or shortly after birth.

The premature atrial or ventricular contraction may be detected visually by careful review of the real-time image of the cardiac cycle, with the observa-tion of discordance of atrial and ventricular activity, or by using M-mode echocardiography to examine cardiac mechanical activity. If the M-mode

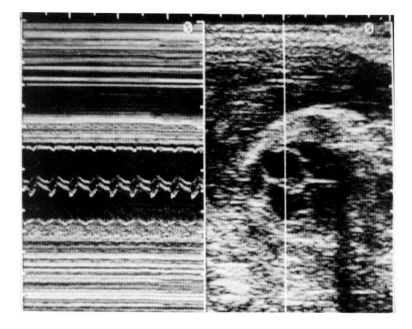

Figure 9-24 Endocardial fibroelastosis may illustrate the general appearance on M-mode echocardiography of fetal cardiomyopathy. The M-mode cursor shown here reveals minimal ventricular sidewall excursion in this very dilated fetal heart.

---

cursor is placed over a ventricle and an atrium, the respective mechanical activity may be simultaneously examined (see Figure 9-13). Either atrial or ventricular premature contractions may be detected.

Pathological consequences are very rare. In the absence of intrauterine growth retardation or signs of hydrops, no alteration in obstetrical management is indicated. If the ectopic beats are frequent, fetal monitoring in labor may be difficult, and fetal scalp blood sampling might be helpful.

Fetal supraventricular tachycardia is a serious abnormality of fetal cardiac rhythm that most often justifies therapeutic intervention. Supraventricular tachycardia may cause a fetal heart rate of up to 300 beats per minute, and atrial flutter can result in rates of over 400 beats per minute. These rhythms may result from an ectopic pacemaker discharging at very rapid rates or from re-entry phenomena at several possible sites.

Supraventricular tachycardia may be constant or intermittent, and may or may not be associated with hydrops. Constant fetal heart rates above 200 beats per minute are considered therapeutic candidates because of the high rate of the development of hydrops, probably due to incomplete ventricular filling.

The diagnosis is made using M-mode techniques that demonstrate a very rapid atrial rate with 1:1 or 1:2 ventricular response (Figure 9-25). Therapeutic success has been reported using maternal digoxin therapy to decrease nodal transmission and therefore slow ventricular rates. Digitalization of the pregnant patient often requires up to double the normal loading dose due to expanded blood volume and more rapid clearing of the drug. It is not recommended that supertherapeutic maternal digoxin levels be sought, but it is often necessary to use larger doses to achieve and maintain the usual therapeutic level. In many reports, it has been necessary to add another of several cardiotropic drugs, including possibly verapamil, propranolol, or quinidine, to gain control of ventricular rate (see also Chapter 14).

Atrioventricular conduction block may be continuous or intermittent and is detected by placing the M-mode cursor over a ventricle and an atrium and noting the dyssynchronous activity (Figure 9-26). Of all the dysrhythmias, it is the most likely to be associated with structural abnormalities. A substantial portion of infants with cardiac conduction block will prove to be the product of pregnancies in women with lupus erythematosus. In these cases, antigen-antibody complexes are found to be deposited in the conduction fibers, and

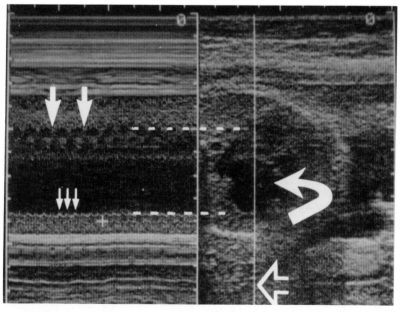

Figure 9-25 Supraventricular tachycardia with incomplete ventricular response is shown here, with the M-mode cursor crossing the left ventricle and the right atrium. The atrial activity (small arrows) is maintaining a rate of about 320 beats per minute, with ventricular response (large arrows) at 160. *Source*: Reprinted from *Practical Obstetrical Ultrasound* (p 126) by J W Seeds and RC Cefalo, Aspen Publishers Inc, © 1986.

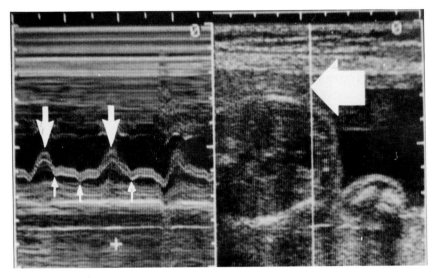

Figure 9-26 Complete heart block may be detected with M-mode echocardiography. (Large arrow indicates M-mode cursor.) Here, atrial activity (small arrows) is seen with no apparent correlation to ventricular activity (large arrows). *Source*: Reprinted from *Practical Obstetrical Ultrasound* (p 128) by JW Seeds and RC Cefalo, Aspen Publishers Inc, © 1986.

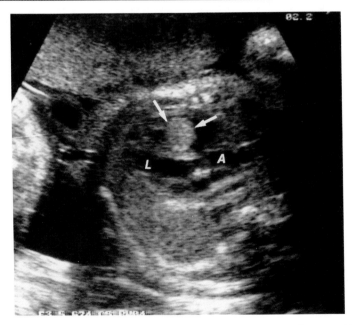

Figure 9-27 This long-axis view shows the left ventricle (L) and aortic outflow tract (A) and a 1.2-cm soft tissue mass within the right ventricle (arrows).

the pathophysiological changes are not reversible. Specifically, a type of immunoglobulin G known as the rho or SSA antibody is associated with fetal conduction block and may be identified in maternal serum.

Cardiac malformations associated with heart block included endocardial cushion defect and atrioventricular canal defects.

The fetus with a heart block may or may not develop signs of pump failure, such as hydrops. Those features of a case that lead to the development of hydrops are not clear. A fetus with complete block with normal growth and development and absence of hydrops may have a reasonable prognosis but may require neonatal placement of a pacemaker. If hydrops develops in utero, the prognosis is very poor. No therapeutic intervention in the case of fetal conduction block with hydrops is known to be helpful.

Intracardiac Tumors

Intracardiac rhabdomyomas are rare soft tissue masses arising as isolated intracardiac tumors or occurring as multiple masses (Figure 9-27). There is a substantial (up to 50%) association between these masses and tuberous sclerosis, an autosomal dominant genetic condition. The pathophysiological significance of the tumors depends on their location and size. Hydrops fetalis can result from large tumors, and rapid growth has been seen. Therefore serial surveillance of fetal growth and development is indicated if such a soft tissue mass is detected and early delivery if fetal growth delay or hydrops is noted.

Acardiac Twin

A rare complication of twin gestation is dysplasia or agenesis of the heart of one twin but with its survival based on retrograde flow through vascular anastomoses in the placenta. There is a spectrum of phenotype, from amorphous tissue with no resemblance to human form to a fairly complete fetus with no functional heart. Most often there are other abnormalities, such as hydrops fetalis, and typically multiple, very large subcutaneous lymphatic cysts (Figure 9-28). The co-twin is usually normal, and management of the pregnancy should focus on the best outcome for the normal co-twin and for the mother.

FURTHER READING

Adams CW. A reappraisal of life expectancy with atrial shunts of the secundum type. *Dis Chest.* 1965; 48:357.

Albert BS, Mellits ED, Rowe RD. Spontaneous closure of small ventricular septal defects. Probability rates in the first five years of life. *Am J Dis Child.* 1973; 125:194.

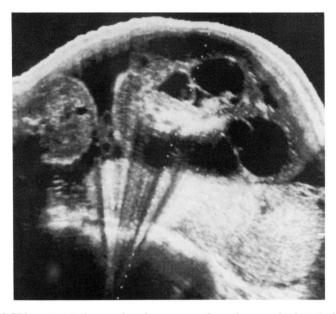

Figure 9-28 This contact static scan of a twin pregnancy shows the normal twin to the left at the midabdomen and a large mass of tissue and cystic spaces to the right, representing an acardiac twin. The large anechoic spaces were the typical subcutaneous lymphatic cysts associated with this condition.

Allan LD, Crawford DC, Anderson RH, Tynan MJ. Echocardiographic and anatomical correlation in fetal congenital heart disease. *Br Heart J.* 1984; 52:542–548.

Allan LD, Crawford DC, Anderson RH, Tynan M. Spectrum of congenital heart disease detected echocardiographically in prenatal life. *Br Heart J.* 1985; 54:523–527.

Allan LD, Tynan M, Anderson RH. Normal fetal cardiac anatomy—A basis for the echocardiographic detection of abnormalities. *Prenatal Diagno.* 1981; 1:131–139.

Anderson RH, Becker AE, Wilcox BR, et al. Surgical anatomy of double outlet right ventricle: A reappraisal. *Am J Cardiol.* 1983; 52:555.

Bender HW, Hammon JW, Hubbard SG, et al. Repair of atrioventricular canal malformation in the first year of life. *J Thorac Cardiovasc Surg.* 1982; 84:515.

Campbell M. Natural history of atrial septal defect. *Br Heart J.* 1970; 32:830.

Chin AJ, Kearne JF, Norwood WI, et al. Repair of complete common atrioventricular canal in infancy. *J Thorac Cardiovasc Surg.* 1982; 84:437.

Copel JA, Pilu G, Green J, Hobbins JC, Kleinman CS. Fetal echocardiographic screening for congenital heart disease: The importance of the four chamber view. *Am J Obstet Gynecol.* 1987; 157:648–655.

Copel JA, Pilu G, Kleinman CS. Congenital heart disease and extracardiac anomalies: Association and indications for fetal echocardiography. *Am J Obstet Gynecol.* 1986; 154:1121–1132.

Danielson GK, Maloney JD, Devloo RA. Surgical repair of Ebstein's anomaly. *Mayo Clin Proc.* 1979; 54:185.

Devore GR. The prenatal diagnosis of congenital heart disease—A practical approach for the fetal sonographer. *J Clin Ultrasound.* 1985; 13:229–245.

Devore GR, Kleinman CS, Donnerstein RL, Platt LD, Hobbins JC. Fetal echocardiography: I, normal anatomy as determined by real-time directed M-mode ultrasound. *Am J Obstet Gynecol.* 1982; 144:249–260.

Devore GR, Donnerstein RL, Kleinman CS, Platt LD, Hobbins JC. Fetal echocardiography: II, the diagnosis and significance of a pericardial effusion in the fetus using real-time directed M-mode ultrasound. *Am J Obstet Gynecol.* 1982; 144:693–701.

Devore GR, Hakim S, Kleinman CS, Hobbins JC. The in utero diagnosis of an interventricular septal cardiac rhabdomyoma by means of real-time directed M-mode echocardiography. *Am J Obstet Gynecol.* 1982; 143:967–969.

Devore GR, Horenstein J, Platt LD. Fetal echocardiography: VI, assessment of cardiothoracic disproportion—A new technique for the diagnosis of thoracic hypoplasia. *Am J Obstet Gynecol.* 1986; 155:1066–1071.

Devore GR, Platt LD. The random measurement of the transverse diameter of the fetal heart: A potential source of error. *J Ultrasound Med.* 1985; 4:335–341.

Devore GR, Platt LD. Use of femur length as a means of assessing M-mode ventricular dimensions during second and third trimesters of pregnancy in normal fetus. *J Clin Ultrasound.* 1985; 13:619.

Devore GR, Siassi B, Platt LD. The use of the femur length as a means of assessing M-mode ventricular dimensions during the second and third trimesters of pregnancy in the normal fetus. *J Clin Ultrasound.* 1985; 13:619–625.

Ebert PA, Turley K, Stanger P, et al. Surgical treatment of truncus arteriosus in the first 6 months of life. *Ann Surg.* 1984; 200:451.

Gertgesell HP Jr, ed. Symposium on fetal echocardiography. *J Clin Ultrasound.* 1985; 13:227–273.

Jatene AD, Fontes VG, Paulista PP, et al. Anatomic correction of transposition of the great vessels. *J Thorac Cardiovasc Surg.* 1976; 72:364.

Jeanty P, Romero R, Cantraine F, Cousaert E, Hobbins JC. Fetal cardiac dimensions: A potential tool for the diagnosis of congenital heart defects. *J Ultrasound Med.* 1984; 3:359–364.

Mustard WT. Successful two stage correction of transposition of the great vessels. *Surgery.* 1964; 55:469.

Natowicz M, Chatten J, Clancy R, et al. Genetic disorders and major extracardiac anomalies associated with the hypoplastic left heart syndrome. *Pediatrics.* 1988; 82:698–706.

Rashkind WF, Miller WW. Creation of an atrial septal defect without thoracotomy: A palliative approach to complete transposition of the great arteries. *JAMA.* 1966; 196:991.

Rastelli GC, Ongley PA, Kirklin JW, et al. Surgical repair of the complete form of persistent common atrioventricular canal. *J Thorac Cardiovasc Surg.* 1968; 55:299.

Rein JG, Freed MD, Norwood WI, et al. Early and late results of closure of ventricular septal defects in infancy. *Ann Thorac Surg.* 1977; 24:19.

Young BK, Katz M, Klein SA. Intrapartum fetal cardiac arrhythmias. *Obstet Gynecol.* 1979; 54:427–432.

Chapter 10

Noncardiac Thoracic Malformations

The sonographic diagnosis of noncardiac anomalies of the fetal chest includes not only the direct visual assessment of chest anatomy but also often the parallel assessment of possible consequential abnormalities of the pregnancy that result from the primary malformation. These include an excess or deficiency of amniotic fluid volume, an abnormality of the relative size of heart or chest to abdomen or long bones, and short limbs that are often associated with thoracodystrophy.

The fetal chest may be examined both longitudinally and transversely. The anatomy and specific imaging techniques for the heart are discussed elsewhere, but it is of some interest to review that a scanplane including the fetal cardiac long axis and providing a clear four-chamber view is slightly oblique to the fetal trunk and chest (see Figures 9-1 and 9-2). Transverse views of the fetal chest show spine, ribs, heart, lungs, and great vessels. The perimeter is slightly oval, with the anteroposterior (A-P) diameter usually the shortest. The lungs are homogeneous in echodensity, similarly to very early placenta. No echolucent or anechoic areas other than cardiac chambers or great vessels belong in the chest. The heart appears slightly to the left of the midline with its long axis directed about 45° inclination to the A-P midline. The A-P midline normally passes through the left atrium, the base of the interventricular septum, and the right ventricle, as mentioned in Chapter 9. Significant displacement of the heart to the right or left suggests the presence of an anomaly such as asymmetrical pleural effusion or right or left diaphragmatic hernia. Significant dislocation of the heart is seen in the case of ectopia cordis (one component of Cantrell's pentalogy).

The normal fetal thoracic circumference (TC) as a function of gestational age (GA) is described by the relationship

$$TC = -0.44 + 0.79 \, (GA)$$

The normal thoracic circumference as a function of abdominal circumference (AC) is described by the relationship

$$TC = 0.37 + 0.93 \, (AC)$$

Using these formulas, tables may be constructed against which individual fetal dimensions might be compared.

NONCARDIAC CHEST MALFORMATIONS

Congenital pleural effusions may also be known as congenital chylothorax or congenital hydrothorax. Fetal pleural effusions may occur as part of a hydropic syndrome or begin as an isolated abnormality. The apparent primary anomaly in isolated fetal hydrothorax is a thoracic duct leak allowing lymph to leak into the pleural space. It is increasingly apparent that once the expansion of the pleural spaces begins, the increase in intrathoracic pressure often causes secondary ascites or even skin edema. This sequence suggests that if discovered late in its evolution, what began as an isolated hydrothorax will be indistinguishable from generalized fetal hydrops.

Congenital pleural effusions appear sonographically as anechoic areas within the chest at the periphery of the lungs (Figure 10-1). The effusions may

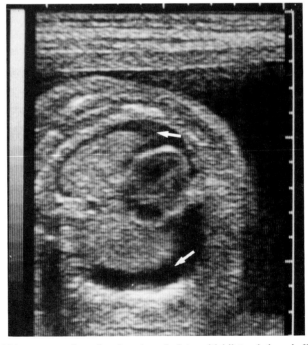

Figure 10-1 This transverse four-chamber view of a fetus with bilateral pleural effusions shows the anechoic fluid (arrows) surrounding the lungs bilaterally.

be symmetrical or asymmetrical (Figure 10-2). If there is significant asymmetry, the mediastinal structures will be seen deviated away from the major accumulation of fluid. A pleural effusion may be discriminated from an intrathoracic cyst by its more diffuse distribution around the lungs rather than by containment within a discrete wall that would result in displacement of adjacent structures.

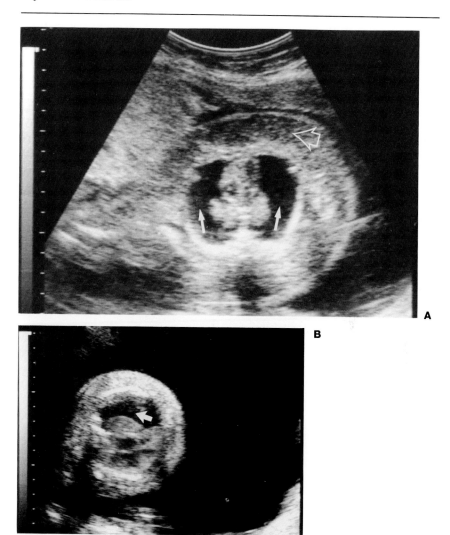

Figure 10-2 A, Severe symmetrical fetal hydrothorax (arrows) is illustrated here. Severe fetal skin edema is also apparent (open arrow). **B,** This sonogram shows a severe left-sided pleural effusion (arrow) in a fetus of 20 weeks' gestational age. After fetal thoracentesis, the effusion did not reaccumulate, but the infant later underwent corrective surgery for a coarctation of the aorta.

Polyhydramnios is a common associated finding of congenital hydrothorax. A decrease in effective fetal ingestion of fluid apparently occurs as a result of the increase in intrathoracic pressure. Fetal urine output is not apparently affected by the decrease in fetal swallowing, because the fetus continues to maintain water balance via the placental interface with its mother.

The clinical presentation of this syndrome is variable. Congenital chylothorax may escape diagnosis until neonatal respiratory embarrassment occurs in an otherwise normal infant following feeding. Thoracentesis results in the aspiration of chylous material that represents intestinal lymphatic drainage. Antenatal clinical presentation may occur late in the third trimester as a rapid growth of uterine size that on sonography is shown to be the result of polyhydramnios. Alternatively, the diagnosis may be made incidentally at the time of sonography for other reasons. The anechoic areas outlining the lungs are most often mild or moderate, and symmetrical in the case of the late gestation. Although there is no clear advantage in this case to antenatal aspiration of the fluid, prompt neonatal aspiration of the pleural fluid may be lifesaving. Delivery should be referred to a center prepared for the special

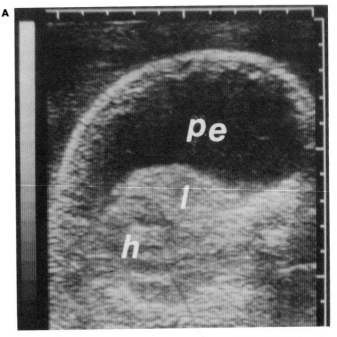

Figure 10-3 A, This severe right-sided pleural effusion (Pe) was associated with polyhydramnios and preterm labor at 30 weeks' gestation. The lung (l) and the heart (h) are also seen. Because of the preterm labor, consideration was given to fetal thoracentesis. **B,** At the time of fetal thoracentesis, the needle (arrow) was seen passing into the effusion (e).

care of such an infant. Antenatal or prompt neonatal aspiration of the thoracic fluid does not guarantee that the infant will not require respiratory support for a period after birth. The pleural fluid aspirated either antenatally or neonatally prior to feeding is not chylous but serous, reflecting the character of intestinal lymph in the absence of fatty digestion.

The diagnosis of congenital hydrothorax may occasionally be made early in gestation, usually at the time of sonography for other purposes. Such observations may be isolated or associated with other malformations such as coarctation of the aorta. Occasionally, antenatal aspiration may be helpful in evaluating the clinical significance of the abnormality (Figure 10-3). Failure of the fluid to reaccumulate after aspiration has been reported, with relatively uncomplicated pregnancy afterward, but unseen associated cardiovascular defects are common and should be diligently searched for. Clearly, such an observation early in gestation should lead to a careful sonographic examination to exclude associated anomalies and consideration of fetal blood sampling or amniocentesis to establish fetal karyotype. Successful fetal karyotypes have also been derived from cell cultures of aspirated fetal pleural fluid.

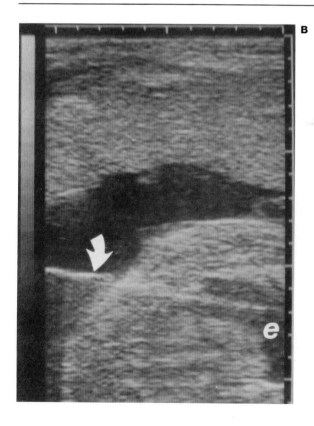

Congenital hydrothorax may also come to diagnosis during the critical gestational period between 26 and 32 weeks. Frequently the pregnancy comes to sonography because of polyhydramnios and rapid fundal growth, or because of the premature labor that results from the polyhydramnios. The effusions may be symmetrical or asymmetrical, and there may or may not be other features of hydrops. The observation that the pleural effusions are of much greater severity than either the skin edema or the ascites suggests the primary nature of the hydrothorax.

Often, the polyhydramnios is severe and the premature labor advanced. Therapeutic options are limited to tocolysis, therapeutic amniocentesis, antenatal thoracentesis, or possibly placement of a continuous diversion catheter. There is interest in antenatal intervention because of the very poor prognosis for a premature infant under 32 weeks' gestation with severe pleural effusions and hydrops fetalis. Tocolysis alone is not a viable option in the case of a significantly overdistended uterus, without efforts to reduce the overdistention. However, therapeutic amniocentesis is not a long-term treatment option either. The risks of inducing infection, rupture of membranes, or placental abruption are significant. Therefore, considerable interest has arisen in either fetal thoracentesis or placement of indwelling catheters draining the effusions to the amniotic cavity.

Experience to date suggests benefit from antenatal drainage of the effusions even if only for a few days or weeks before delivery. The most successful interventions reported have involved the placement or attempted placement of indwelling catheters (Figure 10-4), combined with transient tocolysis, and possibly therapeutic amniocentesis on a limited basis.

The technique most often uses a thin-walled cannula to gain entry into the fetal pleural cavity, followed by the advancement of a small catheter into the space. The effusion then drains into the amniotic cavity. Continuous decompression, decreased polyhydramnios, and fetal survival have all been reported to result from such intervention. It is significant that a reduction of the amniotic fluid volume has been observed following the drainage of such effusions, indicating the dependent relationship of the amniotic fluid excess on the thoracic pressure created by the effusions. Fetal death and failure of catheters have also been reported, however, and therefore preinterventional counseling should include the investigational nature of the treatment and the potential for complications.

DIAPHRAGMATIC HERNIA

Diaphragmatic hernia represents a primary failure of fusion of the leaflets of the diaphragm by the 8th week of embryonic development. Variable displacement of normally abdominal viscera into the chest cavity results.

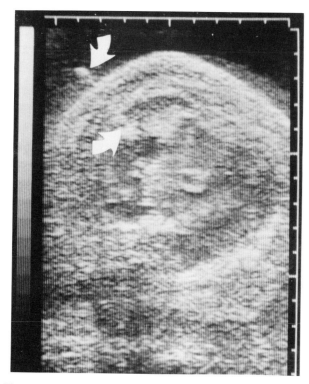

Figure 10-4 The arrows here indicate a Silastic catheter passing from the amniotic cavity into the fetal chest to drain a congenital pleural effusion.

Consequently, lung development may be impaired, and the abdomen presents a smaller, scaphoid appearance.

Ninety percent of congenital diaphragmatic hernias are left-sided, known as Bochdalek's hernias. With left-sided hernias, stomach and small bowel rise to occupy part of the left chest, displacing the mediastinal structures to the right. As a result, sonographically, the heart is seen to lie to the right of the midline, with the left chest filled with disorganized structures of both solid and cystic echotexture (Figures 10-5 and 10-6). Such a disturbance of normal relationships should be readily apparent from the standard four-chamber view. Longitudinal views may show the continuity of the soft tissue of the abdomen with the herniated organs in the chest. These fetuses often demonstrate breathing movements in utero that emphasize the defect by causing reciprocal movement of the herniated viscera on longitudinal scan.

The right-sided hernia may be very difficult to detect antenatally because the fetal liver may splint the defect until after birth, preventing any significant herniation and resultant deviation of normal chest anatomy. In such a case, lung development is more often normal and repair and survival more often

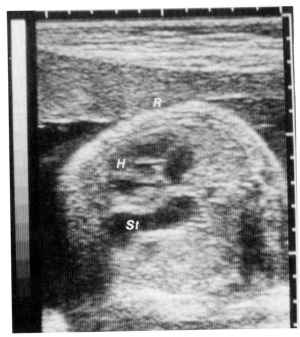

Figure 10-5 This sonogram of a fetus with a left-sided diaphragmatic hernia shows the heart (H) deviated to the right side (R) and the stomach (St) in the chest to the left of the heart.

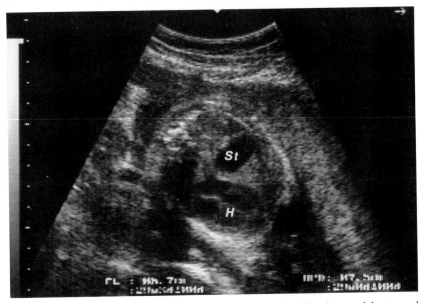

Figure 10-6 Again, here, the heart (H) is deviated to the right side of the chest, and the stomach (St) is seen in the left chest in the case of a left-sided diaphragmatic hernia.

possible. However, in the case of a large right-sided defect, the liver itself may be displaced into the right chest, causing major displacement of mediastinal structures to the left and, typically, severe compression and compromise of lung development (Figure 10-7). In such cases, pulmonary hypoplasia is common, and survival is rare.

Sonography in the case of a diaphragmatic hernia, therefore, shows the mediastinal structures deviated away from the side of the defect. In the case of the left-sided defect, the left chest is filled with mixed solid and cystic structures with a disorganized architecture. With a right-sided hernia, the right chest will be filled with part or all of the liver, with its typical appearance, and there will be severe displacement and compression of the heart and lungs to the left.

Diaphragmatic hernia occurs generally as an isolated defect with a frequency of only 1 to 2 per 1000 births and a low recurrence risk. Although rarely associated with chromosomal or other syndromic conditions, such a diagnosis should lead to a careful search for other malformations and consideration of amniocentesis or fetal blood sampling to establish fetal karyotype.

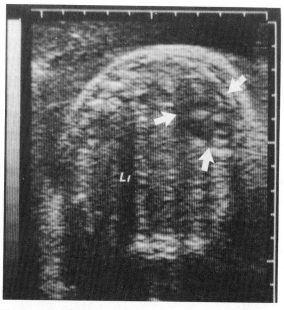

Figure 10-7   This transverse sonogram of a fetal chest shows the fetal heart (arrows) deviated to the left, with the right chest filled with echogenic liver (Li) due to a large right-sided diaphragmatic hernia. *Source*: Reprinted from *Practical Obstetrical Ultrasound* (p 133) by JW Seeds and RC Cefalo, Aspen Publishers Inc, © 1986.

Polyhydramnios may develop late in gestation, complicating obstetrical management or threatening premature labor. This is due probably to the displacement of the mediastinal structures to the right, with deformation and obstruction of the fetal esophagus. Obstetrical management of pregnancies complicated by fetal diaphragmatic hernia is not necessarily altered. There is no clear benefit from cesarean delivery, but delivery should occur in a center prepared for the special care these infants will require, including (usually) ventilator support and pediatric surgical intervention.

Traditionally, long-term functional survival of infants with congenital diaphragmatic hernia has been reported to be only 50%. The usual failure is respiratory, probably due to pulmonary hypoplasia secondary to the compressive effects of the abdominal viscera abnormally located in the chest. Some observers have drawn a vague relationship between antenatal diagnosis and a poorer prognosis, and between the need for a patch graft to close the defect and a poorer prognosis. These observations emphasize a relationship between a very large defect and a poorer prognosis, because it is likely that the larger defects will more often be detected antenatally and the larger defects will more often require patch grafting. Extracorporeal membrane oxygenation (ECMO) is a relatively new technique that may increase the salvage rate of those infants with large defects by allowing prolonged survival after surgical repair despite compromised lung function. Even ECMO is limited to a maximum of 2 weeks, however, and requires the sacrifice of major arterial service to the central nervous system, which is not without the possibility of major complications.

CYSTIC ADENOMATOID MALFORMATION OF THE LUNG

Cystic adenomatoid malformation (CAM) of lung is a primary dysplasia of pulmonary tissue, with a failure of terminal bronchioles to canalize. This results in the physical isolation of these spaces as fluid-filled, nonfunctional tissue. Two visually distinct types are described, based on the size of the cystic spaces, their lobar or uniform distribution in the lung, and the prognosis.

Type I, or lobar CAM of the lung, displays replacement of normal lung tissue by large cysts in a lobar distribution, visually analogous to multicystic renal dysplasia. Sonographically, multiple variable-sized anechoic cystic spaces are seen to replace an entire lobe of the lung (Figure 10-8). Type I CAM is often associated with ascites but is more resectable and survivable than the other major type.

Type II, or diffuse CAM of the lung, results in replacement of the entire lung with microscopic cysts, resulting in echodense, enlarged lungs, visually analogous to polycystic renal dysplasia (Figure 10-9). Type II CAM is also often associated with ascites, but due to its diffuse distribution, resection is not possible, and neonatal or fetal death is expected.

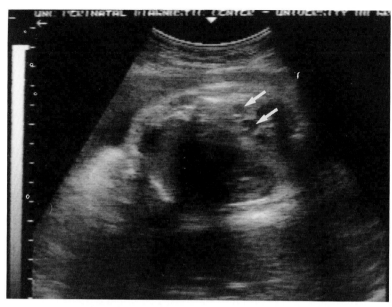

Figure 10-8 Cystic adenomatoid malformation of the lung, type I, results in macroscopic cysts of the lung (arrows), as seen here.

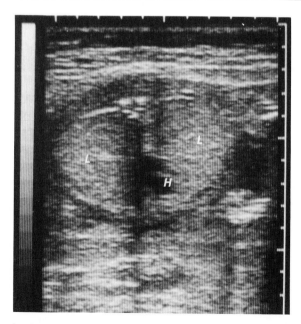

Figure 10-9 Cystic adenomatoid malformation of the lung, type II, results in large, echodense lungs that are clearly disproportionate to the heart and chest as seen here. The lung tissue (L) dwarfs the normal-size-for-dates heart (H).

Cystic adenomatoid malformation occurs as an isolated, sporadic dysplastic defect with a low rate of recurrence. The diagnosis and discrimination of subtype are based on sonographic findings of multiple large cystic spaces within the lung fields, or diffuse enlargement of the lungs relative to the heart, with a diffuse echodense but nonshadowing texture. In the case of type I CAM, antenatal counseling includes a relatively good prognosis for resection and survival, although the surgery required certainly involves significant risk. The antenatal diagnosis of CAM type II, with diffuse involvement of both lungs, represents essentially a lethal malformation, and obstetrical management appropriately centers on maternal welfare. The diagnosis of either type of abnormality will rarely be made in early gestation, and it is not possible to confidently exclude either malformation in early gestation. The polyhydramnios that may complicate either type of CAM may complicate obstetrical management by causing premature labor.

The delivery of an infant with antenatally diagnosed or suspected CAM should occur in a center prepared for the special care and diagnostic and therapeutic evaluation such an infant requires, including ventilator support and pediatric surgery. There is no general basis for recommending cesarean delivery for such a child, though individual cases might benefit depending on chest size or fetal presentation at the time of labor or delivery. Fetal amniotic fluid pulmonary maturity studies should be reliable in the case of type I CAM, since neonatal survival in any case will depend on the normal lung tissue present. In the case of type II CAM, pulmonary maturity studies are not useful, since little or no normal pulmonary tissue is present to contribute to amniotic fluid phospholipid content.

It may be difficult to discriminate type I CAM from various forms of pulmonary sequestration that may also present a sonographic image of multiple cystic structures contained within an isolated segment of lung field. Polyhydramnios and fetal ascites may also complicate such cases, also similar to CAM. Therefore, such a sonographic observation must always be interpreted as possibly diagnostic of either malformation.

PULMONARY SEQUESTRATION SYNDROME

Pulmonary sequestration represents the development of an isolated or sequestered lobe of lung tissue complete with arterial and venous blood supply, completely separate from the remaining pulmonary system. The sequestered tissue may contain cystic structures whose growth may interfere with development of adjacent structures (Figure 10-10). Large pleural effusions may accompany such malformations and cause polyhydramnios. Compression of the normal chest organs may result from extreme effusions, leading to pulmonary hypoplasia and a very poor prognosis.

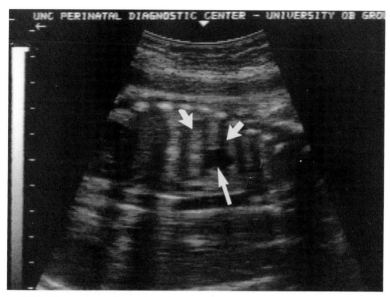

Figure 10-10 The sequestration or isolation of lung tissue with no bronchiolar connection and with an independent vascular supply results in a very variable appearance. Here, both cystic (large arrow) and echogenic soft tissue elements (small arrows) are noted.

Pulmonary sequestration occurs as a very rare sporadic malformation with no known risk of recurrence. Obstetrical management may be complicated by its secondary effects, which include pleural effusion, polyhydramnios, and preterm labor. If delivery can be delayed to a period of reasonable fetal viability, neonatal surgical resection with survival is possible. Early prenatal diagnosis of this condition is not reported, and confident exclusion of such an occurrence in early gestation, therefore, is not possible.

VENTRAL CHEST DEFECTS: CANTRELL'S PENTALOGY

Ventral defects of the chest wall are rare but may be associated with ventral abdominal wall defects. Sternal clefting seen with large upper leaflet ompha-locele, downward displacement of the heart, a pericardial defect, a diaphrag-matic defect, and usually an intracardiac defect are together known as Cantrell's pentalogy. Cantrell's pentalogy is considered a very rare field defect, with the primary anomaly involving the abdominal wall. A field defect represents the influence of a large malformation on the development of adjacent organs.

Cantrell's pentalogy occurs as a rare, sporadic defect with a very low risk of recurrence. Sonographic diagnosis may be made from the standard four-chamber view, as the cardiac outline will be lost inferiorly into the large omphalocele (Figure 10-11). There is variability to the expression of the defect, and complete ectopia cordis may represent an extreme example of this family of anomalies.

Diagnosis early in gestation is reported, and the evaluation should include fetal karyotype by the most expeditious method. Prognosis is not absolute, and survival with milder forms of the lesion has been reported. However, neonatal correction would have to include repair of the abdomen, chest, diaphragm, and whatever intracardiac defect is present (Figure 10-12). Survival would require sufficient pulmonary function to sustain life. There-fore, antenatal counseling cannot confidently predict survival but cannot exclude the possibility either.

Delivery by cesarean is recommended if management for best fetal out-come is desired, due mainly to the large omphalocele and the relatively exposed location of the heart within the sac.

NEONATAL CONSIDERATIONS

Congenital Hydrothorax

Congenital hydrothorax (chylothorax) is an uncommon neonatal condition thought to result from anomalous development of the thoracic duct and cysterni chyli. During early fetal life bilateral thoracic lymphatic ducts form, each attached to a corresponding jugular venous sac. Subsequently the upper third of the right duct and the lower two thirds of the left duct usually obliterate leading to an almost haphazard coupling of the lymphatic trunks and small lymphatic channels. Any disordered development may lead to a variety of lymphatic malformations.

The thoracic duct propels lymph forward toward the jugular venous junctions by a number of mechanisms, including smooth muscle contraction of the lymphatic vessel wall (1) via diaphragmatic excursion, which augments negative intrathoracic pressure, facilitating flow of lymphatic fluid from the cysterni chyli in the abdomen through the thoracic duct; (2) by continuous caudal-to-cranial influx of chyle; and (3) by valves that retard the backflow of chyle in the thoracic duct. Ingested nonsplit fats are absorbed by the intestinal lymphatics and transported in the chyle through the cysterni chyli and thoracic duct to the venous system. Split fats are directly absorbed from the gastrointestinal tract into the portal venous system and transported to the liver. This physiology assumes clinical importance in the nonoperative management of chylothorax. The fat content of chyle has been measured between 0.4 to 4 g per 100 mL of fluid. In addition, significant protein levels are observed in chyle and have been measured between 2.2 and 5.9 g per 100

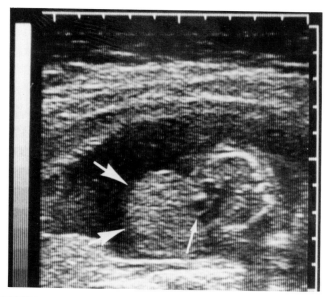

Figure 10-11 This transverse sonogram at 19 weeks' gestation shows a large omphalocele (large arrows) and displacement of the cardiac ventricles into the omphalocele, indicating a defect in the diaphragm and ventral chest wall consistent with Cantrell's pentalogy. *Source*: Adapted with permission from *Prenatal Diagnosis* (1984; 4[6]: 437–441), Copyright © 1984, John Wiley & Sons Ltd.

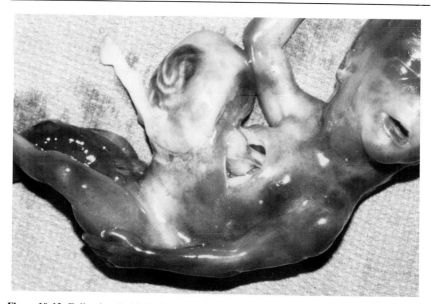

Figure 10-12 Following the birth of the infant scanned in Figure 10-11, the sonographic findings were confirmed. *Source*: Adapted with permission from *Prenatal Diagnosis* (1984; 4[6]: 437–441), Copyright © 1984, John Wiley & Sons Ltd.

mL. Infants with thoracic duct fistulas become rapidly and severely malnourished from unabated loss of fats and proteins. The lymphatic fluid also carries large numbers of lymphocytes. Prolonged loss of lymphocyte-rich lymphatic fluid may be associated with decreased immune competence.

Neonatal Clinical Presentation

When lymphatic fluid accumulates in the pleural space, progressive pulmonary compromise and respiratory distress result. Postnatally, dyspnea, tachypnea, and cyanosis are the most common symptoms. Later inanition occurs from accumulated chyle loss. Unilateral chylothorax may present with mediastinal shift, tachypnea, the use of accessory muscles, and diminished breath sounds and dullness to percussion on the affected side. Chest radiographs confirm massive effusion, pulmonary compression, and mediastinal shift (Figure 10-13). Thoracentesis results in rapid initial improvement, and examination of the pleural fluid may help establish the diagnosis. Infants who are taking milk feedings may have turbid or milky chylous fluid because of the

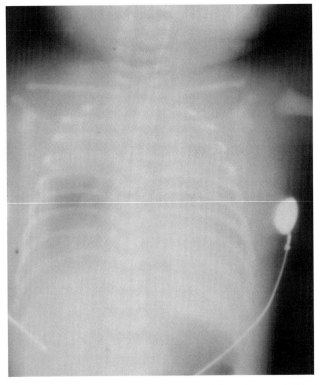

Figure 10-13 This chest radiograph demonstrates massive bilateral congenital hydrothorax in a neonate with respiratory distress.

ingested fat. However, infants who are not being fed enterally or who have had feedings low in fats may have clear chyle because of the lack of ingested fat in the lymphatic fluid.

Neonatal Treatment

Intermittent thoracentesis or thoracostomy tube drainage is usually required for significantly affected infants. The administration of total parenteral nutrition combined with withholding enteral feedings has had a tremendous positive impact on the survival and management of these patients by providing adequate nutrition and minimizing thoracic duct flow until the fistula is healed. Alternatively, enteral feedings low in split fats but high in medium-chain triglycerides have been an effective alternative to total parenteral nutrition for some patients. Selective surgical intervention may be required for infants who have persistent chylothorax despite aggressive nonoperative management. Thoracotomy with ligation of the chylous leak or thoracic duct ligation combined with parietal pleurectomy may be lifesaving for some patients. A relatively new technique of creating a pleuroperitoneal shunt using a one-way valve shunt system has recently been applied to selected patients (Figure 10-14). This technique has been successfully applied in those neonates with either acquired or congenital chylothorax, as long as the infants did not have chylous ascites. Following shunt placement, the peritoneal surface absorbs the lymphatic fluid, thus diminishing the significant fluid, electrolyte, and nutrient losses associated with a chyle fistula. Within several weeks most of the infants have completely recovered, and the shunts have been safely removed. This technique seems to be particularly useful for infants who may not otherwise tolerate thoracotomy.

Most infants with postnatal chylothorax will survive with careful attention to nutritional support, appropriate chest evacuation, and selective surgical intervention.

Congenital Diaphragmatic Hernia

About the 8th week the pleuroperitoneal canal becomes obliterated, separating the thoracic and abdominal cavities. The left pleuroperitoneal canal closes slightly later than the right side, thus explaining the increased number of left diaphragmatic hernias compared with right. When the pleuroperitoneal canal does not close, a posterolateral defect in the diaphragm remains. Failure or delay of closure of the pleuroperitoneal canal leads to herniation of the gut and solid viscera into the pleural cavity. The lung bud fails to mature on the side of herniation, but it may be also possible in some fetuses that the primary abnormality is in the developing lungs, which fail to induce closure of the diaphragm.

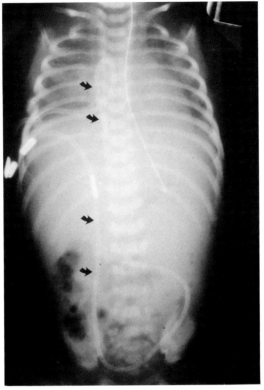

Figure 10-14   A pleuroperitoneal shunt (black arrows) was placed in the infant shown in Figure 10-13. Following surgery, the lung fields rapidly cleared, and the child recovered uneventfully.

The neonate whose chest is prenatally filled with bowel usually has hypoplastic lungs and will present with immediate respiratory distress within the first 24 hours postnatally. As air fills the gastrointestinal tract, further displacement compression of the mediastinum and compression of the contralateral lung will increase respiratory distress. On examination severe dyspnea, tachypnea, retractions, and cyanosis are common. A scaphoid abdomen is frequently observed, along with asymmetry of the chest wall contour and movement. Breath sounds may be diminished or absent on the involved side, and occasionally bowel sounds can be heard through the chest wall. Chest radiographs reveal gas-filled loops of the bowel in the chest on the affected side, combined with a paucity of abdominal gas (Figure 10-15). In addition, there is a significant shift of the trachea and mediastinum to the contralateral hemithorax. Right-sided diaphragmatic defects may be more difficult to diagnose because of more subtle findings on chest radiographs of elevation of the right lobe of the liver into the right hemithorax.

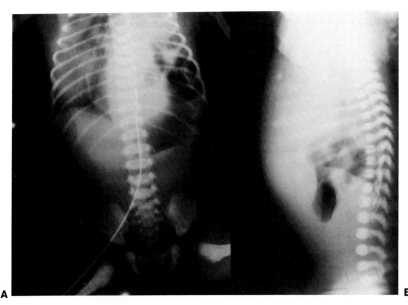

A   **B**

Figure 10-15 A, On the left is an anteroposterior view demonstrating intestine in the left hemithorax, causing a mediastinal shift to the right. The left hemidiaphragm cannot be seen. **B,** The lateral film on the right shows the intestines extending from the abdomen into the chest. The infant has a profoundly scaphoid abdomen.

Associated Anomalies

Most of these patients have significant hypoplasia of the lung, which accounts for the significant morbidity and mortality of this condition. Virtually all of these patients have malrotation of the intestine. In addition, a variety of other lethal and nonlethal anomalies have been recognized in over 20% of these patients, including spinal dysraphism, esophageal atresia, omphalocele, and genitourinary and cardiovascular anomalies. Diaphragmatic hernia has also been associated with trisomies 13 and 18.

Preoperative Treatment

Establishment of an airway and adequate ventilation are of the highest priority in these neonates. If respiratory distress is mild, 100% oxygen by face mask should be started. Bag and mask ventilation should be avoided because distention of the stomach and intestines in the intrathoracic position further compresses the lung. The stomach should be decompressed with an orogastric tube. If respiratory distress is severe, the infant should be intubated and maintained on 100% oxygen. Paralysis with pancuronium may improve ventilation and oxygenation. Using low but effective ventilatory pressures and a rapid respiratory rate (in the range of 50 to 100 breaths per minute) may be necessary. Overly aggressive inflation pressures in the face of hypoplastic and compressed lungs may lead to severe barotrauma and pneumothorax, with diminished patient survival. Sudden cardiovascular collapse during the course of assisted ventilation can occur and may be indicative of a pneumothorax on the contralateral side. A contralateral chest tube should be placed in these patients. Umbilical artery catheter cannulation provides an excellent means of vascular access for infusion of fluids and arterial blood gas monitoring.

Definitive Therapy

Operative intervention with reduction of the abdominal contents back into the abdomen and closure of the diaphragmatic defect is usually performed through a transabdominal approach (Figure 10-16). For right-sided diaphragmatic hernias the transthoracic and transabdominal approaches appear to be equally efficacious. In some patients the diaphragmatic defect is so large that a Gortex patch graft may be necessary to repair this defect. In those patients in whom a Gortex graft is required for diaphragmatic repair, prognosis is much worse. Furthermore, if the abdominal wall cannot be stretched to accommodate the viscera, only the skin is approximated, leaving a large ventral hernia. If the infant survives, the ventral hernia can easily be repaired later.

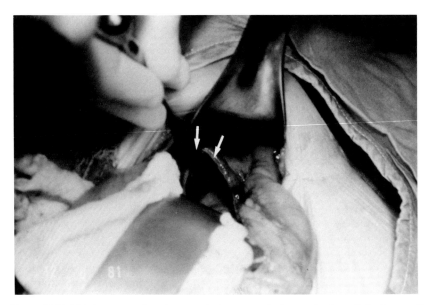

Figure 10-16 This intraoperative photograph shows a typical posterior lateral diaphragmatic defect. The arrows mark the diaphragmatic rim at the edge of the defect. The abdominal viscera have already been removed from the chest.

In some major centers, repair is delayed for very unstable infants with a large diaphragmatic hernia until they have been medically stabilized and have achieved reasonable oxygenation. The relative survival advantages of immediate postnatal repair or delayed repair are not known; however, it appears the latter method preselects for neonates who are capable of surviving.

Postoperative care after diaphragmatic hernia repair consists of appropriate intravenous fluids and careful ventilatory management. Ideally these infants are hyperventilated to achieve a Pco_2 value below 30 mm Hg. Also, inspired oxygen tension is adjusted to keep postductal arterial Po_2 above 100 mm Hg. Pulmonary barotrauma is avoided if at all possible. Continuous pulse oximetry, frequent arterial blood gas sampling, and transcutaneous oxygen measurements are essential for monitoring overall progress and adjusting ventilatory management. Weaning from the ventilator is a slow, laborious process. Even minor changes in the ventilatory rate and oxygen may result in increasing pulmonary hypertension and a return to a persistent fetal circulation, with eventual consequences of increased right-to-left shunting, acidosis, and hypoxemia. Following satisfactory operative correction of the diaphragmatic hernia, a significant number of these patients appear quite stable. During this period the neonates achieve satisfactory ventilation at relatively low pressures and rates. Unfortunately, this "honeymoon" period, which may vary from a few hours to days, may be followed by rapid deterioration with increasing oxygen and ventilatory requirements, reflecting worsening pulmonary hypertension and shunting. Many of these infants succumb to respiratory failure despite the combined use of pulmonary vasodilators and inotropic agents to decrease pulmonary vascular resistance and support systemic blood pressure.

Overall survival in neonates with diaphragmatic hernia remains about 50%, with prognosis being dependent on the severity of lung hypoplasia. One third of these neonates have adequate lung volume and survive, following a benign clinical course (Figure 10-17). One third have severely hypoplastic lungs and die regardless of how aggressive the management. Infants in the middle group initially improve during the "honeymoon" phase, but at least half eventually succumb. This group is the focus of most of the current efforts to improve survival and represents the best candidate group for ECMO. Recent studies indicate that 75% of the infants who initially have a "honeymoon" phase and have subsequent severe deterioration will benefit and survive with ECMO therapy.

For a number of years there has been a growing interest in the concept of prenatal intervention in the fetus with diaphragmatic hernia. Haller and colleagues at Johns Hopkins developed a model mimicking the diaphragmatic hernia by implanting Silastic balloons in the thorax of fetal lambs. Harrison and his colleagues at the University of California, San Francisco, demonstrated that the fetal lambs with simulated diaphragmatic hernias

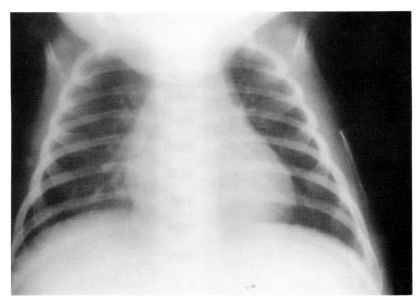

Figure 10-17   Two months after successful repair of a left-sided diaphragmatic hernia, this normal chest radiograph was taken.

would not survive if they were allowed to come to term. The majority of these animals died from respiratory failure and had hypoplastic lungs. However, if antenatal correction of the defect was undertaken in these experimental animals, many animals survived postnatally with normal pulmonary development. Harrison has extended these observations to a small, selected group of human patients and as of June 1989 had one survivor out of six human fetuses who had antenatal correction of a diaphragmatic hernia. The use of this highly controversial and experimental method of management has been too limited as yet for any conclusions except that antenatal correction is now feasible. Furthermore, the efficacy of prenatal correction of diaphragmatic hernia in a human is yet to be established. Significant issues such as controlling premature labor in humans, the risk to both mother and fetus, and the selection of patients for prenatal correction remain to be addressed.

Cystic Adenomatoid Malformation of the Lung

Cystic adenomatoid malformation is a disorder of lung development characterized by an overgrowth of the terminal bronchioles. The embryonic problem responsible for the development of CAM probably occurs prior to the 5th week of conception. An arrest of the joining of the conducting airways derived from the foregut endoderm and the respiratory component, which arises from the mesenchyme that aggregates around the tips of the growing bronchi, may be responsible for the pathological findings that are observed. The pathological classification proposed by Stocker includes three types of CAM. Type I has large cysts, greater than 1.2 cm in diameter. Type II has small cysts, less than 1.2 cm, and is occasionally associated with other anomalies. Type III is primarily solid in nature or may have microscopic cysts. This latter type is associated with a much poorer prognosis.

Any lobe can be involved with CAM, and multilobar involvement is not uncommon. Bilateral involvement is usually associated with a much poorer prognosis and diminished survival. However, one of the authors (R. G. A.) has participated in the management of one survivor who had right upper lobe, left lower lobe, and left upper lobe replacement with adenomatoid malformation. Following pneumonectomy as a neonate and a right upper lobectomy at age 3 years, the child has done well and is currently 7 years old.

Neonatal Presentation

The majority of these neonates present with varying degrees of respiratory distress. Infants with relatively large cysts may have air-fluid interfaces within these cysts that can have a strikingly similar appearance to bowel in the chest on radiographs. Cystic adenomatoid malformation should be considered in the differential diagnosis of infants suspected of congenital diaphragmatic hernia. The major clues that differentiate these two conditions are that the abdomen is not scaphoid in infants with CAM and that the diaphragm can be visualized on chest roentgenogram, along with bowel loops clearly being visualized in the abdomen (Figure 10-18). Initial management consists of appropriate respiratory and mechanical ventilatory support if necessary. Early postnatal lobectomy or even pneumonectomy of the affected tissue is required for most of these patients (Figure 10-19). Prognosis clearly depends on the extent of lung involvement and the degree of pulmonary hypoplasia in the unaffected lung. Occasionally these lesions are diagnosed in older infants or children who have repeated pulmonary infections. Long-term follow-up of these infants following pulmonary resection has revealed satisfactory objective and subjective pulmonary function.

Pulmonary Sequestration Syndrome

The tracheobronchial tree is derived from an outpouching of the embryonic foregut. Pulmonary sequestration arises when there is separation of the segment of the lung or a separate outpouching from the foregut anlage. The timing of the separation is important in that if the sequestered lung tissue arises before pleura formation, the sequestration will be intralobar and surrounded by normal lung tissue. When the sequestration arises after pleural development, it will be invested by its own pleura and will be extralobar and

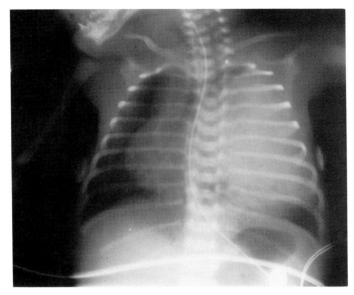

Figure 10-18 A chest radiograph of a symptomatic neonate with a large cystic adenomatoid malformation of the left lower lobe. The bowel is clearly in the abdomen, and a left hemidiaphragm can be seen on this film.

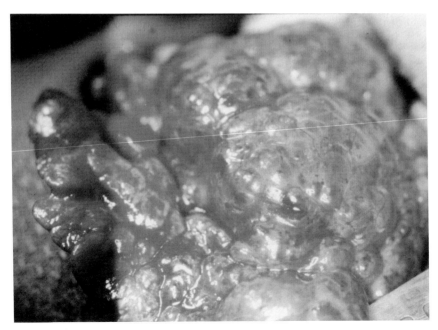

Figure 10-19 At thoracotomy, the left lower lobe was removed. Large fluid- and air- filled cysts replaced normal pulmonary parenchyma.

separate from the remaining pulmonary parenchyma. Although this latter type is similar to an accessory lobe, it does not communicate with a normal airway and has its own systemic blood supply. Pulmonary sequestration is therefore one of several bronchopulmonary foregut malformations, including esophageal duplication, enteric cysts, bronchogenic cysts, and tracheoesophageal fistulas. The unifying pathoembryology here is that this group of anomalies originates from the embryonic foregut.

A male-to-female incidence ratio of 3:1 has been reported for extralobar sequestration. Extralobar sequestration is identified more commonly in the neonate; it is extremely rare for this lesion to involve an entire lung or have bilateral involvement. The location of extralobar sequestration is between the lower lobe and the diaphragm in nearly 75% of the cases. The degree of pulmonary hypoplasia of the uninvolved pulmonary tissue varies with the size of the sequestration. Intralobar sequestration usually affects the lower lobes (approximately 95% of the cases), and the arterial supply is systemic, often arising from the subdiaphragmatic aorta. However, venous effluent in this type of lesion drains into the pulmonary veins for most of the patients.

Associated Anomalies

Extrapulmonary anomalies have been reported to occur in approximately 10% of the children with intralobar sequestration; these include diaphragmatic hernia, congenital heart disease, and renal, skeletal, and craniospinal anomalies. Extralobar sequestration is associated with a much higher frequency of anomalies (reported to be nearly 50%), the most common of which is congenital diaphragmatic hernia. Congenital heart disease and vertebral and chest wall anomalies are also associated with extralobar sequestration.

Neonatal Presentation

The spectrum of symptoms in these neonates is variable. Some children remain asymptomatic until they develop recurrent pulmonary infection or bleeding, which eventually leads to their diagnosis. Others have severe respiratory distress or develop significant congestive heart failure from severe right-to-left shunting postnatally. Pulmonary sequestration has also been associated with nonimmune hydrops. The postnatal diagnosis of extralobar sequestration is corroborated by identifying an intrathoracic mass lesion compressing normal pulmonary parenchyma and associated with a mediastinal shift on chest radiographs (Figure 10-20). Intralobar sequestration is much more difficult to diagnose in the neonate.

Treatment

Resection of the affected pulmonary tissue is the optimal method of therapy (Figure 10-21). Postsurgical prognosis is excellent in those patients without severe pulmonary hypoplasia.

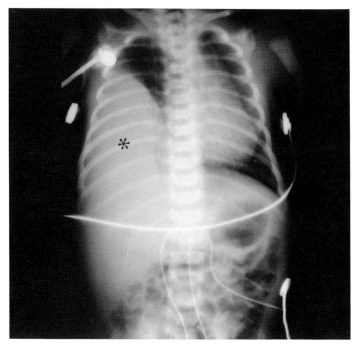

Figure 10-20 A chest radiograph of a neonate with a large extralobar pulmonary sequestration (asterisk), causing mediastinal shift to the left.

Cantrell's Pentalogy

As mentioned above, Cantrell's pentalogy is a complex thoracoabdominal malformation characterized by a distal sternal cleft, epigastric omphalocele, an anterior diaphragmatic defect, pericardial defect, and a cardiac malformation (Figure 10-22). The reported incidence is 1 in 250,000 live births, with no known sex predilection. The variety of cardiac malformations reported include ventricular septal defect (greater than 90%), tetralogy of Fallot (70%), left ventricular diverticulum (approximately 20%), and other lesions including atrial septal defects, tricuspid atresia, cor triloculare, and pulmonic valvular stenosis. The severity of the cardiac abnormality often determines whether the infant will survive or not. Infants born with large omphaloceles require surgical repair in the neonatal period as the best hope for survival. The ventral abdominal wall defect and diaphragmatic defect are repaired concomitantly in these patients. Occasionally the left ventricular diverticulum must be removed to facilitate closure of the diaphragmatic defect. However, the majority of the neonates will not have their intracardiac defects repaired until a much later date, depending on the severity of their lesion and their symptomatology. In those children with Cantrell's pentalogy who have

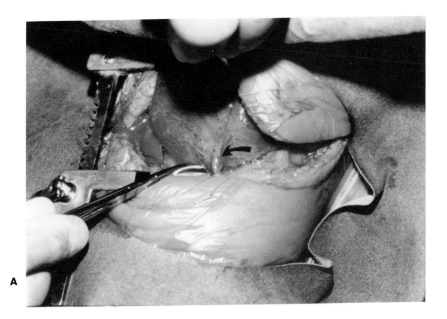

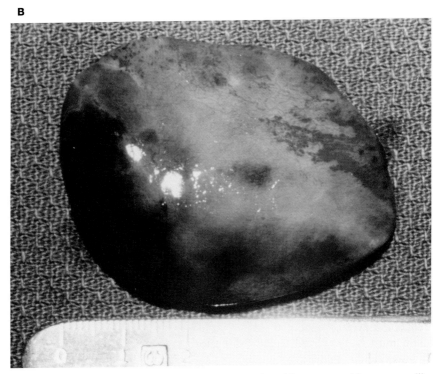

Figure 10-21 A, A systemic blood supply (black arrow) to this sequestered lung was readily identified at thoracotomy. **B,** Gross specimen of the excised extralobar sequestration.

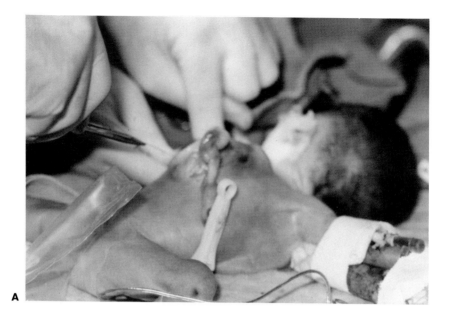

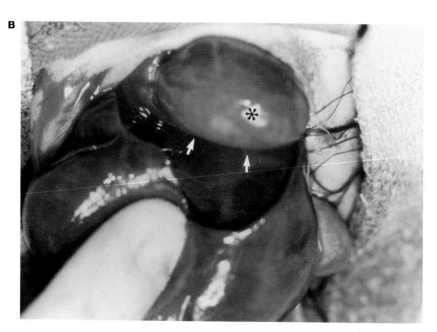

Figure 10-22 A, This premature 1000-g infant had Cantrell's pentalogy, including epigastric omphalocele, diaphragmatic hernia, pericardial defect, bifid sternum, and intracardiac defect. **B,** At surgery, the omphalocele membrane has been removed, the heart is seen protruding through a medial diaphragmatic defect (white arrows), and the surgeon's finger is displacing the liver caudally.

small ventral abdominal wall defects, a single-stage repair of the sternal, diaphragmatic, and cardiac defects has been reported in children 6 months to 11 years of age. Prosthetic materials such as Gortex or Marlex have been useful in repairing some of the larger diaphragmatic and ventral abdominal wall defects. Overall survival for this group of children is reported to be about 50%, and the major determinant of survival is the severity of the cardiac anomaly. Ectopia cordis is a related malformation that may present with a complete sternal defect combined with an exposed heart lying outside the chest wall. The majority of these infants succumb because of severe intracardiac anomalies, although survival has been rarely reported.

Other Mediastinal Masses

Rarely, prenatal diagnosis of other noncardiac intrathoracic lesions is made using maternal-fetal sonography. Although not complete, Table 10-1 lists a variety of anterior, middle, and posterior mediastinal masses that can be identified in neonates. Location in the mediastinum and the nature of these lesions (solid or cystic) provide the most substantial clues for accurately recognizing the specific lesion prenatally. For example, a solid posterior mediastinal mass is usually a neurogenic tumor; a multicystic structure in the anterior mediastinum is likely to be a cystic hygroma (a form of lymphangioma). Prognosis varies with each of these lesions, although survival with excellent quality of life following surgical removal is possible (Figure 10-23). Obstetrical management is rarely altered for these patients. Occasionally a large intrathoracic cyst may be aspirated if it is felt that it contributes to pulmonary hypoplasia.

Table 10-1 Differential Diagnosis of Mediastinal Masses in Neonates

1. Anterior mediastinal masses
   Teratoma
   Intrathoracic goiter
   Thymic lesions
   Lymphangioma
   Diaphragmatic hernia of Morgagni
   Pericardial cyst
   Bronchogenic cyst

2. Middle mediastinal masses
   Bronchogenic cyst
   Pericardial cyst

3. Posterior mediastinal masses
   Neurogenic tumor
   Neuroenteric cyst
   Esophageal duplication
   Anterior meningocele
   Pulmonary sequestration
   Diaphragmatic hernia

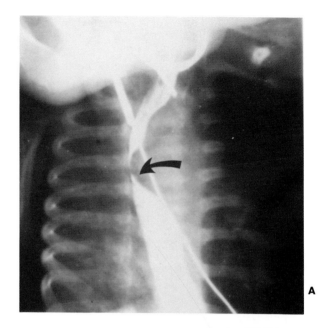

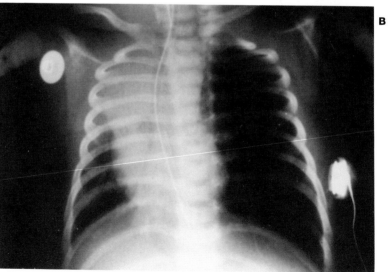

Figure 10-23 A, The radiograph here shows indentation of the midesophagus (arrow) by a mediastinal mass. **B**, This film shows severe air trapping in the left lung, mediastinal shift, and right upper lobe atelectasis. **C**, At surgery, a large bronchogenic cyst compressing the left main bronchus was successfully excised.

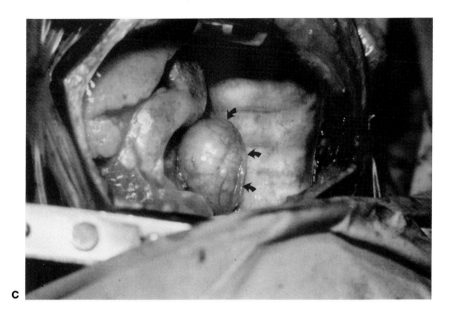

C

FURTHER READING

Adzick NS, Harrison MR, Glick PL, et al. Diaphragmatic hernia in the fetus: Prenatal diagnosis and outcome in 94 cases. *J Pediatr Surg.* 1985; 20:357–361.

Asher JB, Sabbagha RE, Tamura RK, et al. Fetal pulmonary cyst: Intrauterine diagnosis and management. *Am J Obstet* Gynecol. 1985; 151:97.

Azizkhan RG, Canfield J, Alford BA, et al. Pleuroperitoneal shunts in the management of neonatal chylothorax. *J Pediatr Surg.* 1983; 18:842–850.

Cantrell JR, Haller JA, Ravitch MM. A syndrome of congenital defects involving the abdominal wall, sternum, diaphragm, pericardium and heart. *Surg Gynecol Obstet.* 1958; 107:602–614.

Chitkara U, Rosenberg J, Chervenak FA, et al. Prenatal sonographic assessment of the fetal thorax: Normal values. *Am J Obstet Gynecol.* 1987; 156:1069–1074.

Haller JA, Golladay ES, Pickard LR, et al. Surgical management of lung bud anomalies: Lobar emphysema, bronchogenic cysts, cystic adenomatoid malformations, and intrapulmonary sequestration. *Ann Thorac Surg.* 1979; 28:33–43.

Harrison MR. The fetus with a diaphragmatic hernia. *Pediatr Surg Int.* 1988; 3:15–22.

Johnson A, Callan NA, Bhutani VK, et al. Ultrasonic ratio of fetal thoracic to abdominal circumference: An association with fetal pulmonary hypoplasia. *Am J Obstet Gynecol.* 1987; 157:764–769.

Kitagawa M, Hislop A, Boyden EA, Reid L. Lung hypoplasia in congenital diaphragmatic hernia. *Br J Surg.* 1971; 58:342–346.

Lange IR, Manning FA. Antenatal diagnosis of congenital pleural effusions. *Am J Obstet Gynecol.* 1981; 140:839.

Langham MR, Krummel TM, Bartlett RH, et al. Mortality with extracorporeal membrane oxygenation following repair of congenital diaphragmatic hernia in 93 infants. *J Pediatr Surg.* 1987; 12:1150–1154.

Nimrod C, Davies D, Iwanicki S, et al. Ultrasound prediction of pulmonary hypoplasia. *Obstet Gynecol.* 1986; 68:495.

Nishibayashi SW, Andrassy RJ, Woolley MM. Congenital cystic adenomatoid malformation: A 30-year experience. *J Pediatr Surg.* 1981; 16:704.

Randolph JG. Chylothorax. In: Welch KJ, Judson GR, Ravitch MM, O'Neal JA, Rowe MI, eds. *Pediatric Surgery.* 4th ed. Chicago: Yearbook Medical Publishers; 1986: 654–656.

Reece EA, Lockwood CJ, Rizzo N, et al. Intrinsic intrathoracic malformations of the fetus: Sonographic detection and clinical presentation. *Obstet Gynecol.* 1987; 70:627–632.

Sieber WK. Lung cysts, sequestration and bronchopulmonary dysplasia. In: Welch KJ, Judson GR, Ravitch MM, O'Neal JA, Rowe MI, eds. *Pediatric Surgery.* 4th ed. Chicago: Yearbook Medical Publishers; 1986: 645–654.

Skiptunas SM, Weiner S. Early prenatal diagnosis of asphyxiating thoracic dystrophy (Jeune's syndrome) *J Ultrasound Med.* 1987; 6:41.

Stocker JT, Madewell JE, Drake RM. Congenital cystic adenomatoid malformation, classification and morphology. *Spectrum Human Path.* 1977; 8:156.

Vain NE, Swanner OW, Cha CC. Neonatal chylothorax: A report and discussion of nine consecutive cases. *J Pediatr Surg.* 1980; 15:261–265.

Chapter 11

Fetal Intestinal Obstruction and Other Abdominal Masses

EMBRYOLOGY

The fetal intestinal tract may be arbitrarily divided for purposes of discussion into derivatives of the foregut, derivatives of the midgut, and derivatives of the hindgut. Derivatives of the foregut include the pharynx, the lower respiratory system, the esophagus, the stomach, the duodenum, the liver and pancreas, and the biliary system. Derivatives of the midgut include the small intestine (including most of the duodenum), the cecum, the ascending colon, and the majority of the transverse colon. The hindgut is seen as the precursor to the distal transverse colon, the descending colon, the sigmoid colon, the rectum, and part of the anal canal.

The major precursor to the fetal digestive system is known as the primitive gut, which is itself derived from the dorsal aspect of the yolk sac. As the early disklike embryo begins to form cranial, tail, and lateral ventral folds that curl into the yolk sac, the most dorsal aspect of the yolk sac is incorporated into the embryo and forms the primitive gut. This process of ventral folding to produce a more three-dimensional embryo with an internal cavity begins about 24 days postmenstrual and is well developed by 28 days postmenstrual. The primitive gut at this time remains connected to the remaining yolk sac through the yolk stalk.

The initially short esophagus separates from the laryngotracheal tube with the development of a tracheoesophageal septum and lengthens with the cranial growth of the embryo. Faulty development of the septum results in esophageal atresia and the commonly associated tracheoesophageal fistula. During the 5th and 6th weeks, the stomach dilates and rotates to the right, or clockwise, resulting in the development of the lesser sac from the attached celomic membrane.

The duodenum is derived from both foregut and midgut, with the junction being just distal to the opening of the bile duct. During the 5th and 6th weeks, the lumen of the duodenum is typically occluded, apparently due to proliferation of lining epithelium. Normally, by the end of the 8th week, recanalization has occurred, but failure to re-establish the lumen results in clinical duodenal

243

atresia. Typically, the obstruction is located just distal to the origin of the bile duct. The pancreas grows from both a ventral and a dorsal outgrowth from the proximal segment of the primitive duodenum. During rotation and growth, these two primordia fuse to form the normally singular pancreas. Failure to fuse or abnormal fusion can result in dual development or an annular (circumferential) pancreas.

Between the 6th and 11th weeks postmenstrual, the midgut undergoes 270° rotation in a counterclockwise direction as you face the embryo. This results in the caudal gut coming to overlie the duodenum. This process occurs at least in part within what will become the proximal umbilical cord. By the end of the 10th week, the process is completed, and the midgut has normally been retracted into the peritoneal cavity, with closure of the umbilical ring. Failure of the gut to retract in this manner results in omphalocele, with variable quantities of viscera remaining within the proximal umbilical cord, covered by a two-layer membrane consisting of peritoneum and amnion.

Obstruction of the midgut can result from malrotation with a volvulus or vascular accidents resulting in randomly placed atresias.

FETAL INTESTINAL TRACT

The fetal intestinal tract is not only preparing for birth and for its role in digestion and absorption after birth but begins functioning as early as 14 weeks' gestation in the ingestion and absorption of amniotic fluid, including dissolved and suspended matter in the fluid that is of nutritional value. It is estimated that approximately 17% of the effective nutrition of the fetal period is absorbed from ingested amniotic fluid. This is the basis for the observation of growth retardation associated with congenital obstruction of the upper gut.

Obstruction may occur at any level of the gut, as noted above, including the esophagus, the duodenum, the jejunum, the ileum, or the large intestine. Obstruction can result from failure of recanalization, as in the case of the duodenum, resulting in malfunction from the 8th week onward, or may result from acute events during a later fetal period, such as vascular failure, volvulus, or intussusception, causing an acute malfunction or obstruction.

Obstruction of the upper fetal intestinal tract can be complex, such as is seen in the common association of esophageal atresia with tracheoesophageal fistula, and require prompt and appropriate neonatal intervention to produce an optimal outcome. Furthermore, proximal intestinal obstruction can be associated with cytogenetic abnormalities, such as the estimated 30% frequency of Down syndrome associated with duodenal obstruction. Obstruction of the large intestine can be purely mechanical, such as that resulting from volvulus, or it can be associated with congenital disease, illustrated by the common (50%) association of meconium ileus with cystic fibrosis.

Clinical manifestations of fetal intestinal obstruction are rare in early gestation, and diagnosis of intestinal obstruction is unlikely before 24 weeks, even though it may be shown that effective function of the fetal intestinal tract begins much earlier. The most common clinical manifestation of fetal intestinal obstruction is polyhydramnios. Typically the polyhydramnios associated with esophageal obstruction is detected between 24 and 32 weeks. This observation of what appears to be late detection of the consequences of a primary malformation may be due to alternative routes of amniotic fluid equilibrium, such as transcutaneous reabsorption or decreased fetal urine production.

The normal fetus produces about 5 mL of urine per kg of weight per hour. This amounts to as much as 450 mL per day at term. If the fetus doesn't remove a comparable volume, then polyhydramnios can result. Therefore, the most common indication for ultrasound that results in the detection of fetal intestinal obstruction is a fundal measurement that is large for dates. At sonography, the observation of a fetus with dimensions appropriate for dates and a visual excess of amniotic fluid should then prompt a careful examination of the fetus for signs of intestinal obstruction.

NORMAL SONOGRAPHIC ANATOMY

Normally the fetal abdomen on transverse scan is circular in shape, tapering in size slowly from the diaphragm to the pelvis (Figure 11-1). In the upper abdomen, the liver occupies up to 60% of the area of the transverse scanplane, with perhaps the upper pole of the stomach appearing on the left side (Figures 11-2 and 11-3). Below the liver and stomach, the intestinal mass presents a relatively homogeneous, echodense appearance, without shadowing. At the periphery of the peritoneal cavity closest to the transducer, there is often a thin echolucent rim that may suggest ascites, but if this does not extend around to the dependent side of the abdomen, it is not ascites but rather a pseudoascites that is a normal observation resulting from echo dropout at those fetal tissue interfaces.

ESOPHAGEAL OBSTRUCTION

The classic association of polyhydramnios with absence of a visible stomach on repeated scan should lead to suspicion of esophageal obstruction, most often due to atresia (Figure 11-4). However, since up to 60% of cases of esophageal atresia are associated with tracheoesophageal fistulas that might allow some fluid to gain access to the stomach, the presence of a visible stomach may be misleading and does not perfectly exclude esophageal atresia.

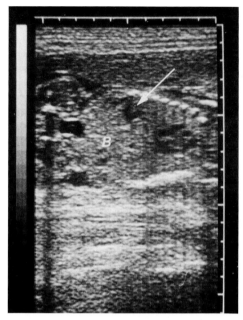

Figure 11-1 This frontal view, with a scanplane of about the midaxillary line, illustrates the echotexture of the normal fetal abdomen. The stomach (arrow) is in the upper left quadrant, and the bowel (B) presents a mixed, vague texture. *Source*: Adapted from *Practical Obstetrical Ultrasound* (p 40) by JW Seeds and RC Cefalo, Aspen Publishers Inc, © 1986.

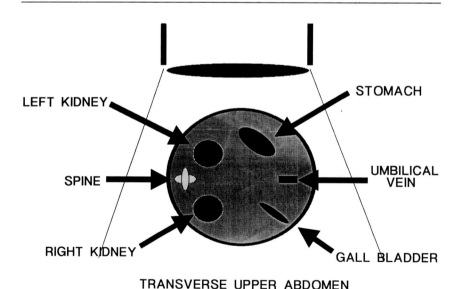

Figure 11-2 The essential elements of transverse fetal abdominal anatomy are shown in this drawing, though not all of them will necessarily be found in the same scanplane.

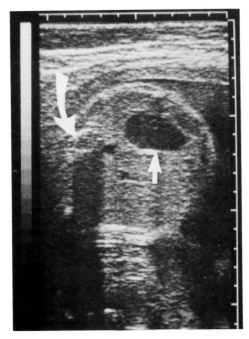

Figure 11-3 A transverse sonogram of the upper fetal abdomen shows the spine (curved arrow) to the left and the stomach (straight arrow) in the left upper abdomen.

Functional obstruction of the esophagus secondary to myotonic dystrophy or other congenital muscle dystrophy may also lead to polyhydramnios, but usually with a visible stomach. Therefore, although it might be expected that polyhydramnios based on esophageal obstruction or dysfunction would result in absence of stomach on a scan, it is not a uniform finding.

DUODENAL OBSTRUCTION

Polyhydramnios associated with the sonographic observation of two anechoic (cystic) masses of the upper fetal abdomen indicates the possibility of duodenal obstruction (Figure 11-5). The two masses represent the dilated stomach, narrowing to the pylorus of the stomach, then dilating again to the duodenum proximal to the site of obstruction. Although atresia is the most likely explanation, this picture might also result from intraluminal duodenal webs or an annular pancreas (Figures 11-6 and 11-7). It is essentially impossible to distinguish these diagnoses antenatally, and they must be included in the diagnosis. The distinction between atresia and intraluminal webs is largely academic, since both appear to result from defective recanalization

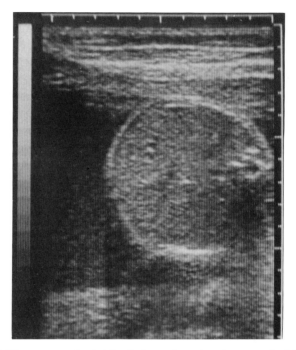

Figure 11-4 The transverse fetal abdominal scan shown here in a case of polyhydramnios at 32 weeks' gestation shows no stomach fluid. Although a diagnosis of esophageal obstruction should be suspected, it is not proven.

during the 8th week, and both show a strong (33%) association with aneuploidy in the form of trisomy 21.

Clinical management is not immediately altered by the diagnosis of duodenal atresia. A careful sonographic search for any associated malformations should be performed. Either amniocentesis or fetal blood sampling to establish fetal karyotype is indicated. The diagnosis of trisomy 21, in most clinical settings, however, does not allow alteration of clinical management either.

The polyhydramnios is common and often complicates care by leading to premature labor, but any consideration of tocolysis or therapeutic amniocentesis must take into account the chronic nature of the problem and the gestational age. Premature labor in the context of this diagnosis past 32 weeks may not be best treated by tocolysis. It is unlikely that either tocolysis or therapeutic amniocentesis will result in long-term benefit. Significant polyhydramnios secondary to duodenal atresia with premature labor before 25 weeks' gestation is unlikely to benefit from tocolysis. However, if short-term benefit is desired in order to achieve specific goals, such as glucocorticoid administration to the mother to accelerate fetal lung maturity, this must be weighed against the potential morbidity of any tocolytic protocol.

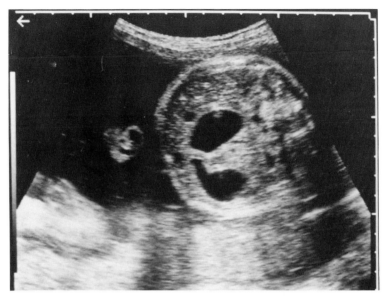

Figure 11-5 The two echo-free (black) masses in this transverse upper abdominal view of a fetus with polyhydramnios represent the dilated stomach, narrowing to the pylorus of the stomach, and the dilated duodenum proximal to duodenal atresia.

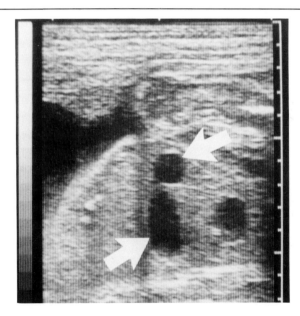

Figure 11-6 The paired cystic structures (arrows) seen on this oblique scan of the fetal abdomen in a case of polyhydramnios were the result of intraluminal duodenal webs. *Source*: Reprinted from *Practical Obstetrical Ultrasound* (p 139) by JW Seeds and RC Cefalo, Aspen Publishers Inc, © 1986.

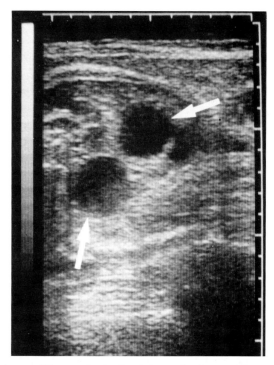

Figure 11-7 Another possible cause for duodenal obstruction is an annular pancreas, which was found to be the case in this infant with paired upper abdominal fluid-filled masses (arrows). *Source*: Reprinted from *Practical Obstetrical Ultrasound* (p 138) by JW Seeds and RC Cefalo, Aspen Publishers Inc, © 1986.

Duodenal obstruction should not alter the method of delivery. There is no theoretical or empirical benefit to the fetus from abdominal delivery. Referral for delivery at a center prepared for the delivery of such an infant and the subsequent surgical care may be beneficial and should be considered. Planned delivery as the result of an induction of labor may facilitate optimal care by allowing the greatest organization of the neonatal team.

ILEAL AND JEJUNAL OBSTRUCTION

Congenital obstruction of the small intestine may result from malrotation during the embryonic period, with resulting volvulus, or from vascular failure at any time, resulting in cell death and atresia if an early event or functional failure and necrosis if a late one.

Small bowel obstruction may also result in polyhydramnios, but this consequential event is more likely if the obstruction is more proximal in location. Distal ileal obstructions are less likely to result in polyhydramnios

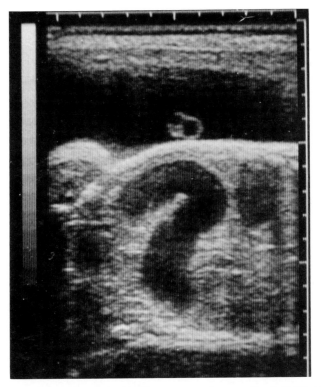

Figure 11-8 Polyhydramnios resulted in this sonogram of a serpentine fluid-filled loop of small bowel, in a case of jejunal atresia.

due to sufficient absorption by the functional bowel. The intermediate level of absorption characteristic of these obstructions also typically results in the late development of polyhydramnios when it is seen, and therefore the late diagnosis of the condition.

The sonographic appearance of jejunoileal obstructions is one of polyhydramnios with a dilated anechoic (fluid-filled) serpentine mass in the fetal abdomen (Figure 11-8). The stomach may or may not be seen to be dilated. The dilated bowel may achieve a diameter of up to 1 to 2 cm, but rupture is rare.

LARGE BOWEL OBSTRUCTION

Obstruction of the large bowel is most often the result of meconium ileus, which is associated with cystic fibrosis half the time. Vascular atresias and volvulus can also be seen. Clinical events are uncommon unless there is consequential dysfunction such as in the case of meconium ileus with rupture and meconium peritonitis with small bowel dysfunction. In such a case, polyhydramnios is a common observation.

The sonographic appearance of meconium ileus is that of a large-diameter colon containing the typically echogenic meconium, often with a small peritoneal effusion (Figure 11-9). In the case of rupture, a large area of mixed solid and cystic echotexture is seen, often with hyperperistaltic small bowel adjacent to it (Figures 11-10, and 11-11). Late in this process, the meconium induces a peritonitis, with inflammation and calcification (Figure 11-12).

Meconium ileus with rupture and peritonitis is typically a late-gestation complication, and delivery is indicated if the pregnancy is near term or fetal lung maturity is documented. Prompt exploration with repair can be lifesaving. Although meconium ileus is less often associated with aneuploidy, fetal blood sampling or amniocentesis may be offered to clarify this issue before delivery.

The method of delivery is not necessarily altered by this diagnosis; however, if delivery appears necessary due to the acute fetal condition but the

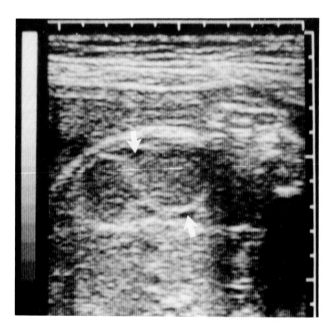

Figure 11-9 Meconium ileus resulted in perforation and mild chemical peritonitis in this fetus. The peritoneal fluid (arrows) was inflammatory.

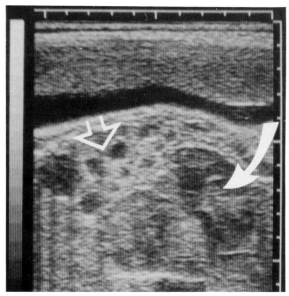

Figure 11-10 Bowel perforation often results in meconium extravasation and the formation of a meconium pseudocyst, as seen here. The small intestine (open arrow) was hyperperistaltic, but the area of the pseudocyst (curved arrow) showed no movement. This baby had cystic fibrosis.

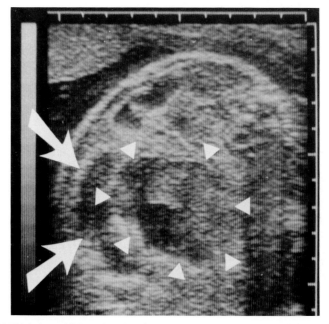

Figure 11-11 This infant with bowel perforation and a meconium pseudocyst (triangles) also had cystic fibrosis. Arrows point to areas of hyperperistalsis.

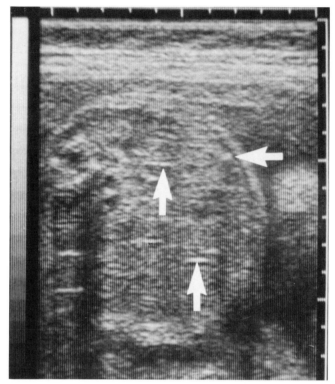

Figure 11-12 Chronic meconium peritonitis commonly results in calcification, as seen in this transverse sonogram of the fetal abdomen (arrows). *Source*: Reprinted from *Practical Obstetrical Ultrasound* (p 141) by JW Seeds and RC Cefalo, Aspen Publishers Inc, © 1986.

cervix is unfavorable, cesarean delivery may be indicated. Delivery at a referral center prepared for the special care such an infant requires is indicated.

NEONATAL CARE OF INTESTINAL OBSTRUCTION

Fetal intestinal obstruction is a broad category of life-threatening problems that require rapid and logical evaluation to sort out a variety of surgically correctable disorders. The diagnosis may or may not have been made or suspected antenatally, making it critical for the neonatal team to be alert to the possibility of such problems.

Classic symptoms of intestinal obstruction in neonates include vomiting, abdominal distention, and failure to pass meconium. These symptoms provide helpful information in determining the site and the likely cause of obstruction. For example, nonbilious emesis implies the patient has a preampullary obstruction, whereas bilious emesis occurs in infants with postampullary obstruction. The onset of emesis is generally more rapid in infants with proximal intestinal obstruction. Maternal polyhydramnios, as noted above, is often associated with complete proximal intestinal obstruction (esophageal atresia, duodenal or jejunal obstruction); partial obstructions or distal obstructions less often result in excess amniotic fluid.

Neonates with meconium ileus, meconium peritonitis, or anorectal atresia may present with significant abdominal distention at birth. Rapid distention developing soon after birth may be seen in neonates with tracheoesophageal fistula or intestinal perforation. Furthermore, delayed distention may occur in infants with distal intestinal obstruction. The gas pattern on the abdominal radiograph should be carefully observed. In general, the more distal the obstruction, the greater the number of dilated loops of intestine.

Esophageal Atresia

Esophageal atresia results from faulty separation of the trachea and esophagus, which normally occurs between the 24th and 31st days of gestation. Although a variety of specific anomalies can occur, the most common type (approximately 90%) is an esophageal atresia with a blind upper pouch and a tracheoesophageal fistula (TEF) to the distal esophagus. In 5% to 8% of the infants, there is an isolated esophageal atresia without TEF. The next most common defect is an isolated TEF (H-type) without esophageal atresia. Other defects, such as esophageal atresia with a proximal TEF or a combined proximal and distal TEF, are very rare, occurring in less than 1% of all cases.

Prenatal diagnosis of esophageal atresia is suspected in 10% of cases and only when polyhydramnios is seen in conjunction with a small or absent fetal stomach. These findings are more likely to be found in the fetus with esophageal atresia and no distal TEF. Postnatally, the diagnosis is suspected when an orogastric tube cannot be passed into the stomach. A chest radiograph demonstrating the curled orogastric tube in the proximal blind esophageal pouch is diagnostic (Figure 11-13). Barium contrast studies are usually unnecessary and may be dangerous because of the potential aspiration of the contrast material (Figure 11-14). Air is an excellent contrast agent and when injected through a tube often outlines the proximal esophageal pouch beautifully on radiography. These neonates clinically present with excess salivation, choking, and respiratory distress with feedings. Air in the bowel confirms the presence of a distal TEF.

Associated Anomalies

There is a significant association of other anomalies in infants with esophageal atresia. These are most easily remembered in the use of the acronym "VACTERL": *V*, vertebral anomalies; *A*, anorectal anomalies; *C*, cardiac

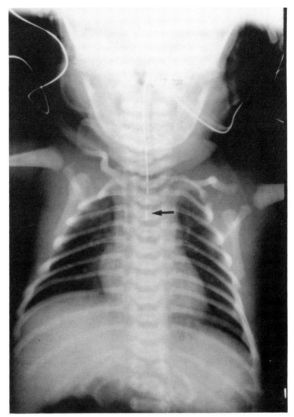

Figure 11-13 Chest radiograph of a neonate with esophageal atresia. The orogastric tube is lodged in the upper blind esophageal pouch (arrow). Air in the stomach and distal gastrointestinal tract confirms the presence of a distal tracheoesophageal fistula.

defects; *T*, TEF; *E*, esophageal atresia; *R*, renal anomalies; *L*, limb anomalies. These defects may be seen individually or together. Chromosomal anomalies such as trisomies 13, 18, and 21 are identified in a small but significant percentage of these patients.

Management

These infants are at high risk for aspiration, which occurs by two mechanisms. In the first, the proximal blind esophagus leads to aspiration of pooled oral secretions and is best managed by suctioning the oropharynx and esophagus using a Replogle tube specially designed for this purpose. The second, more important mechanism of aspiration results from gastric distention as air passes through the TEF. High intragastric pressure leads to reflux of gastric contents into the tracheobronchial tree. Therefore, vigorous assisted ventilation should be avoided to minimize forcing air into the gastro-intestinal tract. The infant should be placed prone with the head elevated at least 25° to 30° to minimize gastroesophageal reflux and to facilitate postural drainage of oral secretions. Intravenous hydration and antibiotic therapy are important for optimal management.

Operative Repair and Prognosis

Surgical repair consists of a right thoracotomy, extrapleural dissection, division and closure of the TEF, and anastomosis of the esophageal segments (Figure 11-15). Gastrostomy is reserved for occasions when primary repair has been difficult or is delayed due to severe prematurity, severe lung disease, or long-gap atresia. More than 90% of these infants survive, and when mortality occurs it is almost always related to associated anomalies or extreme prematurity. Up to 65% of these children have pathological gastroesophageal reflux, and nearly one third will require a fundoplication. Despite these and other problems, most of these children will lead normal and productive lives.

Duodenal Obstruction

Newborn infants with complete duodenal obstruction present with bilious emesis or bile-stained gastric aspirate. Abdominal distention is limited to the upper abdomen. The infant may or may not pass meconium. Incomplete obstruction may present as feeding intolerance and intermittent bilious vomiting. Meconium and flatus are usually passed. The primary initial concern is to differentiate the potentially lethal entity of intestinal malrotation and midgut volvulus from other anatomic obstructions such as duodenal atresia, stenosis, or webs.

Associated Anomalies

Malrotation is often an isolated anomaly; however, it can be seen in conjunction with other anomalies such as omphalocele, gastroschisis, and diaphragmatic hernia. Trisomy 21 occurs in up to 30% of neonates with duodenal atresia, stenosis, or annular pancreas.

Management

When a proximal intestinal obstruction is suspected in the neonatal period, an orogastric tube should be placed, the stomach emptied, and 30 mL of air injected into the stomach. Supine and lateral chest and abdominal radiographs are useful in the initial evaluation of the infants. In normal infants gas should progress well along the small bowel during the first 2 hours after birth.

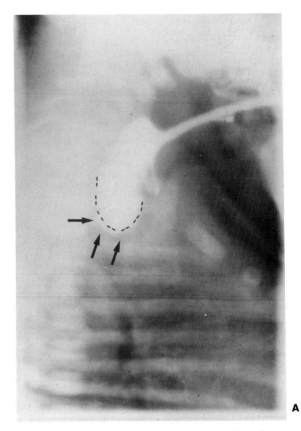

A

Figure 11-14 A, This contrast study shows barium filling the blind upper esophageal segment. The dotted line and arrows outline the esophageal boundaries. **B**, Aspirated barium (arrows) following a barium swallow is apparent on this chest radiograph of a neonate with esophageal atresia with fistula.

Within 6 hours gas should have reached the cecum, and by 12 hours the entire colon should be filled. Therefore, within a few hours after birth an estimate of the level of intestinal obstruction can be made. If air outlines the stomach and duodenum only, complete duodenal obstruction indicative of duodenal atresia or a completely obstructing malrotation is present (Figure 11-16). Malrotation is the most likely diagnosis when air can be seen distal to the obstruction. If there is any reason to delay surgical repair (e.g., respiratory distress), an upper gastrointestinal contrast study or contrast enema should be performed to rule out intestinal malrotation (Figure 11-17). If not treated early, the consequences of malrotation with volvulus can be devastating, with infarction of the entire midgut from jejunum to transverse colon (Figure 11-18). When duodenal atresia, web, or stenosis is clearly diagnosed,

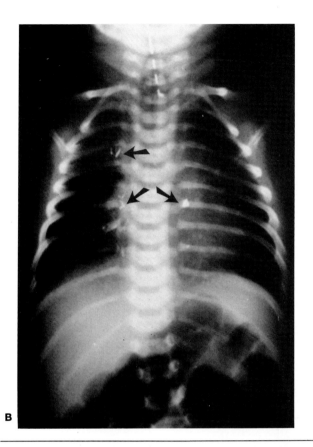

B

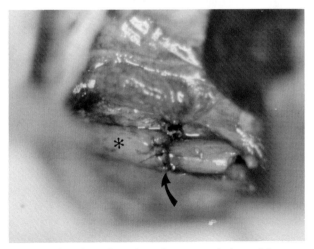

Figure 11-15   Intraoperative view of esophageal anastomosis (arrow) in a neonate with esophageal atresia. The proximal esophagus is marked with an asterisk.

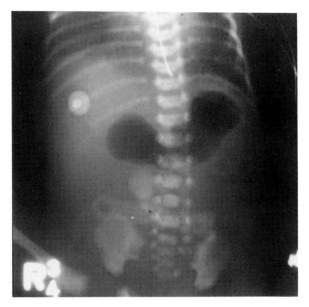

Figure 11-16   The radiographic "double bubble" typical of complete duodenal obstruction is seen here. There is absence of distal bowel gas.

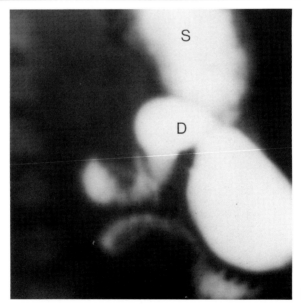

A

Figure 11-17   A, This upper gastrointestinal contrast study demonstrates malrotation and volvulus. The stomach (S) and duodenum (D) are marked. The corkscrew appearance of the distal duodenum and proximal jejunum is characteristic for volvulus. **B,** The same infant at laparotomy. Obstruction of the duodenum (D) by Ladd's bands (large arrows) is apparent. The cecum (C) with appendix (small arrow) lies on the midabdominal surface.

an orogastric tube is passed and placed on suction and definitive repair is performed electively at the earliest opportunity.

Operative Repair and Prognosis

Duodenal atresia and annular pancreas are repaired with a duodenostomy or duodenojejunostomy (Figure 11-19). Duodenal stenosis and webs are corrected by duodenoplasty. Most of these infants will have a period of proximal gastrointestinal dysfunction until motility returns to normal, lasting from 2 to 4 weeks. Total parenteral nutrition (TPN) has significantly reduced morbidity and mortality. When these lesions occur as isolated anomalies, the prognosis is excellent.

Children with malrotation and volvulus require a Ladd procedure, which consists of derotation of the volvulus, lysis of the obstructing peritoneal bands, appendectomy, and resection of any gangrenous intestine. Prognosis for these infants depends on the extent of intestinal resection required. If the child is left with a short bowel, a prolonged period of malabsorption may occur. Here again, TPN will allow the infant to grow until satisfactory adaptation of the remaining bowel has occurred.

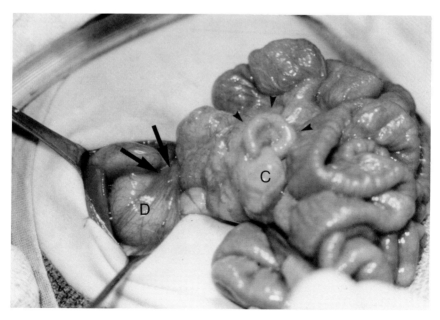

B

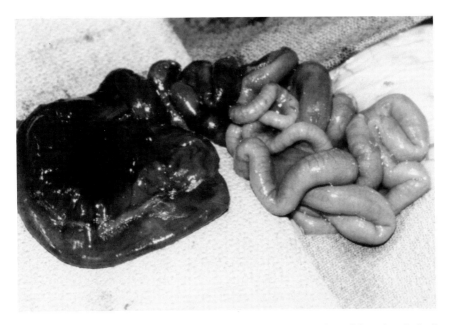

Figure 11-18   Gross specimen showing the segmental infarction of small bowel typical of volvulus.

Small Intestinal Atresia

This group of intestinal obstructions includes jejunal and ileal atresias, multiple atresias, and intestinal stenosis (Figure 11-20). The etiology of most of these lesions is an in utero vascular accident. These infants present with abdominal distention and emesis of feedings or bile. The diagnosis is relatively easy to make from abdominal radiographs, which may show multiple loops of dilated bowel on supine views and air-fluid levels on lateral decubitus views (Figure 11-21). All the visible intestinal loops are of comparable size, so one cannot easily differentiate small from large intestines on the radiographs. However, no contrast studies are required, especially if urgent surgery is planned. Occasionally atresias occur because of in utero midgut or segmental volvulus (Figure 11-22). If a delay in operative correction is necessary, an upper gastrointestinal contrast study is warranted to ensure that the duodenal "C loop" is in the appropriate location.

Management

During the initial management, orogastric decompression is necessary to prevent aspiration. Intravenous hydration and electrolyte replacement are

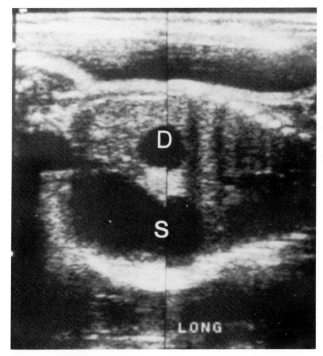

A

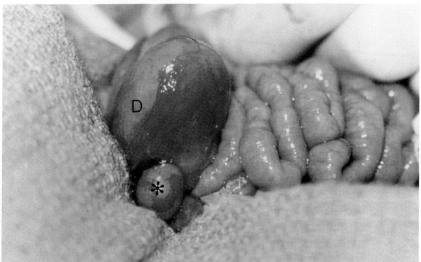

B

Figure 11-19 A, This oblique longitudinal composite antenatal sonogram demonstrates duodenal obstruction at 30 weeks' gestation. The fluid-filled stomach (S) and proximal duodenum (D) are clearly distended. **B,** After birth, the proximal obstructed duodenum (D) and duodenal atresia were verified at laparotomy. The bowel distal to the atresia (asterisk) is very small. A duodenostomy was performed, and the infant had an unremarkable recovery.

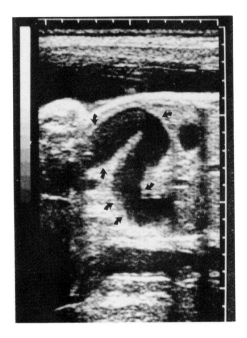

A

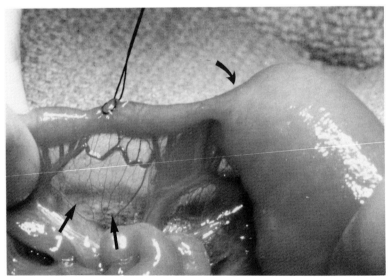

B

Figure 11-20 A, Coronal longitudinal sonogram of a 32-week fetus with jejunal atresia. The dilated bowel is outlined by small arrows. Polyhydramnios was the basis for the ultrasound examination. **B,** After birth, the diagnosis of jejunal atresia was confirmed at laparotomy (arrow). The mesenteric vasculature in the region of the atresia is abnormal, supporting the intrauterine vascular accident etiology of bowel atresias. The pursestring suture marks the site where patency of the distal bowel was evaluated by intraluminal insertion of methylene blue–stained saline.

needed to compensate for excess and obligatory fluid losses. Additional resuscitation depends on the condition of the infant. If ventilatory support is required, intubation is preferable to mask ventilation to avoid further gastric and intestinal distention with its considerable risk of regurgitation and aspiration. Antibiotics are routinely administered because of the increased risk of sepsis.

Intestinal atresias are corrected by celiotomy and primary anastomosis when possible (Figure 11-23). Proximal jejunal atresia may require tapering of the proximal jejunal segment to prevent functional obstruction at the anastomosis. Approximately 15% of these neonates will have multiple atresias, with the length of functional bowel being the critical prognostic factor. In addition, 15% will have cystic fibrosis; therefore, all infants with jejunoileal atresia should have a sweat chloride test at 6 weeks of age.

Prognosis

If the bowel anastomosis is functional and adequate intestinal length remains, survival chances are excellent. However, if short bowel or malabsorption complicates recovery, prolonged dependence on TPN or elemental enteric formulas may be required until intestinal adaptation has occurred.

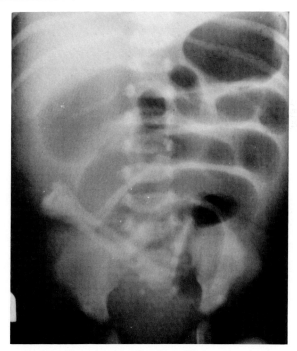

Figure 11-21 This abdominal film shows the dilated loops of bowel and lack of distal intestinal gas that are typical findings of small intestinal obstruction.

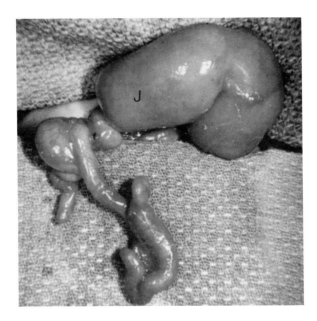

Figure 11-22 Antenatal midgut volvulus caused this jejunal atresia (J) and functional loss of the entire small bowel.

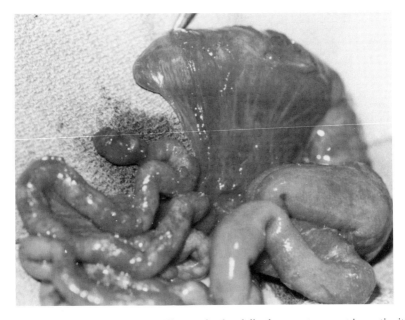

Figure 11-23 Ileal atresia at surgery. The proximal and distal segments are not in continuity.

Meconium Ileus

Meconium ileus is the term applied to neonatal intestinal obstruction seen in infants with cystic fibrosis. Cystic fibrosis results from a disorder of exocrine gland function. A number of organ systems are adversely affected in these patients, including the pancreas, lung, intestine, biliary tract, sweat glands, and reproductive organs. The clinical manifestation in the neonate relates to hyperviscous mucus secretion in the intestine and abnormally sticky, dehydrated meconium, which obstructs the distal ileum. Exocrine pancreatic insufficiency is already present at birth in most affected infants. The lungs are normal at birth, but progressive pulmonary disease occurs as a result of inspissated mucus plugging and secondary infection in the smaller airways.

Two forms of meconium ileus are recognized, simple and complicated. Simple meconium ileus, as its name implies, is a straightforward meconium obstruction of the mid-ileum, with the intestinal lumen being otherwise patent. These neonates present with abdominal distention, bilious vomiting, and failure to pass meconium. The markedly dilated mid-ileum is filled with thick, tenacious meconium. Distal to the obstruction, the distal ileum is narrow and contains hard pellets of gray meconium, giving the bowel a beaded appearance (Figure 11-24). The colon is very small and unused in these neonates. Complicated meconium ileus, the second form, is causally associated with several additional serious problems, including in utero volvulus, intestinal atresia, meconium peritonitis, and meconium pseudocyst, all of which arise from the primary underlying disorder. In addition to these symptoms, these infants may present with progressive abdominal distention, respiratory distress, abdominal wall erythema and edema, and in some cases signs of severe hypovolemia. Nearly 50% of patients will demonstrate this second type of meconium ileus.

Meconium ileus should be suspected when there is disparity in the size of distended bowel loops, a soap bubble appearance of the intraluminal contents, and lack of air-fluid levels in the distended bowel on upright radiographs (Figure 11-25). When diffuse calcifications are seen on abdominal radiographs, meconium peritonitis resulting from intrauterine intestinal perforation is likely. Meconium pseudocyst is seen as a discrete mass with a rim of dense calcification. Approximately one third of cases of complicated meconium ileus have no recognizable radiographic features that distinguish them from simple meconium ileus.

Management and Prognosis

Hyperosmolar water-soluble contrast enemas under fluoroscopic guidance have been effective in relieving the meconium obstruction in simple meconium ileus in about 60% of affected infants (Figure 11-26). A contrast enema

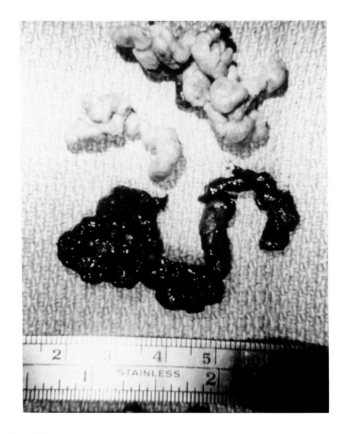

Figure 11-24 Light gray and hard beaded meconium (above) and rubberlike tenacious green meconium from an infant with meconium ileus.

---

also differentiates other causes of large bowel obstruction, including meconium plug, small left colon syndrome, colonic atresia, and Hirschsprung's disease. Adequate intravenous hydration is critical for these neonates, as the hyperosmolar contrast material can precipitate shock.

When necessary, operative treatment focuses on complete evacuation of the meconium obstruction. The intestine is irrigated through an enterostomy with saline or a 2% *N*-acetylcysteine solution. Some infants require an intestinal resection with primary anastomosis or temporary enterostomy. Pulmonary infection, malabsorption, recurrent obstruction, and rectal prolapse are common complications in this group of children. Early postnatal survival is now in the 70% to 80% range at 1 year. After infancy the outlook depends on the severity and progression of the pulmonary disease.

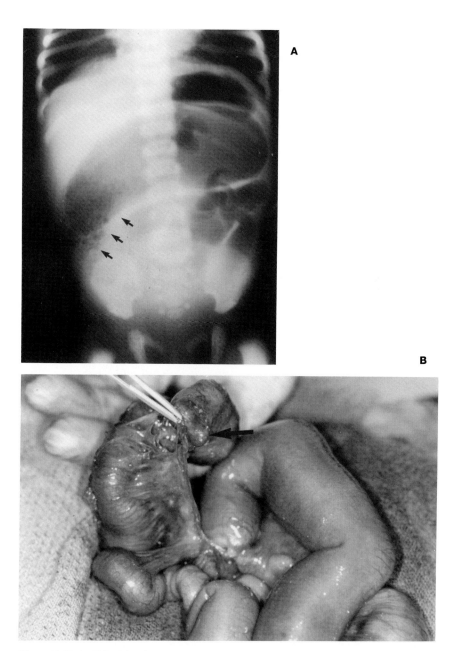

Figure 11-25 A, This abdominal radiograph from an infant with meconium ileus shows the soap bubble appearance of the meconium (small arrows) in the obstructed dilated small bowel. **B,** Meconium ileus at surgery. This infant has developed ileal atresia as a result of meconium ileus. There are dense inflammatory adhesions encasing the distal bowel, held by the forceps. Nearly 30% of patients have this complex form of meconium ileus.

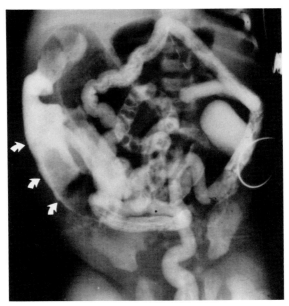

Figure 11-26 A contrast enema in an infant with simple meconium ileus. Contrast refluxes from the microcolon into the dilated meconium-filled distal ileum (arrows).

Meconium Peritonitis

Meconium peritonitis occurs in 1 in 35,000 live births. The most common etiology is in utero intestinal perforation that results from intestinal obstruction. Obstruction with perforation may follow meconium ileus, volvulus, atresia, or intestinal bands. Intraperitoneal meconium causes a giant cell foreign body reaction, dense fibroblastic proliferation, and calcifications in the peritoneal cavity (Figure 11-27). Calcifications are seen in two thirds of all cases and are clearly helpful in establishing a diagnosis. In some infants the perforation has sealed antenatally. The indication for surgical repair is intestinal obstruction or persistent intestinal perforation, occurring in 85% (Figure 11-28). The aim of surgical treatment is to remove devitalized tissue, preserve adequate intestinal length, and re-establish enteric continuity. A primary intestinal anastomosis can be performed in some infants; others may require a temporary enterostomy. Current long-term survival is approximately 70%.

Colonic Obstruction

Although colonic obstruction can be detected by antenatal ultrasound, most infants with the condition will initially present with symptoms in the neonatal period. Delayed or absent meconium passage is characteristic for

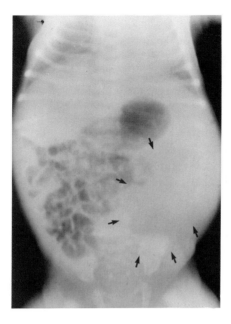

Figure 11-27 This abdominal radiograph of a neonate with a large meconium cyst (black arrows) does not demonstrate the commonly observed calcifications.

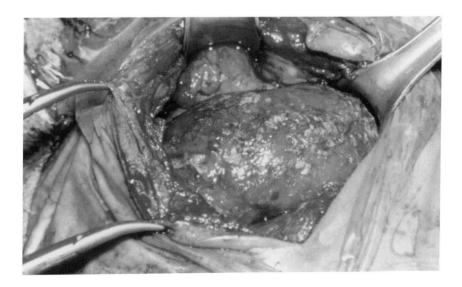

Figure 11-28 Operative view of a large meconium cyst and peritonitis. Resection of the cyst and primary intestinal anastomosis were possible here.

Table 11-1 Prenatal Diagnosis of Abdominal Masses

1. *Solid tumors*
   Renal: Mesoblastic nephroma, Wilms' tumor
   Hepaticobiliary: Hepatoblastoma, adenoma, hamartoma, hemangioma,
      lymphangioma
   Retroperitoneal: Neuroblastoma, ganglioneuroma, teratoma

2. *Nonrenal cystic masses*
   Hepaticobiliary: Liver cyst, choledochal cyst
   Gastrointestinal: Duplication anomalies, mesenteric cysts, omental cysts,
      junction obstruction, omphalomesenteric cysts, jejunoileal atresia,
      meconium cysts, meconium ileus syndrome
   Genital: Ovarian cysts, hydrometrocolpos

3. *Renal cystic masses*
   Polycystic kidney disease, multicystic kidney, multicystic nephroma,
      ureteropelvic junction obstruction, urachal cyst, ureterovescicle, ureterocele,
      hydronephrosis/hydroureter, urethral valves, urethral atresia, prune belly,
      ureteral duplication, anomalies, megacystis/megaureter

most of these disorders, which are listed in Table 11-1. Gradually increasing abdominal distention followed by feeding intolerance and vomiting is common. Meconium plug and small left colon syndrome may be indistinguishable from meconium ileus in presentation. In fact, 15% of infants with meconium plug will later have a positive sweat test for cystic fibrosis. Furthermore, at least 10% of the infants thought to have meconium plug or small left colon syndrome will have Hirschsprung's disease. Therefore, all of these infants should have a suction rectal biopsy to rule out Hirschsprung's disease or should be closely followed for several months to ensure there is normal bowel function.

Hirschsprung's disease most frequently presents in the newborn period, but its symptoms often evolve more gradually than those of colonic atresia. The majority of these patients have aganglionosis in the rectosigmoid colon, although the entire colon and occasionally the small intestine can be involved. Nearly 95% of infants with Hirschsprung's disease will not pass meconium in the first 24 hours. However, early stool passage does not eliminate Hirschsprung's disease completely because a few of these children later develop life-threatening enterocolitis, which manifests as abdominal distention, obstipation, fever, and foul-smelling diarrhea.

Associated Anomalies

Meconium plug may be seen in patients with cystic fibrosis or Hirschsprung's disease. Small left colon syndrome is more common in infants of diabetic mothers. Infants with trisomy 21 have a higher incidence of Hirschsprung's disease.

Management

Abdominal radiographs are important initial diagnostic studies for differentiating these distal obstructions from more proximal lesions. Disparity of bowel loop size and a very large air-filled loop are frequently seen in colonic atresia and Hirschsprung's disease. A contrast enema is mandatory to differentiate the various causes of distal ileal and colonic obstruction (Figure 11-29). If the contrast study is not diagnostic but is suspicious of Hirschsprung's disease, a rectal biopsy should be performed to confirm the diagnosis. The presence of a transition zone in the colon on barium enema or failure of the barium to be evacuated after 24 hours is highly suggestive of the diagnosis. When meconium plugs or small left colon syndrome are present, hyperosmolar water-soluble contrast enemas, fluoroscopically guided, are usually effective in restoring normal meconium passage.

Orogastric suction to prevent aspiration and strict attention to appropriate intravenous hydration are important for all these neonates. Rectal tube placement and warm saline enemas may help evacuate a dilated sigmoid colon in Hirschsprung's disease and might be lifesaving for an infant with overwhelming sepsis and enterocolitis who requires stabilization prior to emergency operation. Broad spectrum antibiotics to cover gram-negative and anaerobic organisms should be administered.

Operative Procedures and Prognosis

If the contrast enemas fail to alleviate the obstruction in small left colon syndrome, a temporary colostomy is indicated. Eventual enteric continuity and long-term survival are the rule.

Infants with established Hirschsprung's disease need an enterostomy, usually a colostomy, placed in the most distal bowel that has ganglion cells (Figure 11-30). Once the child is several months old, a definitive pull-through procedure (Soave, Duhamel, or Swenson operation) can safely be performed. The purpose of these procedures is to bring bowel-containing ganglion cells down to the anorectal junction in order to restore normal bowel function. More than 90% of these patients have excellent long-term results and are without incontinence.

Restoration of intestinal continuity is the primary objective in patients with colonic atresia. Primary resection and anastomosis can be achieved in many infants with segmental involvement. However, if the entire distal colon is atretic, a colostomy is constructed. At 9 months to 1 year of age, reconstruction with an abdominoperineal pull-through can be performed. Survival and functional outlook for these infants are excellent if there are no other serious anomalies.

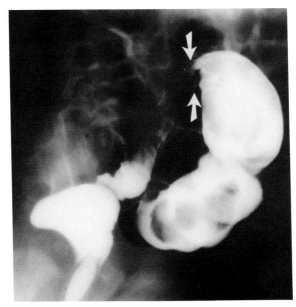

Figure 11-29 This contrast enema in a child with Hirschsprung's disease demonstrates a transitional zone in the sigmoid colon (arrows).

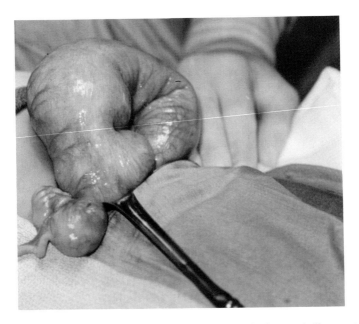

Figure 11-30 The distal rectosigmoid colon of an infant with Hirschsprung's disease, at surgery. The dilated bowel has ganglion cells and will function normally when not obstructed.

Anorectal Malformations

Anorectal malformations occur in approximately 1 in 5000 live births. This constellation of anomalies includes cloacal malformations, anorectal agenesis, rectal atresia, anal agenesis, and anal stenosis. These lesions often are associated with rectovaginal or rectovestibular fistulas in females and rectourethral or perineal fistulas in males (Figure 11-31). The vast majority of these lesions are diagnosed only after birth. Infants with a high lesion, such as anorectal agenesis with rectourethral fistula, are treated initially with a diverting colostomy. Complete reconstruction with a perineal pull-through procedure is performed when the infant is several months old. However, a low imperforate anus with anovestibular fistula may be definitively repaired in the newborn period.

Associated Anomalies

Associated anomalies are common, particularly genitourinary malformations and all of the VACTERL association anomalies mentioned previously in the section on esophageal atresia.

Prognosis

Prognosis for survival is good but often is related to the severity of other anomalies. Fecal continence following reconstructive procedures varies with the level of the anorectal malformation and the presence of sacral anomalies. Patients with low and intermediate anorectal lesions generally have good functional outcomes. Infants with high lesions have often had fecal incontinence following reconstruction; however, newer operative procedures appear to offer hope for improved functional outcome for these children.

ABDOMINAL MASSES: GENERAL CONSIDERATIONS

Prenatal ultrasonography occasionally reveals the presence of an intra-abdominal mass in the fetus not clearly associated with the gastrointestinal tract. The differential diagnoses of intra-abdominal masses in the fetus and neonate are extensive (Table 11-1). The differential diagnosis can be narrowed down to a few specific lesions by (1) identifying the precise location of the mass within the abdomen or, preferably, establishing the organ of origin, (2) determining whether the lesion is solid or cystic, and (3) visualizing a recognizable consequence of a lesion on adjacent or distant systems.

Masses arising from abnormalities in the urinary tract account for the majority (over 60%) of abdominal masses prenatally identified (see detailed discussion in Chapter 13). After birth, careful physical examination is a crucial part of the postnatal evaluation of the infant with an intra-abdominal

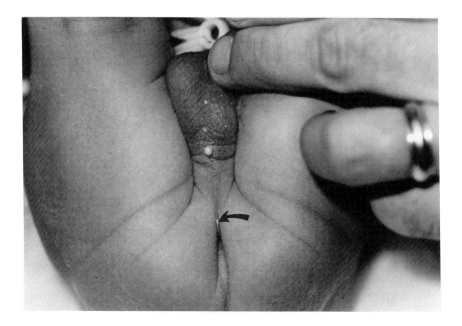

Figure 11-31 This infant has a high imperforate anus and a rectoperineal fistula (arrow). Mucus pearls are present in the scrotal raphe.

mass. Palpation defines the location and size of the lesion as well as its mobility and consistency. A bimanual rectal and abdominal examination may reveal pelvic masses as well as a degree of pelvic involvement. Inspection of the vaginal and urethral openings is important to rule out hydrometrocolpos or other lesions.

In the neonate, abdominal ultrasonography has replaced the intravenous urogram as a primary screening and diagnostic modality. Abdominal ultrasound provides significant information about the size and the organ of origin of the mass. In addition, the solid or cystic nature of masses can be readily determined. Some patients may require additional diagnostic studies, including contrast-enhanced CT scans, magnetic resonance imaging, radionuclear scans, and contrast gastrointestinal studies prior to planned surgical procedures.

Fortunately, the vast majority of perinatally diagnosed abdominal masses are benign, but early postnatal evaluation and treatment remain essential for optimal care. The majority of these babies are born asymptomatic, allowing time for a thorough evaluation and appropriate planning for intervention. Urgent operation may be indicated in some neonates for bleeding, perforation, or ischemic necrosis.

Solid Neoplasms

Renal Tumors

Mesoblastic nephromas and Wilms' tumors are the most common renal neoplasms in the neonate. Mesoblastic nephroma, the more common of the two lesions in this age group, is generally benign. Infants almost uniformly do well following surgical removal (Figure 11-32). Perioperative diagnostic imaging modalities may not distinguish between mesonephric blastoma and Wilms' tumor (Figure 11-33). Although Wilms' tumor is malignant, long-term survival following surgery is excellent for the majority of infants, with rates reported to be greater than 90%. However, a much poorer prognosis obtains for patients with unfavorable histological types (e.g., anaplasia, sarcomatous Wilms' tumor).

Neurogenic Tumors

Neuroblastomas occur in 1 in 10,000 births and are the most common intra-abdominal tumor of childhood. Neuroblastoma is a highly malignant, nonencapsulated tumor that commonly metastasizes to bone marrow, bone, lymph nodes, liver, and skin. These tumors originate from neural crest ectoderm and may arise at any point along the adrenal-sympathetic chain. The tumors usually produce catecholamines; therefore, screening for catecholamines and their metabolites is useful to establish the diagnosis. Seventy-five percent of these tumors are retroperitoneal, with the majority arising in the adrenal gland (Figure 11-34A and 11-34B). The tumors can extend into the spinal canal through the intervertebral foramen and may be responsible for significant neurological deficits, such as paraplegia (Figure 11-34C). Treatment for early stage (I and II) lesions by surgical extirpation results in long-term survival in 90% of infants. Young infants with metastatic disease to the liver, bone marrow, and skin have a superior survival rate compared with older children with the same extent of disease (75% versus 15%). The reason for this survival advantage is that many tumors undergo spontaneous maturation and regression in small infants. However, children of any age with metastatic disease to the bone have an extremely poor prognosis even with chemotherapy, with a survival rate of less than 15% at 3 years.

Hepatic Neoplasms

In the neonate solid hepatic tumors are usually benign. These lesions include hamartomas, adenomas, hemangiomas, or lymphangiomas and may not need specific surgical treatment. Prognosis is very good for most patients even if surgical excision is required. Hepatoblastoma is the most common

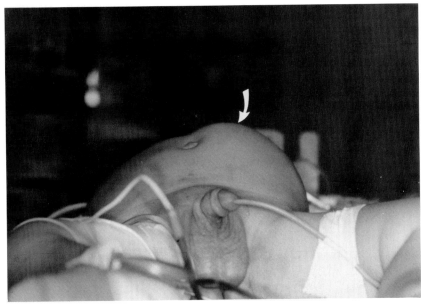

A

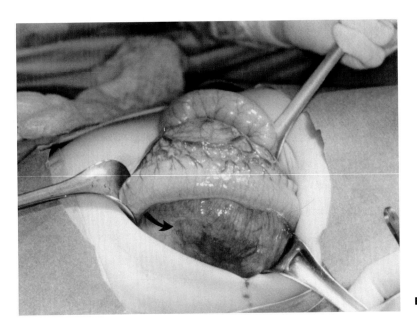

B

Figure 11-32 A, This 3-month-old infant has an obvious large abdominal mass (arrow).
B, At laparotomy in the same infant, a large mesoblastic nephroma (arrow) was excised; the
child is well at 2 years of age.

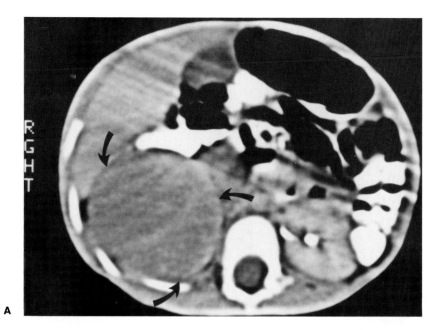

A

B

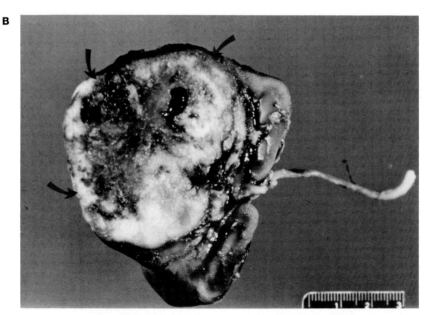

Figure 11-33 A, This tomographic study of a child with a Wilms' tumor shows the right kidney very distorted and replaced with tumor (arrow). Normal left kidney function remains. **B**, The tumor was excised and divided to show the relationship of the tumor (arrows) to the normal kidney parenchyma (on the right side of specimen).

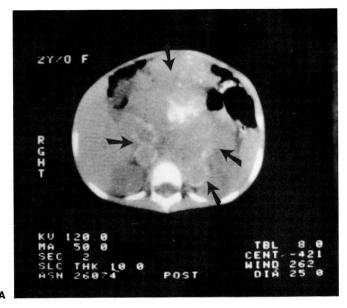

A

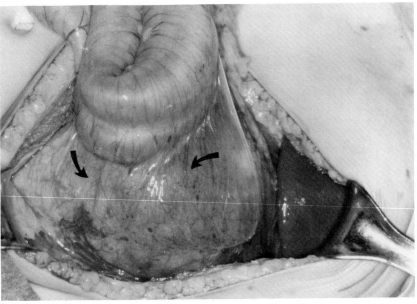

B

Figure 11-34 A, This tomographic study shows a large adrenal neuroblastoma (arrows) extending across the midline of this infant. **B,** At surgery the tumor, which proved to be unresectable, is seen displacing the colon (arrow). **C,** This sagittal magnetic resonance image shows a pelvic neuroblastoma extending into the spinal canal (arrow).

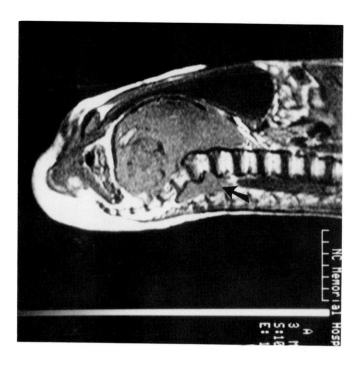

C

malignant hepatic tumor in infancy (Figure 11-35). Prognosis is excellent for those patients who have complete resection of the tumor followed with chemotherapy (greater than 90% 2-year survival). When the tumor cannot be totally excised, the prognosis is very poor (less than 15% 2-year survival).

Nonrenal Cystic Masses

Liver and Biliary Tree

Postnatal ultrasound and CT imaging studies confirm the diagnosis of benign liver cysts. Symptomatic hepatic cysts are best treated with surgical excision or marsupialization. The prognosis is very good following surgical treatment of these very rare lesions.

Choledochal cysts are extremely rare cystic dilatations of the extrahepatic biliary system (Figure 11-36). Young infants will often present with obstructive jaundice, acholic stools, and hepatomegaly. Abdominal ultrasonography is the best screening study in the postnatal period as it provides valuable information about the status of the intrahepatic ducts and the liver (Figure 11-37). Preoperative 99 diisopropyl iminodiacetic acid (DISIDA) Tc 99m scintigraphy is very useful for examining biliary excretion in these

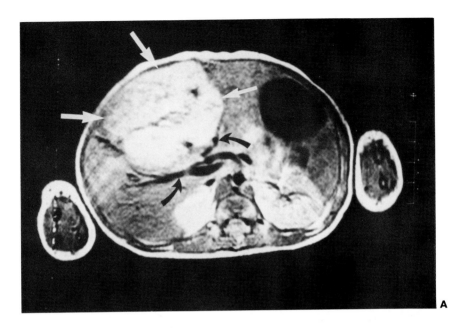

A

Figure 11-35 **A**, Magnetic resonance imaging shows this hepatoblastoma (straight arrows) involving the central liver in a 3-week-old infant. The liver vasculature (curved arrows) is enhanced by this technique. **B**, The gross tumor at surgery. Trisegmentectomy was required to excise the tumor. **C**, Hamartomas of the liver have a gross appearance similar to many malignant hepatic neoplasms, as demonstrated here. Localized surgical resection of this hamartoma cured the patient.

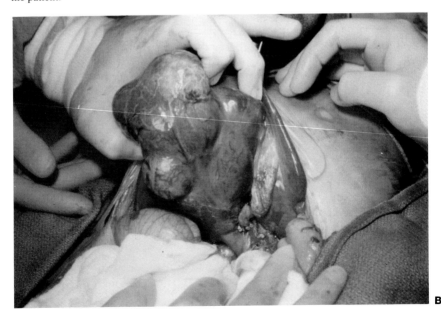

B

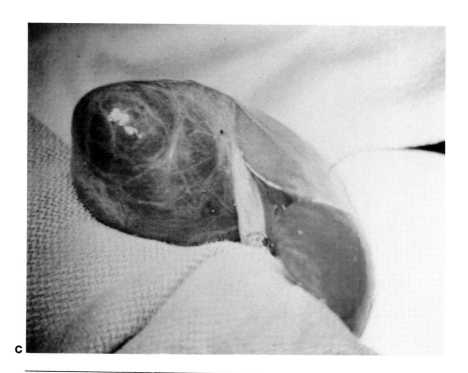

c

patients (Figure 11-38). Operative excision of the choledochal cyst with a Roux-en-Y hepaticojejunostomy usually provides a lifelong cure. If operative therapy is performed later in childhood, severe cirrhosis is likely to occur, which may adversely alter prognosis and ultimate survival. Retained portions of choledochal cyst mucosa may undergo malignant degeneration 10 to 20 cystojejunostomy. Therefore, complete excision of choledochal cyst mucosa is recommended to prevent this late consequence.

Mesenteric and Omental Cysts

The etiology of mesenteric and omental cystic lesions is thought to be related to anomalies of the lymphatic system in the abdomen. Mesenteric and omental cysts can be unilocular or multiloculated (Figure 11-39). The majority of patients are born asymptomatic. Rarely, these lesions are associated with symptoms of intestinal obstruction or massive abdominal distention or ischemia secondary to torsion of the mass. Surgical resection is the therapy of choice, with prognosis being excellent.

Ovarian Cysts

The prenatal diagnosis of ovarian cyst is usually serendipitous (Figure 11-40A). Postnatal abdominal ultrasonography will confirm the prenatal find-

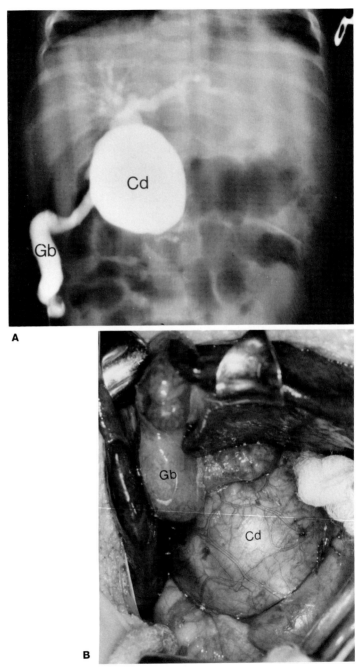

Figure 11-36 A, Intraoperative cholangiography through the gallbladder (Gb) demonstrates this choledochal cyst in a 2-month-old infant. **B,** At surgery, the cyst was excised and the biliary system drained by a hepaticojejunostomy.

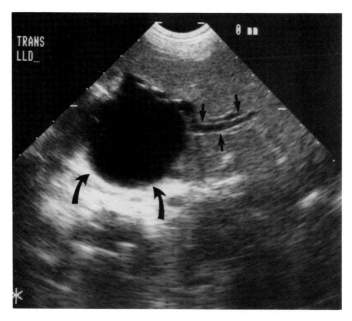

Figure 11-37 Preoperative abdominal ultrasound in the same patient shows a cystic structure at the edge of the liver and dilated intrahepatic bile ducts (arrows).

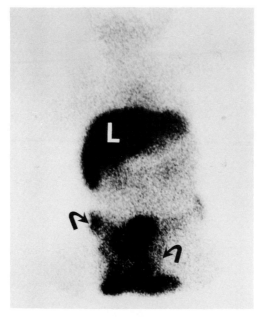

Figure 11-38 Preoperative DISIDA Tc 99 scintigraphy shows hepatic function (L) but no biliary excretion in this infant. Renal and enteric excretion of the radionucleotide is evident (arrows).

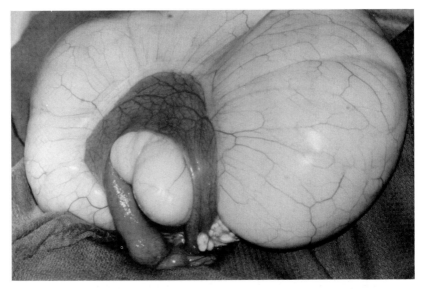

Figure 11-39   The multiloculated chylous mesenteric cyst seen here at surgery was causing intestinal obstruction.

ings. Most infants with ovarian cysts are generally asymptomatic; however, torsion of the enlarged ovarian mass may occur (Figure 11-40B). It has been reported in autopsy studies of newborn females that nearly 50% of female infants have cystic ovaries at birth. From this information it is presumed that maternal and placental hormones play a role in the pathogenesis of ovarian cysts in the fetus. Several authors have reported that prenatally diagnosed ovarian cysts that were followed postnatally with ultrasonography disappeared without surgical intervention. These patients corroborate the possibly hormone-based etiology of ovarian cysts in the fetus. Surgical excision of the ovarian cyst may be required if symptoms of ovarian torsion are present or the lesion does not disappear over several months (Figure 11-41).

Duplication Cysts

The vast majority of masses arising from the gastrointestinal tract in infants are cystic in nature. Duplication cysts of the gastrointestinal tract occur anywhere between the mouth and the rectum but are most commonly found in the terminal ileal and cecal regions. Many of these lesions cause no symptoms but can lead to intestinal obstruction and bleeding. On physical examination these masses are mobile and firm. Preoperative ultrasonography and contrast gastrointestinal studies provide the most useful imaging diagnostic information (Figure 11-42). Surgical excision is curative in these patients (Figure 11-43).

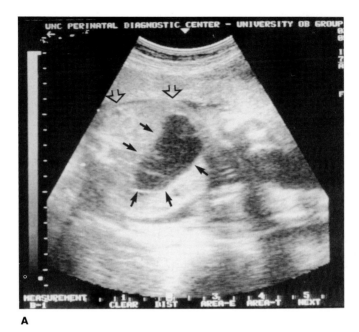

A

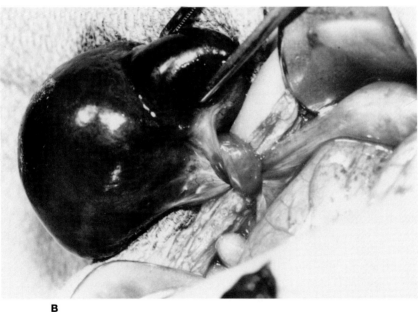

B

Figure 11-40 A, This transabdominal sonogram at 34 weeks' gestation shows a discrete intra-abdominal cystic mass (black arrows) that proved to be an ovarian cyst. **B,** Torsion of the enlarged cystic ovary occurred in this neonate, and oophorectomy was required.

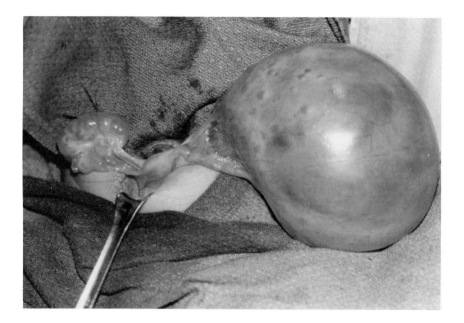

Figure 11-41 The ovarian cyst shown here at surgery did not resolve spontaneously postnatally. Ovarian cystectomy with preservation of considerable normal ovarian tissue was possible.

Hydrometrocolpos

The female neonate can develop a large pelvic mass as a result of an imperforate hymen or vaginal atresia. The presence of a large cystic pelvic mass in the female warrants careful evaluation of the perineum and vaginal area. Identification of a bulging perineum and an absent vaginal orifice is clearly diagnostic in most patients. Ultrasonography is useful to identify whether there is evidence of urinary tract obstruction secondary to this large pelvic mass. Direct needle injection of a contrast medium through the perineum may also provide final confirmation of the diagnosis. When newborn infants present with this problem, it is related to the accumulation of vaginal and cervical secretions, which are stimulated by maternal hormones. In the case of imperforate hymen, simple incision of the obstructing membrane provides adequate drainage of the hydrometrocolpos. On the other hand, with vaginal atresia a more complex reconstruction may be necessary for cure. In achieving surgical correction of these lesions, injury to the adjacent and often distorted urethra must be avoided.

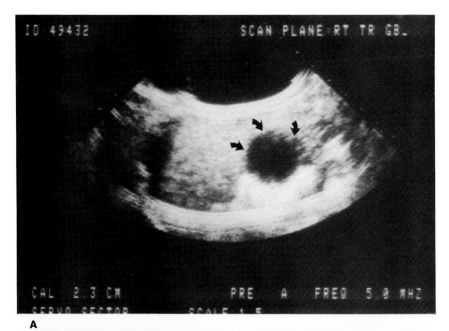

A

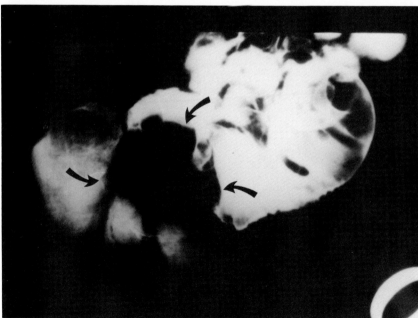

B

Figure 11-42 **A**, An intra-abdominal cystic mass (arrows) is demonstrated by this preoperative abdominal ultrasound. **B**, Preoperative intestinal contrast studies show a filling defect in the ileocecal region typical of a duplication cyst (arrows).

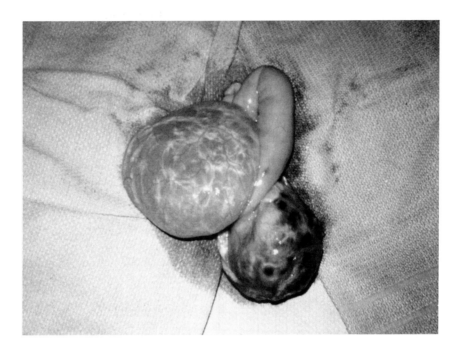

Figure 11-43 A duplication cyst at surgery. Surgical excision was performed, and the patient enjoyed an uncomplicated recovery.

FURTHER READING

Adelman S, Benson CD, Hertzler JH. Surgical lesions of the ovary in infancy and childhood. *Surg Gynecol Obstet.* 1975; 141:219.

Aiken J. Congenital intrinsic duodenal obstruction in infancy. A series of 30 cases treated over a 6 year period. *J Pediatr Surg.* 1966; 1:546.

Boley S. An endorectal pullthrough operation with primary anastomosis for Hirschsprung's disease. *Surg Gynecol Obstet.* 1968; 127:353.

Bower RJ, Sieber WK, Kieswetter WB. Alimentary tract duplication in children. *Ann Surg.* 1978; 188:669.

Copel JA, Cullen M, Green JJ, Mahoney MJ, Hobbins JC, Kleinman CS. The frequency of aneuploidy in prenatally diagnosed congenital heart disease: An indication for fetal karyotyping. *Am J Obstet Gynecol.* 1988; 158:409–413.

D'Angio GJ, Evans AE, Breslow N, et al. The national Wilms' tumor study: Biology and management of Wilms' tumor. In: Levine AS, ed. *Cancer in the Young.* New York: Masson Publishing Co: 1982; 633–663.

D'Angio GJ, Evans AE, Koop CE. Special pattern of widespread neuroblastoma with a favorable prognosis. *Lancet.* 1971; 1:1046.

Davidson PM, Auldist AW. Contemporary surgical treatment for choledochal cysts. *Pediatr Surg Intern.* 1987; 2:157–160.

deLorimer AA, Fonkalsrud EW, Hays DM. Congenital atresia and stenosis of the jejunum and ileum. *Surgery.* 1969; 65:819.

Filston HC, Izant RJ. *Surgical Neonate: Evaluation and Care.* 2nd ed. Norwalk, Conn: Appleton-Century-Crofts, 1985.

Filston HC, Kirks DR. Malrotation—The ubiquitous anomaly. *J Pediatr Surg.* 1981; 16:614–620.

Filston HC, Rankin JS, Kirks DR. The diagnosis of primary and recurrent tracheoesophageal fistulas: Value of selective catheterization. *J Pediatr Surg.* 1982; 17:144.

Gaudin J, Le Trequilly C, Parent P, et al. Neonatal ovarian cysts. Twelve cysts with antenatal diagnosis. *Pediatr Surg Intern.* 1988; 3:158–168.

Grosfeld JL, Baehner RL. Neuroblastoma: An analysis of 160 cases. *World J Surg.* 1980; 4:29.

Grosfeld JL, Ballantine TVN, Shoemaker R. Operative management of intestinal atresia and stenosis based on pathological findings. *J Pediatr Surg.* 1979; 14:369.

Hartung RW, Kilcheski TS, Greaney RB, Powell RW, Evertson LR. Antenatal diagnosis of cystic meconium peritonitis. *J Ultrasound Med.* 1983; 2:49.

Hashimoto BE, Filly RA, Callen PW. Fetal pseudoascites: Further anatomic observations. *J Ultrasound Med.* 1986; 5:151.

Howell CG, Otherson HB Jr, Kiviat NE, et al. Therapy and outcome in 51 children with mesoblastic nephroma: A report of National Wilms' Tumor Study. *J Pediatr Surg.* 1982; 6:826.

Jassani MN, Gauderer MWL, Fanaroff AA, Fletcher B, Merkatz IR. A perinatal approach to the diagnosis and management of gastrointestinal malformations. *Obstet Gynecol.* 1982; 59:33–39.

Kim SH. Choledochal cyst: Survey by the surgical section of American Academy of Pediatrics. *J Pediatr Surg.* 1981; 16:402.

Lauer JD, Cradock TV. Meconium pseudocyst: Prenatal sonographic and antenatal radiologic correlation. *J Ultrasound Med.* 1982; 1:333.

Lilly JR. Surgical treatment of choledochal cyst. *Surg Gynecol Obstet.* 1979; 149:36.

Louhimo I, Lindahl M. Esophageal atresia: Primary results in 500 consecutively treated patients. *J Pediatr Surg.* 1983; 18:219.

Mahour GH, Wogu GU, Siegel SE, et al. Improved survival in infants and children with primary malignant liver tumors. *Am J Surg.* 1983; 146:236–240.

Mollit DL, Ballantine TVN, Grosfeld JL. Mesenteric cysts in infancy and childhood. *Surg Gynecol Obstet.* 1978; 147:182.

Nelson LH, Clark CE, Fishburne JI, Urban RB, Penry MF. Value of serial sonography in the in utero detection of duodenal atresia. *Obstet Gynecol.* 1982; 59:657–659.

Olsend MM, Luck SR, Loyd-Still J, Raffensperger JG. The spectrum of meconium disease in infancy. *J Pediatr Surg.* 1982; 17:479.

Pena A. Posterior sagittal anorectoplasty: Results in the management of 332 cases of anorectal malformations. *Pediatr Surg Intern.* 1988; 3:94–104.

Pena A, deVries PA. Posterior sagittal anorectoplasty: Important technical considerations and new applications. *J Pediatr Surg.* 1982; 17:796.

Pretorius DH, Drose JA, Dennis MA, Mandester DK, Manco-Johnson ML. Tracheoesophageal fistula in utero: Twenty-two cases. *J Ultrasound Med.* 1987; 6:509.

Randolph JG, Altman RP, Arensman RM, et al. Liver resection in children with hepatic neoplasms. *Ann Surg.* 1978; 187:599–605.

Skoll MA, Marquette GP, Hamilton EF. Prenatal ultrasonic diagnosis of multiple bowel atresias. *Am J Obstet Gynecol.* 1987; 156:472–473.

Swenson O, Sherman JO, Fisher JH. Diagnosis of congenital megacolon: An analysis of 501 patients. *J Pediatr Surg.* 1973; 8:587.

Chapter 12

Fetal Ventral Wall Defects

Although rare (approximately 1 in 3500 to 5000 live births), fetal ventral wall defects, including omphalocele and gastroschisis, are prenatally detectable malformations that require accurate identification and thoughtful management to achieve optimal outcome.

An omphalocele is a failure of the embryonic abdominal folds to meet in the midline and form a normal umbilical ring by the end of the 4th week postovulation. As a result, a variable amount of abdominal viscera develops within the proximal umbilical cord, covered by a two-layer membrane of peritoneum and amnion (Figure 12-1). The mass of extra-abdominal tissue is located in the midline, and the umbilical cord attaches to it. The umbilical vessels may be traced through the extra-abdominal tissues into the fetal abdomen.

Gastroschisis, on the other hand, describes a through-and-through defect of the abdominal wall, usually to the right side and slightly above the umbilicus. The exact embryopathology of gastroschisis is not as clear as that of omphalocele. Gastroschisis may result from abnormal involution of the right umbilical vein or from rupture of the umbilical ring in the 8th week. Whatever the exact mechanism, small bowel easily extrudes through the resulting hole in the abdominal wall and continues to develop outside the abdominal cavity (Figure 12-2).

The incidence of omphalocele (1 in 5000) is roughly twice that of gastroschisis (1 in 10,000), although there is some indication that the incidence of gastroschisis may be increasing.

Congenital defects of the fetal abdominal wall are not familiar to the lay public, and considerable explanation is necessary when such a malformation is diagnosed or suspected. Although similar in location and even occasionally in appearance, there are significant differences between these two malformations in terms of prognosis for successful repair and unimpaired survival. Through a brief review of the nature, embryology, sonographic appearance, and prognosis for infants with these types of birth defects, perhaps the tragedy of pregnancy termination of a fetus with a repairable defect can be avoided. A simple but methodical approach to the evaluation of the fetus with a ventral wall malformation will provide the parents and the clinician with the information necessary for appropriate management decisions.

EMBRYOLOGY

Omphalocele

During the 4th embryonic week, the lateral aspects of the discoid fetus fold ventrally to enclose the embryonic coelom. Typically, two lateral folds migrate to meet a cephalic fold and a caudal fold, to form the umbilical stalk by 28 days postconception. Failure of this event results in failed closure of the abdominal wall and an omphalocele. Bowel and often other abdominal viscera, including even liver, will be found within the omphalocele, which can be of widely variable size but generally the size of an omphalocele remains constant in a given individual. Malrotation of the intestine is expected, since the gut cannot return to the peritoneal cavity and form a secondary attachment to the dorsal wall. The majority of cases involve the lateral folds and lead

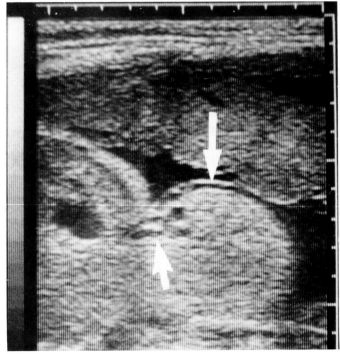

Figure 12-1 This transverse sonogram of the abdomen of a fetus at the level of the umbilicus shows a large soft tissue mass attached to the midline, with a covering membrane (vertical arrow) and umbilical vessels traversing the mass to the fetus (short arrow). *Source*: Reprinted from *Practical Obstetrical Ultrasound* (p 134) by JW Seeds and RC Cefalo, Aspen Publishers Inc, © 1986.

to a large, isolated omphalocele. Defective migration or formation of the cephalic fold can result not only in an omphalocele of the upper abdomen but also defects in the diaphragm and pericardium, and even displacement of the heart. Caudal fold omphaloceles can be associated with persistent cloacal complexes and bladder exstrophy.

Gastroschisis

During the 5th week postconception, shortly after the body folds mentioned above normally form the umbilical ring, the lengthening intestine migrates into the proximal umbilical stalk, where further growth and development occur until the intestine's return to the peritoneal cavity by the end of the 10th embryonic week. Failure of the intestine to return to the abdominal cavity has been viewed as the basis for congenital umbilical hernia, often

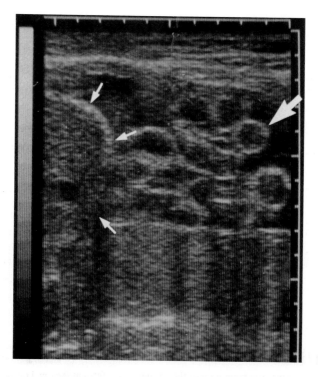

Figure 12-2 Gastroschisis in the third trimester presents this picture of free-floating loops of small bowel (large arrow) within amniotic fluid, and minimal disruption or distortion of the fetal abdominal wall contour (small arrows). *Source*: Reprinted from *Practical Obstetrical Ultrasound* (p 137) by JW Seeds and RC Cefalo, Aspen Publishers Inc, © 1986.

associated with malrotation. Defective migration into the umbilical stalk due to unknown causes has been proposed as one possible explanation for gastroschisis. A rupture at the base of the umbilicus, possibly related to concurrent involution of the right umbilical vein, might allow the herniation of the small intestine through a defect.

CLINICAL PRESENTATION

Clinical Signs and Symptoms

Neither omphalocele nor gastroschisis results in clinical abnormalities in early pregnancy. No change in fundal growth or maternal clinical physiology is typically noted prior to 28 weeks' gestation. Later in pregnancy, uterine size might be large or small for dates. In the case of gastroschisis, associated bowel atresias or torsion of entrapped bowel may result in fetal malabsorption of amniotic fluid and subsequent polyhydramnios and increased uterine size for dates. Conversely, in the absence of such a bowel obstruction and polyhydramnios, the fetal growth retardation often noted in association with gastroschisis may result in a fundal height less than expected for a given gestational age. It is likely that fewer than one third of cases will come to clinical attention because of abnormalities of uterine height.

Maternal Serum Alpha-Fetoprotein Screening

Maternal serum alpha-fetoprotein (MSAFP) screening offers promise for the early detection of pregnancies complicated by ventral wall defects. Approximately three out of four cases of ventral wall malformations will result in an elevated MSAFP. The elevation of MSAFP is likely related to the high levels of alpha-fetoprotein in fetal peritoneal fluid and the transudation or leakage of alpha-fetoprotein into the amniotic fluid. The sensitivity of MSAFP screening appears to be somewhat higher for gastroschisis than for omphalocele, probably because of the more direct leakage of peritoneal contents through the wall defect.

High-resolution ultrasound is able to detect and characterize the large majority of cases of either malformation. A few cases of both omphalocele and gastroschisis, though, are sufficiently small to escape sonographic detection.

Routine Ultrasound Screening

Routine screening of prenatal patients with ultrasound or ultrasound examination for other unrelated indications will result in the detection of a majority of cases of ventral wall defects. The sensitivity of ultrasound screening for ventral wall defects in a low-risk population, however, depends on the skill and experience of the operator as well as methodical attention to detail. The sensitivity of the technique will be higher in the case of a high-risk patient population examined by an operator with significant experience in searching for anomalies than in the case of a low-risk population examined for other reasons by a clinician not experienced in the diagnosis of malformations.

Careful imaging of the fetal umbilical insertion site (Figures 12-3 and 12-4) is a critical step in sensitive screening for these malformations. An omphalocele, even a small one, is essentially a malformation of the umbilical insertion. The result can be an obvious soft tissue mass extending from the lower anterior midline of the fetal abdomen (Figure 12-5), or simply a small soft tissue bulge of the proximal umbilical cord (Figure 12-6). The early appearance of gastroschisis is not obviously distinct from that of omphalocele,

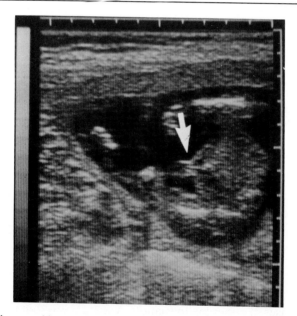

Figure 12-3 The normal fetus, on transverse scan at the umbilicus, looks like this. The umbilical attachment (arrow) is sharp, clean, and easily seen. *Source*: Reprinted from *Practical Obstetrical Ultrasound* (p 42) by JW Seeds and RC Cefalo, Aspen Publishers Inc, © 1986.

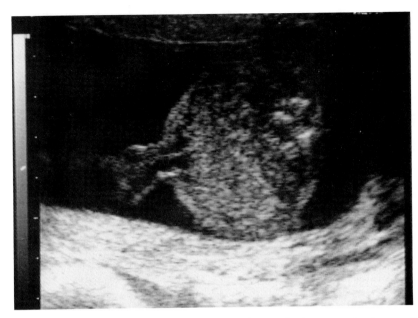

Figure 12-4   Later in gestation, the umbilical attachment site is even easier to see with ultrasound, as shown here.

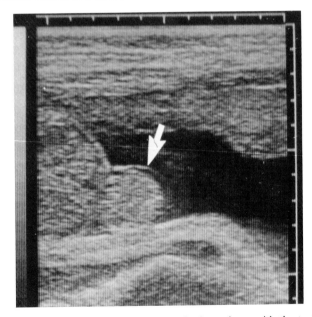

Figure 12-5   An omphalocele in early pregnancy is shown here, with the typical covering membrane (arrow). Note that the membrane is not seen in the vertical dimension due to its simple structure.

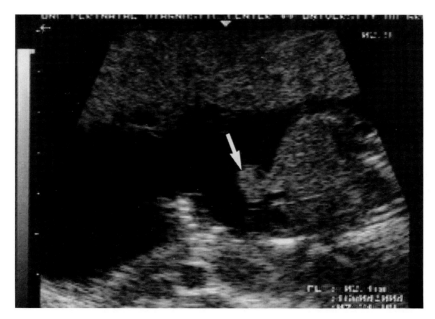

Figure 12-6 The omphalocele shown here (arrow) is very small, and remained small throughout pregnancy. The karyotype was normal, no other anomalies were found, and neonatal repair was successful. Despite the small size, the potential for associated anomalies and aneuploidy is unchanged.

---

because the bowel often assumes a rather discrete shape (Figure 12-7), similar to omphalocele but without the covering membrane. Furthermore, in the case of omphalocele, the abdominal wall contour is distorted, and there is no separate umbilical insertion. With gastroschisis, on the other hand, the umbilical insertion site can usually be seen.

Typically, the appearance of omphalocele does not change with the growth and development of the fetus. The mass late in pregnancy is similar to the mass in early pregnancy, changed only by the normal growth expected. Gastroschisis, on the other hand, often changes its appearance dramatically with advancing gestational age. Early in gestation bowel dilatation is rare, and the bowel wall appears thin and unremarkable (Figure 12-8). However, between 24 and 28 weeks in most cases, perhaps as a result of increasing oncotic tonicity of the amniotic fluid, a typical subserosal inflammatory reaction occurs in the extracelomic bowel that results in thickening of the bowel wall and a characteristic rough or fluffy appearance (Figure 12-9). This inflammatory response also often results in a matting together of the external bowel and even functional obstruction and proximal dilatation. Late in gestation the appearance of two or more populations of external bowel of significantly different caliber may be an indication for delivery (Figure 12-10).

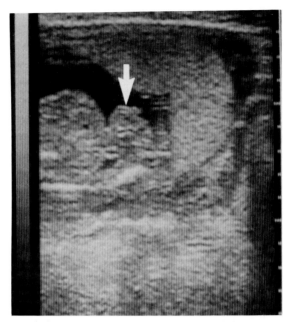

Figure 12-7 Early in gestation, the herniated loops of small bowel in the case of gastroschisis shown here may simulate an omphalocele, because they are grouped closely together. No membrane, however, is seen. *Source*: Reprinted from *Practical Obstetrical Ultrasound* (p 136) by JW Seeds and RC Cefalo, Aspen Publishers Inc, © 1986.

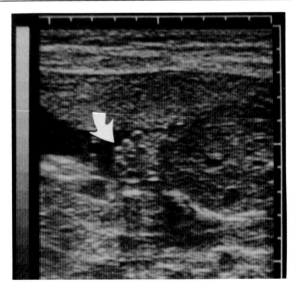

Figure 12-8 Even by 24 weeks' gestation, the caliber of the external small intestine is unremarkable, as the inflammatory reaction has not yet occurred. The small bowel here (arrow) is not inflamed.

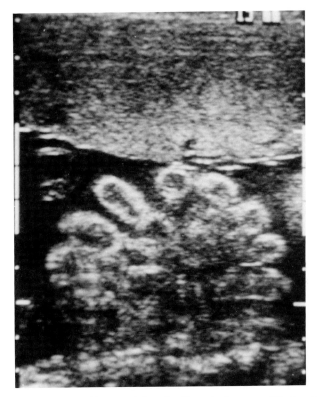

Figure 12-9   By 32 weeks, and in many infants by 28 weeks, because of the increasing osmolar tonicity of the amniotic fluid, a subserosal inflammation occurs in the external bowel that causes thickening and a fuzzy appearance on scan, as seen here.

CLINICAL IMPLICATIONS OF DIAGNOSIS

It is of more than academic interest to discriminate gastroschisis from omphalocele. The rate of aneuploidy associated with omphalocele varies widely but appears to be at least 30%. Other major associated anomalies have been reported to accompany 40% to 70% of cases of omphalocele. These include aneuploidy, genetic syndromes, midline defects, and cardiac defects. In contrast, gastroschisis is not associated with any increase in the probability of aneuploidy, and only a modest increase in the probability of other structural defects. The detection of a ventral wall defect, therefore, should include a careful evaluation to discriminate these two possible diagnoses.

If during the sonographic examination of a fetus, a low ventral midline soft tissue mass is discovered, there is a discrete covering membrane, the abdomi-

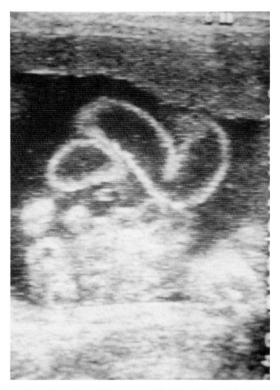

Figure 12-10 Obstruction of portions of the externalized small bowel in the case of gastroschisis can occur either because of the inflammatory reaction described above or due to secondary or associated atresias. The dilated bowel shown here is such a case.

nal wall contour is seen to be lost, and the umbilical cord is seen to attach to the midline mass, omphalocele may be confidently diagnosed. A careful search for other malformations, including neural tube defects, cardiac defects, gastrointestinal obstructions, and genitourinary defects, should be immediately undertaken. Fetal karyotype analysis should be offered by the most appropriate method. In the case of omphalocele with no other associated malformations and a normal karyotype, the prognosis can be very good, but it must be remembered that unseen anatomic defects may await delivery for detection. It is appropriate to be optimistic if a careful search fails to detect other problems, but it is also appropriate to be honest with the patient about the limitations of ultrasound and the possibility of genetic conditions that might escape sonographic detection.

In the case of omphalocele detected in midtrimester, karyotype may be offered using amniocentesis or fetal blood sampling in order to facilitate the rapid provision of important cytogenetic information. In later pregnancy, fetal karyotype can also be useful in planning obstetrical management. In the case of the diagnosis of lethal aneuploid conditions, such as trisomy 13 or 18, obstetrical management most often can focus on maternal welfare. However, if the fetal karyotype is normal and a careful search reveals no other malformations, management decisions must be based on the assumption of neonatal salvage, repair, and survival.

If the ultrasound examination shows free-floating loops of small bowel in the amniotic cavity with no covering membrane (Figure 12-11), and a normal umbilical insertion can be found nearby, gastroschisis is the most likely diagnosis. Fetal karyotype is not considered necessary if the diagnosis is confident and based on optimal sonographic observations, but a detailed sonographic examination of the heart and abdomen is indicated. Some intracardiac defects have been reported in association with gastroschisis as well as bowel atresias and other obstructions.

CLINICAL MANAGEMENT

Careful attention to uterine growth and serial ultrasound monitoring of amniotic fluid volume and fetal growth are basic elements of appropriate prenatal care of a pregnancy complicated by a fetal ventral wall defect. Fetal

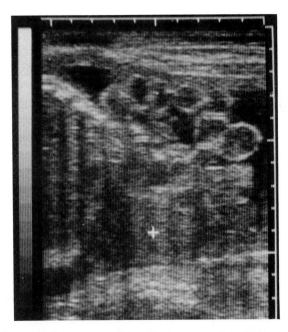

Figure 12-11 This typical appearance of free-floating loops of small bowel outside the fetal abdomen should lead to the diagnosis of gastroschisis.

bowel obstruction, either from atresia, torsion, or compression, can lead to polyhydramnios, preterm labor, and perinatal loss if not detected early. Prematurity is a leading cause of perinatal loss in most reports. If bed rest is not sufficient to prolong pregnancy in such a case, consideration might be given to tocolysis or even therapeutic amniocentesis. Serial ultrasound evaluations at no less than 2-week intervals can be helpful in the early detection of fetal bowel obstruction or abnormalities of fetal growth. Intrauterine growth retardation complicates about 20% of cases of omphalocele and up to 70% of cases of gastroschisis. This association supports the thesis that in the normal case, fetal bowel absorption contributes significantly to fetal nutrition.

ROUTE AND TIMING OF DELIVERY

In general, in either type of ventral wall defect, the older, larger, and more mature a baby is at birth, the better the prognosis for successful repair and survival. Premature labor and premature birth unfortunately complicate many cases, due in large part to polyhydramnios.

Some observers have suggested that sonographic surveillance of gastroschisis is beneficial to detect the development of the serosal inflammation and matting of the bowel as an indication for early delivery, but this is controversial.

Although it seems reasonable to assume that abdominal delivery might reduce the risk of trauma to exposed viscera in the case of ventral wall defects, few reports support cesarean as a beneficial method of delivery by itself. There is some information that suggests that in the case of the large omphalocele with liver exstrophy, cesarean delivery improves survival, but no evidence exists supporting abdominal delivery of the baby with gastroschisis for other than obstetrical indications unless obstruction and dilatation are noted.

CARE FOLLOWING PRENATAL DIAGNOSIS

A careful search for major associated anomalies, including establishing fetal karyotype, is usually performed following the detection of a ventral abdominal wall defect. A chromosomal abnormality or multiple fetal anomalies may significantly influence parental decisions regarding pregnancy termination prior to viability or may alter the course of obstetrical management in the last trimester. A fetus with a giant omphalocele and no other detectable anomalies has an excellent prognosis with surgical correction and would likely be delivered by cesarean section to minimize trauma to the liver. On the other hand, the parents may opt for pregnancy termination when the fetus has a lethal trisomy 13 detected before the 20th week of gestation. In addition, vaginal delivery may be the most appropriate mode of delivery of such an infant during the last trimester.

The role of the pediatric surgeon as discussed in Chapter 5 is important in the prenatal counseling of parents. Based on the type and extent of the abdominal wall defect and associated anomalies, the surgeon should portray what the parents can realistically expect as far as prognosis and long-term quality of life are concerned. The timing and nature of medical or surgical interventions along with major risks and complications should be discussed with the parents. The excellent prognosis for infants with either gastroschisis or isolated omphalocele needs to be emphasized. This is an excellent opportunity for the surgeon and parents to establish a meaningful relationship well before the emotional and physical turmoil of the delivery. Although prenatal counseling does not eliminate parental anxiety and feelings of helplessness, it does provide the parents with important information and time that allow them to begin to cope with this stress prior to the perinatal period.

Clinical Presentations

As described above, the infant born with gastroschisis has eviscerated small and often large bowel herniated through a defect in the abdominal wall, which usually lies just to the right of the umbilicus. In contrast to the omphalocele, there is no amniotic peritoneal sac covering the exposed viscera. The liver is always situated in the abdominal cavity, although the testes or ovaries and fallopian tubes may be found outside the abdominal cavity. The bowel typically appears thickened, edematous, and foreshortened secondary to the chemical peritonitis of the intrauterine exposure to amniotic fluid (Figure 12-12). Approximately 15% of these children have associated intestinal atresias that are most likely related to intrauterine mesenteric vascular accidents. In addition, all infants with gastroschisis have intestinal malrotation because normal midgut rotation (see the embryology discussion in Chapter 11) is prevented by the intestinal herniation.

Prematurity has been reported in as high as 60% of this population of children and has been attributed to a number of factors, including maternal polyhydramnios. In addition, a large proportion (70%) will be very small for gestational age, presumably because there is interference of amniotic fluid absorption from the immotile fetal gut. In animal studies fetal amniotic fluid ingestion and absorption may account for up to 15% of fetal growth.

The infant with the omphalocele has a somewhat different appearance in that the viscera that lie outside the abdominal cavity are covered by a two-layer membrane consisting of peritoneum and amnion. In the typical central omphalocele where the lateral abdominal folds have improperly developed, liver, spleen, and intestines are commonly found in the sac. In some cases

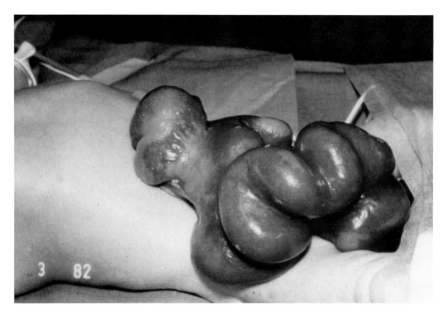

Figure 12-12   The bowel of this neonate with gastroschisis is edematous and inflamed due to chronic intrauterine exposure to amniotic fluid.

virtually all of the liver mass and intestines are located within the sac, creating a tremendous abdominal-visceral disproportion (Figure 12-13). If failure of the cephalic abdominal fold has occurred, then an omphalocele may also include an associated sternal defect, severe cardiac defects, and diaphragmatic and pericardial defects. This constellation of defects is known as the pentalogy of Cantrell (Figure 12-14). If the caudal abdominal fold has not properly developed, cloacal exstrophy and omphalocele coexist. In cloacal exstrophy there is a failure of hindgut development associated with imperforate anus and emptying of the distal ileum into the exstrophied bladder (vesicointestinal fissure; Figure 12-15). Other major genitourinary and craniospinal defects have been associated with this entity.

As stated earlier in this chapter, up to 70% of infants with omphaloceles will have significant additional anomalies, including major chromosomal anomalies in 30% to 40%. Prenatal diagnostic information, such as karyotype and detection of additional anomalies, is very helpful to the neonatology and surgical teams managing the infant after birth. However, even if karyotype is normal, a careful postnatal survey of the infant for additional anomalies, particularly cardiac anomalies, undetected antenatally is necessary. For example, omphalocele may be a somatic component of the Beckwith-Wiedeman syndrome, which is characterized by severe hypoglycemia and visceral macrosomia and is not detectable antenatally.

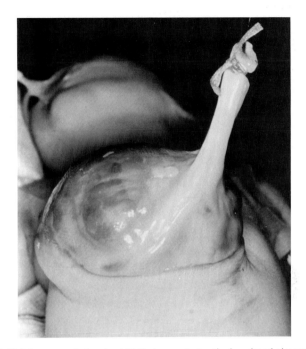

Figure 12-13 This large omphalocele at birth demonstrates the herniated viscera covered by a thin membrane.

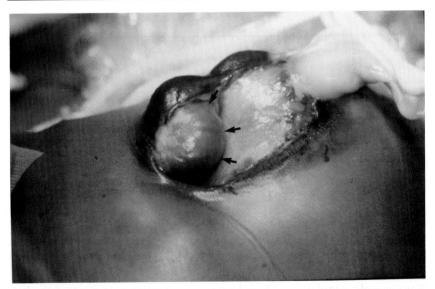

Figure 12-14 This neonate had the classic pentad of Cantrell's pentalogy, including epigastric omphalocele, cardiac anomalies, and sternal, diaphragmatic, and pericardial defects. Here, the heart is seen (arrows) protruding through the abdominal wall defect.

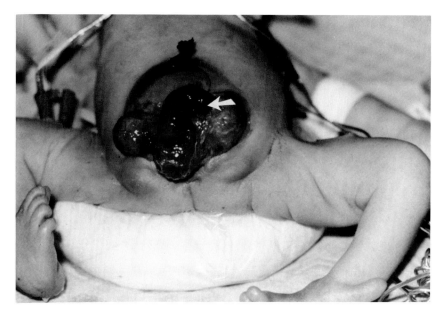

Figure 12-15 Cloacal exstrophy in a neonate. The exposed bladder halves are separated by a ridge of prolapsed terminal ileum and cecal tissue (arrow). Omphalocele and imperforate anus accompany the bladder and intestinal anomalies.

Occasionally infants are born with the omphalocele membrane ruptured before or during delivery. There is usually a sac remnant, which allows the clinician to distinguish these infants from those with gastroschisis (Figure 12-16). However, the initial management of these infants is exactly the same.

Initial Stabilization

Initial management can be broken down into five major areas: (1) protection of the exposed viscera or sac with moist and sterile dressings; (2) prevention of mesenteric vascular or caval obstruction by ensuring that the exposed viscera or sac is not twisted or kinked (the infant should be placed in the right lateral decubitus position to take the weight off the diaphragm and prevent traction on the bowel or liver); (3) prevention of evaporative heat loss by enclosing the lower two thirds of the baby's body in a sterile plastic intestinal bag (Figure 12-17); (4) intestinal decompression with an orogastric tube, preferably a 10 French Replogle sump tube, to prevent aspiration and intestinal distention; and (5) preservation of intravascular volume with intravenous cannulation and hydration.

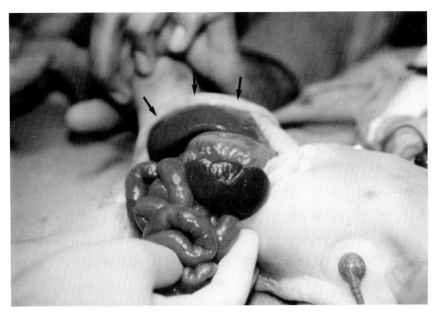

Figure 12-16 This infant had a ruptured omphalocele at term. The omphalocele membrane (arrows) is partially separated from the abdominal wall, exposing the viscera. The intestines are edematous and inflamed, as is also seen with gastroschisis.

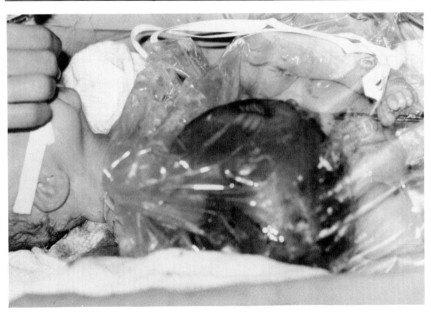

Figure 12-17 Here a sterile plastic intestinal bag is used to protect the viscera of an infant born with a large abdominal wall defect. These bags prevent heat loss and desiccation of the viscera.

The infant with the gastroschisis or the ruptured omphalocele has a large surface area of inflamed intestine, which leads to rapid fluid and heat losses. These infants are particularly predisposed to severe hypovolemic shock, with attendant complications of poor perfusion. They may require initial bolus doses of lactated Ringer's solution, 20 mL/kg, and require intravenous fluids at up to 3 to 4 times normal maintenance rates to maintain euvolia. Urine output measured at 1.5 to 2 mL/kg/h is indicative of satisfactory resuscitation. Infants with intact omphaloceles usually do not have the same massive fluid requirements and may only require maintenance fluid volumes.

In both conditions, blood cultures are taken and such antibiotics as ampicillin and gentamicin are administered. Definitive postnatal management needs to be carried out in a tertiary care setting with a multidisciplinary team of pediatric surgeons, neonatologists, and pediatric anesthesiologists.

Definitive Surgical Treatment

Infants with gastroschisis and ruptured omphalocele require relatively urgent surgical repair; however, preoperative stabilization of the infant's fluid status is crucial for the safe delivery of anesthesia. After appropriate stabilization, approximately 60% to 75% of these infants can be repaired by primary closure (Figure 12-18). The limitations of primary closure include high intra-abdominal pressure, which interferes with effective ventilation

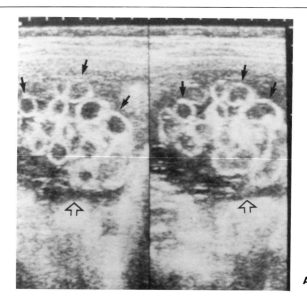

A

Figure 12-18 A, Antenatal sonography showing gastroschisis in a 30-week fetus. Note the echogenic fluid-filled bowel loops (small arrows) and the relatively intact abdominal wall (open arrow). **B,** The same infant at birth. In this photograph, an exposed testis is seen (arrow). **C,** Several months following primary repair of the infant shown above, the excellent result is evident.

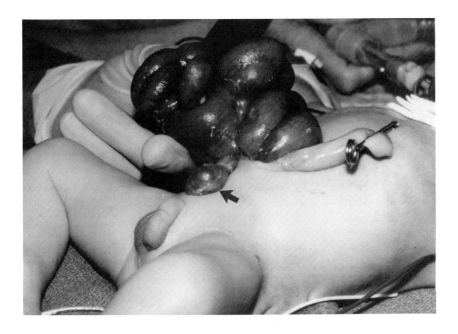

B

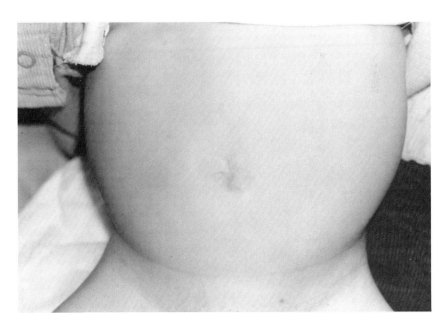

C

and impedes intestinal or renal perfusion. In some cases, although a primary closure has been performed, the infant will manifest acidosis, poor urine output, and hypoventilation. In these circumstances the abdomen should be reopened; otherwise, intestinal infarction and death may result. Those infants who cannot be closed primarily are repaired in stages, with construction of a prosthetic Silastic pouch sutured to the fascia to house the viscera (Figure 12-19). Over several days the intestines are sequentially reduced back into the abdominal cavity. The measurement of intra-abdominal pressures and the clinical status of the infant help guide the rapidity with which the viscera are reduced and the timing of subsequent closure of the abdominal wall. These infants require intensive monitoring and often need a period of postoperative ventilatory support. Total parenteral nutrition is important for survival until gastrointestinal function returns.

Although the primary closure of small- or medium-sized omphaloceles is quite feasible, the infant with a large, intact omphalocele with a herniated globe-shaped liver provides a tremendous clinical challenge (Figure 12-20A and 12-20B). In these patients primary closure is impossible, and misguided,

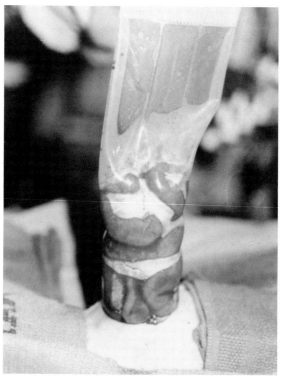

Figure 12-19 This Silastic hood, sutured to the fascia, is used to protect the intestinal viscera for several days until the abdominal cavity can accommodate the intestines.

excessively vigorous attempts at primary closure are associated with visceral injury and circulatory collapse, respiratory distress, and intestinal infarction. As in the gastroschisis infant, staged closure with prosthetic Silastic materials has provided the most successful method of handling even the most difficult patients (Figure 12-20C). Even following staged reduction, there may be a residual ventral hernia that is best dealt with when the child is older and the abdominal cavity is significantly larger. Infants with large defects may need a longer interval of time between the placement of the silo and successful closure of the abdominal wall (Figure 12-20D). As time passes, there is an increased chance of infection, with separation of the silo from the abdominal wall. Other techniques are also available, including extensive mobilization of the lateral abdominal flank skin to cover these defects (Figure 12-20E).

Nonoperative management of intact omphaloceles using 0.5% solutions of alcohol or mercurochrome have been applied to infants who have other life-threatening anomalies that take priority over the omphalocele repair, or for infants with lethal anomalies such as trisomy 13. Nonoperative techniques are associated with a 35% to 40% mortality, primarily due to associated anomalies. Recently the mercurochrome technique has fallen into disfavor and is now infrequently used because of the significant incidence of mercury poisoning in these patients.

Prognosis

Currently approximately 95% of infants with gastroschisis survive to lead normal lives without permanent disabilities. Prior to the advent of TPN many of these infants died from malnutrition and sepsis due to prolonged intestinal dysfunction. Chemical serositis of the intestine, mentioned above, leaves the bowel edematous, thickened, and with poor motility. Weeks may go by before the infant can tolerate any enteral feedings. Furthermore, some of these infants may have extensive intestinal losses as a result of atresias or postnatal intestinal ischemic necrosis. With prolonged TPN, adequate adaptation of the intestinal tract in many of these children is possible.

The prognosis of the infant with omphalocele primarily depends on the extent of associated anomalies. Infants with lethal chromosomal defects, severe cardiac anomalies, or pulmonary hypoplasia usually do not survive. The overall survival rate among infants with omphalocele is approximately 70%. Once closure of the omphalocele has been achieved in the infant with no other major defects, long-term problem-free survival is the rule. Even children born with a giant omphalocele, with its severely restricted peritoneal area and eviscerated globular liver, are likely to survive.

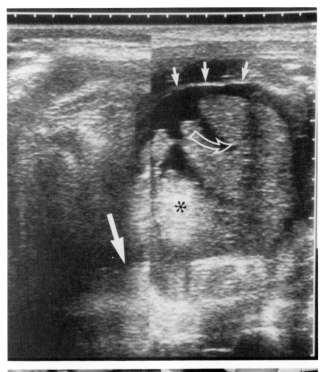

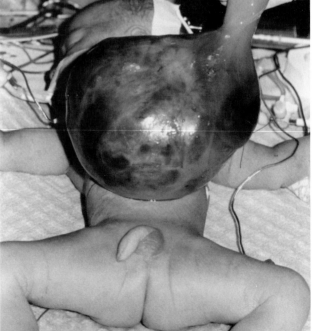

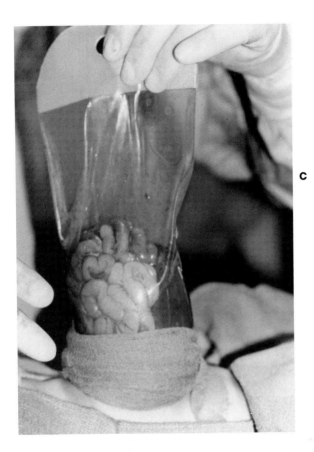

C

Figure 12-20 A, This prenatal sonogram of a fetus at 30 weeks' gestation shows a large omphalocele (small white arrows). The globular liver is evident (open arrow), and the intestines are seen within the sac (asterisk). **B**, Following cesarean delivery, the infant with a giant omphalocele presents a tremendous clinical challenge. **C**, The Silastic silo seen here was used to protect the liver and intestines while they were slowly squeezed into the abdominal cavity. **D**, Two weeks after beginning treatment, the bowel and liver are almost completely within the abdomen. The base of the silo is separating from the fascia (black arrows) due to infection and increased intra-abdominal pressure. **E**, Lateral abdominal releasing incisions (arrows) were used to mobilize adequate skin and subcutaneous tissue to cover the liver. A residual ventral hernia will be closed at a later date. ▶

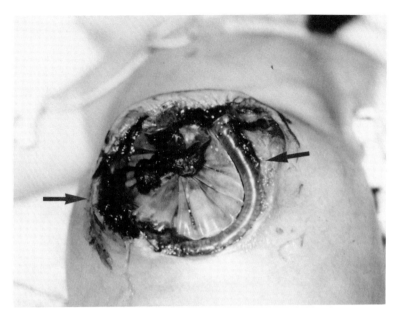

D

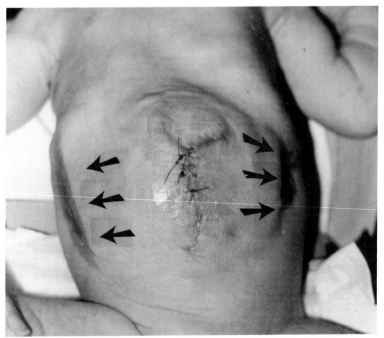

E

FURTHER READING

Cantrell JR, Haller JA, Ravitch MM. A syndrome of congenital defects involving the abdominal wall, sternum, diaphragm, pericardium and heart. *Surg Gynecol Obstet.* 1958; 107:602.

Carpenter MW, Curci MR, Dibbins AW, Haddow JE. Perinatal management of ventral wall defects. *Obstet Gynecol.* 1984; 64:646.

Filston HC. Gastroschisis—Primary fascial closure. The goal for optimal treatment. *Ann Surg.* 1983; 197:260.

Kirk EP, Wah RM. Obstetric management of the fetus with omphalocele or gastroschisis: A review and report of one hundred twelve cases. *Am J Obstet Gynecol.* 1983; 146:512.

Mayer T, Black R, Matlak ME, Johnson DG. Gastroschisis and omphalocele. An eight year review. *Ann Surg.* 1980; 192:783.

Schaffer RM, Barone C, Friedman AP. The ultrasonographic spectrum of fetal omphalocele. *J Ultrasound Med.* 1983; 2:219.

Schuster SR. A new method for the staged repair of large omphaloceles. *Surg Gynecol Obstet.* 1967; 125:837.

Sukarochana K, Sieber WK. Vesicointestinal fissure revisited. *J Pediatr Surg.* 1978; 13:713.

Chapter 13

Urinary Tract Malformations

EARLY DEVELOPMENT

The permanent fetal kidneys begin to develop in the 5th week of embryonic life in the form of a metanephric bud growing out of the mesonephric duct into metanephric mesoderm. The metanephric bud, through successive branching, gives rise to the renal pelvis, calices, and collecting tubules and induces formation from the metanephric mesoderm of the metanephric tubules, which eventually give rise to the glomeruli and the proximal and distal convoluted tubules. The distal convoluted tubule must contact and become confluent with a collecting tubule for the system to become functional. Failure of the metanephric bud to form at all gives rise to renal agenesis, and failure of the distal convoluted tubule to become confluent with a collecting tubule results in congenital polycystic kidney disease.

Initially quite close together in the fetal pelvis, these early kidneys gradually rise in the abdomen and attain their normal adult position by the 9th week. Urine formation begins between 10 and 12 weeks' gestation. Between the 5th and 8th weeks, the urorectal septum separates the urogenital sinus from the rectum. The urogenital sinus is to become the urinary bladder. Early in this process, it is continuous with the allantois, which later regresses to become the urachus. Rarely, the allantois persists, giving rise to a urachal fistula or cyst; either would occur along the track from the apex of the bladder to the umbilicus. Congenital abnormalities of the urinary tract fall into the two broad categories of agenesis/dysplasia and obstructive uropathy. We review the sonographic appearance of the normal fetal urinary tract at various gestational ages, the sonographic appearance of the more common malformations, and briefly review experience with antenatal treatment of some of the obstructive uropathies.

THE NORMAL FETAL URINARY TRACT

The earliest sonographic visualization of the fetal kidneys may be made at 10 to 12 weeks using endovaginal ultrasound. The kidneys appear to be circular organs on either side of the spine in the dorsal aspect of the transabdominal scanplane. The echotexture of the kidneys is similar to that of surrounding tissues. The urinary bladder is generally not apparent at this early age. By 16 weeks' gestation, the kidneys may be visualized as echolucent compared to surrounding tissues (Figure 13-1), and the urinary bladder is almost always visible as an anechoic area in the lower anterior midline of the fetal pelvis (Figure 13-2). If not seen, repeat examination in 1 hour will usually reveal its presence. The sonographic appearance of the kidneys remains vague through the midtrimester (Figure 13-3), but with the normal fat deposition of the last trimester, the kidneys are more easily seen, as they are outlined by the typical echogenic rim of fat (Figure 13-4). Urine filling the renal pelves may or may not be apparent (Figure 13-5). By midpregnancy, the urinary bladder should almost always be seen with careful scanning. The visualization of a fetal bladder is strong evidence for the presence and functioning of fetal kidneys, although it has been reported that a fetal bladder may be found with careful scanning in the case of renal agenesis. The bladder in such a case probably contains tissue transudate only. The kidneys may be

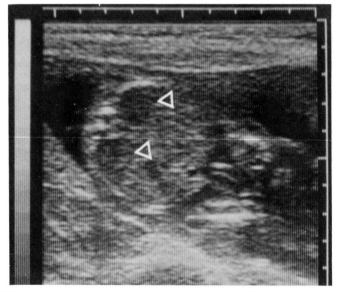

Figure 13-1 This transverse abdominal sonogram of a fetus at 16 weeks illustrates the typical appearance of fetal kidneys (triangles) at this age. *Source*: Reprinted from *Practical Obstetrical Ultrasound* (p 44) by JW Seeds and RC Cefalo, Aspen Publishers Inc, © 1986.

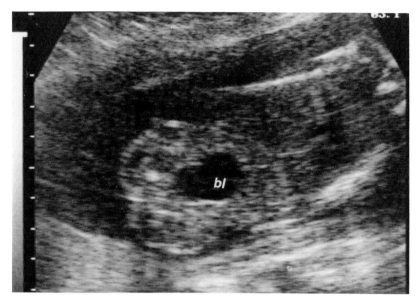

Figure 13-2   The fetal bladder (bl) shown on this coronal view of the pelvis of an 18-week fetus should always be seen with extended observation of a midtrimester fetus.

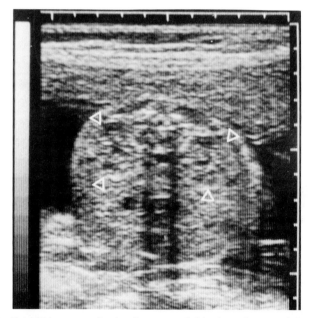

Figure 13-3   Fetal kidneys remain visually unremarkable through most of the midtrimester (triangles).

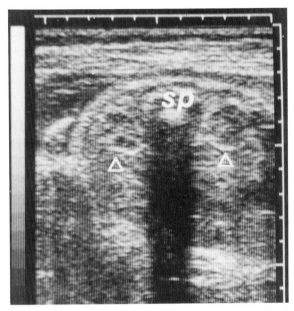

Figure 13-4 By the third trimester, fetal kidneys (triangles) are sonographically highlighted by the deposition of perirenal fat. The fetal spine (SP) casts a typical acoustic shadow.

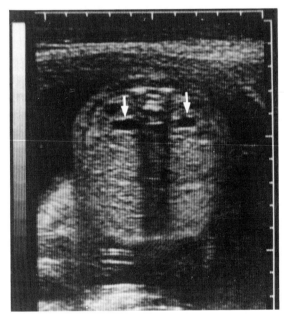

Figure 13-5 The fetal renal pelves are often visually prominent, as noted here (arrows), but are considered normal if they measure less than 5 mm.

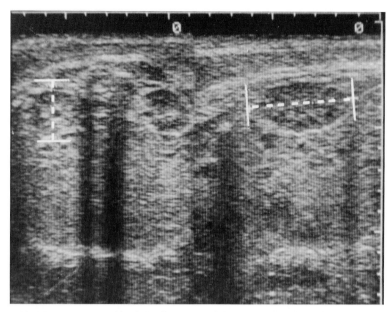

Figure 13-6 Measurement of both the diameter and the length of the fetal kidneys is illustrated here in this third trimester fetus.

measured both in their anteroposterior and longitudinal aspects (Figure 13-6). Normative data are available for judging this growth (Table 13-1), but the diagnosis of major congenital disease of the fetal kidneys rarely, if ever, depends on the detection of an anomaly of dimensions alone. In almost every case of significant congenital renal disease, there is clear visual evidence of dysfunction or anatomic malformation, such as urine accumulation above an obstruction or severe oligohydramnios. It may be useful in some cases to look at the kidney length to femur length ratio to avoid possible confusion from inaccurate gestational age data.

The urinary bladder may be measured and the volume estimated using the formula for the volume of an ellipsoid (volume = length × width × depth × 0.5233). Fetal urine output may be estimated by comparing serial estimates of volume. Experience suggests that this estimation technique actually underestimates bladder volume by about 10%, but this error should be constant, and therefore interval differences should be fairly accurate. In addition, visual estimation of amniotic fluid volume is a significant monitor of fetal urinary tract function after 18 weeks' gestational age.

Amniotic fluid is a physiologic extension of the urinary tract after 20 weeks' gestation. In early pregnancy, amniotic fluid is a product of multiple sources, including transudation across the fetal skin, cord, and membranes, but beginning with the first fetal urine production at 10 to 12 weeks, fetal urine

Table 13-1 Femur Length, Kidney Length, and FL/KL Ratio at Various Gestational Ages

Gestational Age (wks)	Femur Length (mm)	Kidney Length (mm)	Ratio
24	42	24	0.57
25	45	25	0.55
26	48	26	0.54
27	50	27	0.54
28	53	27	0.51
29	55	28	0.51
30	57	29	0.51
31	60	30	0.50
32	62	30	0.48
33	64	31	0.48
34	67	32	0.48
35	69	33	0.48
36	71	34	0.48
37	73	35	0.48
38	76	36	0.47
39	78	37	0.47
40	80	38	0.47

becomes a constituent, and if there is not a functional, patent fetal urinary tract by 20 weeks' gestation, amniotic fluid is absent. Therefore, ultrasound examination at 19 to 20 weeks showing normal amniotic fluid is strong, but not absolute, evidence for the absence of significant congenital renal disease. An important exception to this observation is congenital polycystic renal dysplasia, since several cases demonstrating normal appearance and normal amniotic fluid volume at midpregnancy have been reported.

SCREENING FOR CONGENITAL URINARY TRACT DISEASE

History of the previous birth of a child with congenital renal disease justifies referral for targeted ultrasound examination between 16 and 18 weeks' gestation. Some dysplasias and obstructive uropathies have specific recurrence patterns, and early antenatal detection offers the parents management options and referral for prepared delivery at a center ready to offer the special help many of these infants require.

Clinical screening of pregnancy in the absence of a history of the possible presence of a urinary tract malformation is primarily in the form of sensitive clinical monitoring of the growth of the uterus. Between 20 and 34 weeks, the height of the uterus in centimeters above the symphysis is approximately equal to the number of weeks of gestation (Figure 13-7). A discrepancy of 4 cm or more either greater than or less than expected suggests either an error in gestational age assignment or an abnormality of amniotic fluid volume that might relate to a urinary tract anomaly. Severe oligohydramnios may result from renal agenesis, bilateral dysplasia, or obstructive uropathy. Unrecognized rupture of membranes might also produce such an appearance (Figure 13-8). Therefore, finding a uterus significantly smaller than expected justifies performing an ultrasound examination to confirm gestational age and judge the adequacy of amniotic fluid. Polyhydramnios, as well, can result from urinary tract malformation (Figure 13-9). A ureteropelvic junction obstruction can result in extreme dilatation of the fetal renal pelvis on the affected side or the growth of a perinephric retroperitoneal urinoma. Both can cause distortion or displacement of fetal bowel, to the point of impairing normal bowel function and result in polyhydramnios. Therefore, with polyhydramnios a careful sonographic evaluation of the fetal urinary tract is in order.

Biochemical screening for urinary tract anomalies is available in the form of MSAFP screening. A significant proportion of pregnancies with elevated MSAFP will be complicated by severe oligohydramnios that is the result of fetal urinary tract malformation or dysplasia. The mechanism of the relationship is unclear, but the clinical common denominator appears to be the

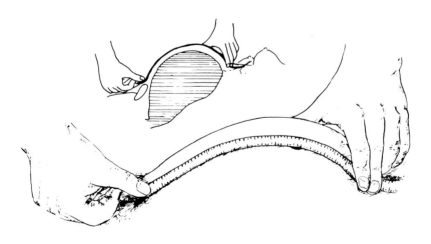

Figure 13-7 The curvilinear measurement of uterine fundal height, illustrated here, is a good clinical screen for both amniotic fluid volume and fetal growth. The fundal height in centimeters should equal gestational age in weeks, ± 4 cm. *Source:* Reprinted from *Practical Obstetrical Ultrasound* (p 90) by JW Seeds and RC Cefalo, Aspen Publishers Inc, © 1986.

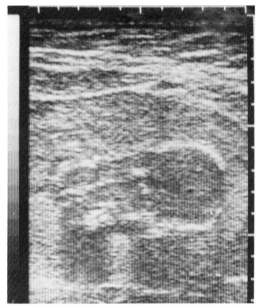

Figure 13-8 A uterus small for dates and the sonographic appearance of absent amniotic fluid seen here indicate serious urinary tract pathology or ruptured membranes and an empirically poor prognosis.

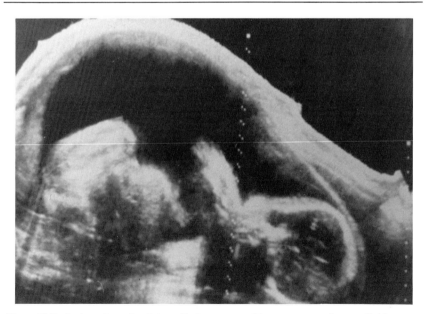

Figure 13-9 A uterus large for dates with the sonographic appearance of excess fluid, as seen here, indicates the clinical diagnosis of polyhydramnios and should lead to a careful fetal examination for malformation.

oligohydramnios. The prognosis for survival for these infants is poor, but in a significant proportion of the babies even a careful autopsy fails to reveal an anatomic abnormality.

AGENESIS

As discussed above, failure of the metanephric bud to form or failure of the outgrowth to encounter the necessary metanephric mesoderm results in renal agenesis. The incidence is about 1 to 2 per 1000, with a slight male preponderance and a recurrence risk of 3% if the first affected child is male, and possibly 10% if the first affected child is female. Diagnosis may be made by detection of a uterine fundal growth lag, elevated MSAFP, or at the time of ultrasound for other indications. At the time of ultrasound, the typical appearance after 18 weeks is that of severe oligohydramnios, extreme fetal crowding, and occasionally fetal death, probably from cord compression (Figure 13-10). Prior to 18 weeks, variable volumes of fluid may be present from sources other than fetal urine, and serial scanning is necessary to confirm the gradual loss of this fluid. Late in pregnancy, it may be difficult to distinguish a case of renal agenesis from severe oligohydramnios of other origins, such as that associated with intrauterine growth retardation or unrecognized rupture of membranes. A careful sonographic evaluation aimed at identification of kidneys or significant bladder filling is the most reliable method of confirming the diagnosis. Difficulty may be encountered, however, because the absence of fluid diminishes the clarity of the images in most cases. Adrenal hyperplasia, combined with the more globular shape of the adrenal glands in the case of renal agenesis, can create confusion and suggest the presence of kidneys on scan when in fact there are none. Furthermore, although bladder filling is good evidence for the presence of functioning kidneys, occasionally a small bladder can be seen when there is no renal function. Tissue transudate, as noted above, is presumably responsible for this.

The typical appearance of a neonate with renal agenesis is the result of prolonged growth and development in a uterus without adequate amniotic fluid. The head is brachycephalic, with flattening of the face (Figure 13-11). Distal joints appear deformed with arthrogryposis, and pulmonary hypoplasia is the rule (Figure 13-12). Neonatal death occurs shortly after birth from ventilatory failure. These characteristics result from oligohydramnios and therefore would be expected in the case of severe long-standing oligohydramnios from other causes as well. Antenatal management, if renal agenesis is confidently diagnosed, can focus on maternal welfare since neonatal survival is not possible. However, if the diagnosis cannot be confidently made, management for best fetal outcome is generally recommended. Termination of pregnancy if the diagnosis is made in early pregnancy is a possible option.

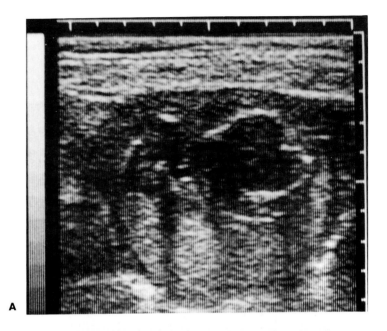

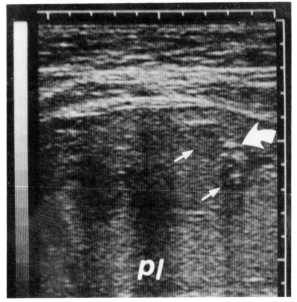

Figure 13-10 A, In the case of severe oligohydramnios in early gestation, it may be difficult to confidently establish the presence or absence of kidneys. In the fetus seen here, no kidneys were present at autopsy. *Source*: Reprinted from *Practical Obstetrical Ultrasound* (p 91) by JW Seeds and RC Cefalo, Aspen Publishers Inc, © 1986. **B,** A similar picture of severe oligohydramnios in a case of unusual aneuploidy, with an isochromosome X karyotype but with nonfunctional kidneys (small arrows) present. The fetal spine (large arrow) is to the right.

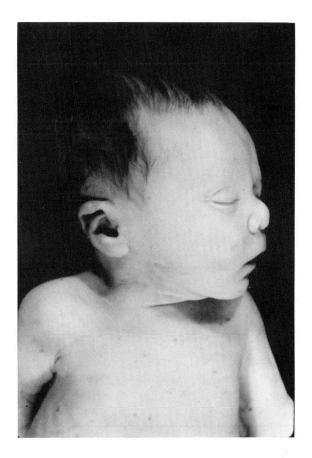

Figure 13-11 The typical Potter's syndrome appearance, with flattening of the face and nose, brachycephaly, and distal arthrogryposis.

The diagnosis of renal agenesis made late in pregnancy may be dealt with in some institutions with induction of labor, given the lethal nature of the malformation.

RENAL DYSPLASIA

Potter, in 1964, divided renal dysplasia into four categories:

1. Type I: infantile polycystic dysplasia
2. Type II: multicystic dysplasia
3. Type III: adult polycystic dysplasia
4. Type IV: secondary cystic dysplasia

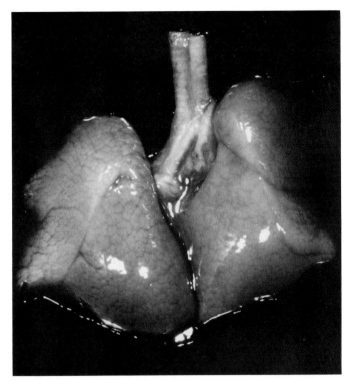

Figure 13-12 The pulmonary hypoplasia seen here and associated with renal agenesis and any condition resulting in severe, long-standing oligohydramnios is characterized by low lung weight (less than 2% of total wet body weight), and a low radial alveoli count if the fetus is born near term.

Infantile Polycystic Dysplasia

Infantile polycystic dysplasia is a very rare disorder, occurring with a frequency of about 1 in 50,000 and demonstrating an autosomal recessive Mendelian inheritance pattern with a 25% recurrence risk. The expression of the disease may result in a spectrum of renal involvement, from near total replacement with severe oligohydramnios, Potter's facies, and pulmonary hypoplasia with neonatal death, to only partial replacement with survival for variable periods and variable associated liver disease and morbidity.

The fetal kidneys appear echodense and enlarged as a result of the replacement of the parenchyma with thousands of tiny cysts (Figure 13-13). The calyces and renal pelves are normally formed. As mentioned above, polycystic dysplasia results from failure of the collecting tubules to connect to the distal convoluted tubules, with dilatation of the distal convoluted tubules creating vast numbers of microscopic cysts. Therefore, the kidneys are large

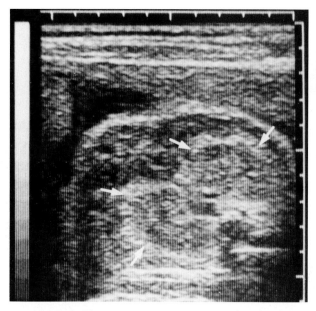

Figure 13-13 Infantile polycystic renal dysplasia seen antenatally results in enlarged, echodense kidneys as seen here (arrows), because of multiple 1- to 2-mm cysts. *Source*: Reprinted from *Practical Obstetrical Ultrasound* (p 153) by JW Seeds and RC Cefalo, Aspen Publishers Inc, © 1986.

and echodense, but shadowing is not seen. Typically both kidneys are affected throughout, but cases of partial involvement have been reported, and several cases of affected pregnancies that looked normal with normal amniotic fluid early in gestation have been reported. It is not possible, therefore, to confidently exclude polycystic dysplasia in early pregnancy. In the case of full expression of the condition, severe oligohydramnios, absent bladder filling, and the typical Potter's appearance would be expected, with failure to survive.

Multicystic Dysplasia

Multicystic dysplasia is the more common type of renal dysplasia seen in antenatal diagnosis clinics, occurring in about 0.1 to 1 in 1000 pregnancies, with a male predominance. Four fifths of these cases are unilateral, with a normal contralateral kidney, normal bladder filling, and normal amniotic fluid volume. The appearance in multicystic dysplasia is that of an enlarged kidney filled with large macroscopic anechoic cysts (Figure 13-14). These cysts are not interconnected, as in the case of severe caliectasis from distal

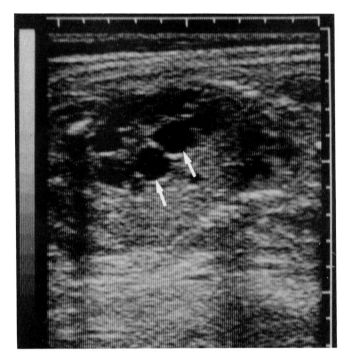

Figure 13-14 Multicystic renal dysplasia, in contrast to polycystic dysplasia, results in multiple large unconnected cystic spaces replacing the affected kidney (arrows).

obstruction, and are of variable size. The cysts will grow with time and can achieve quite large size (Figure 13-15). In about one in five cases, both kidneys are affected, with the expected result of severe oligohydramnios, absent bladder filling, and a Potter's phenotype (Figure 13-16). In the rare association of multicystic dysplasia on one side and agenesis on the other, the result is similar (Figure 13-17). Multicystic dysplasia appears to fall into a polygenic/multifactorial inheritance pattern. The recurrence risk is about 2% to 4%. Multicystic dysplasia may be seen as a part of several autosomal recessive syndromes, including Meckel's syndrome, making genetic consultation desirable in the case of the birth of an infant with this condition.

Antenatal management is not usually altered by this diagnosis. In the majority of unilateral cases, the outcome of the pregnancy is not affected by the diagnosis, although in the case of bilateral disease or agenesis on the contralateral side, the outcome is neonatal death. In the rare case, the affected kidney achieves such size as to alter the amniotic fluid equilibrium, and the result is polyhydramnios. In that case management is largely based on obstetrical considerations. The method of delivery is not altered based on this diagnosis.

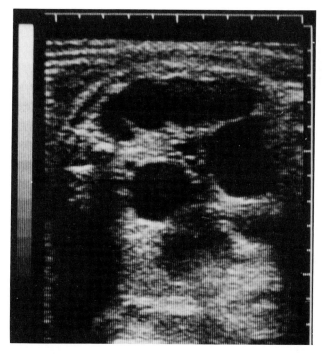

Figure 13-15   The growth of the cysts in a case of multicystic dysplasia is apparent in this sonogram performed 10 weeks after the image of Figure 13-14.

Neonatal Care of Multicystic Kidney: Management and Prognosis

The neonatal diagnosis of multicystic kidney (MCK) can be confirmed or strongly suggested by ultrasonography. An MCK does not function and has no potential for recovery. A voiding cystourethrogram (VCUG) is desirable in these patients to look for associated genitourinary anomalies such as contralateral vesicoureteral reflux and contralateral urteropelvic junction (UPJ) obstruction. A renal scan differentiates the MCK from pyelocaliectasis. A urinary catheter placed in the bladder will prevent the mimicking of function when there is associated vesicoureteral reflux. Sometimes MCK has a similar sonographic appearance to UPJ obstruction. At birth, almost all UPJ obstructions will have some functional capacity, although they can also be associated with parenchymal cysts or dysplasia. Since there is no potential for recovery, elective nephrectomy is usually recommended for these patients (Figure 13-18). The most common complication of retaining a nonfunctioning MCK is hypertension. Another rare but concerning complication is the development of malignant neoplasms in the retained kidney. To date there have been at least seven reported cases of malignant neoplasms such as

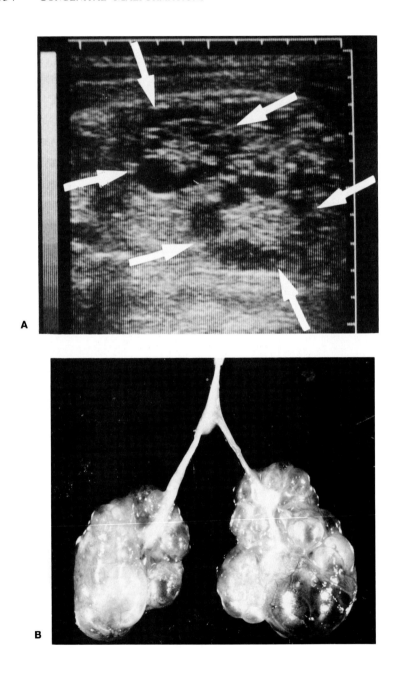

Figure 13-16 **A**, Bilateral multicystic renal dysplasia results in both kidneys (arrows) being replaced by macroscopic cysts. **B**, The kidneys of a fetus with bilateral multicystic dysplasia show the typical grapelike appearance.

Wilms' tumor in these kidneys. If there are no other associated genitourinary anomalies, the patient with a solitary MCK has an excellent prognosis.

Adult Polycystic Dysplasia

Adult polycystic dysplasia is a rare autosomal dominant cystic dysplasia that is typically not clinically apparent until adulthood, although occasional cases are reported in childhood. Antenatal diagnosis is rare but has been reported, with the antenatal appearance described as being similar to that of infantile polycystic dysplasia, with enlargement of the kidneys and echogenic parenchyma.

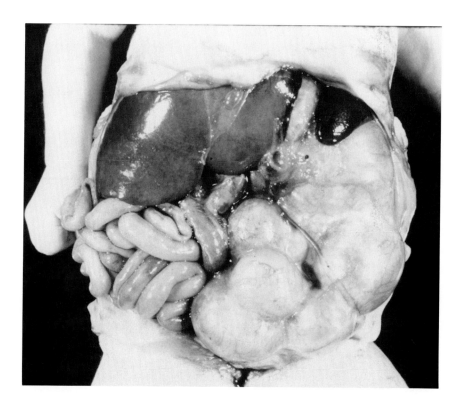

Figure 13-17 The single multicystic kidney of an infant with unilateral multicystic dysplasia and contralateral agenesis.

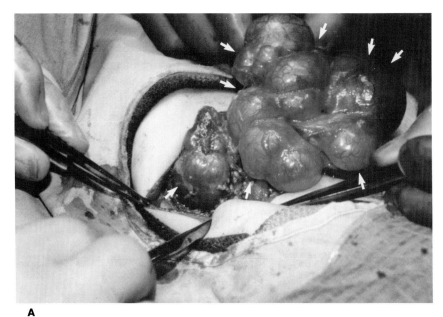

A

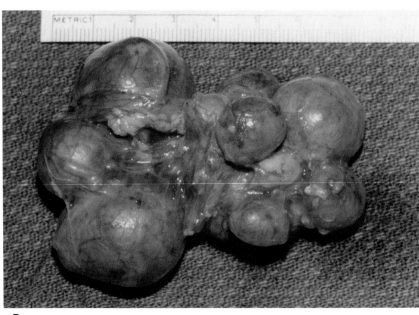

B

Figure 13-18 A, Unilateral multicystic kidney (arrows) at laparotomy. Nephrectomy and subsequent recovery were uneventful. **B,** Excised kidney from same patient.

Secondary Cystic Dysplasia

Urethral atresia primarily results in obstruction of the urinary tract. In such a case the kidneys develop a form of cystic dysplasia instead of hydronephrotic caliectasis. In early pregnancy they appear either small or normal in size, but echodense relative to the surrounding tissues instead of echolucent as would normally be the case (Figure 13-19). As pregnancy progresses, cortical cysts develop and grow to variable size (Figure 13-20). The kidneys are usually enlarged and contain subcortical cysts of variable size and location (Figure 13-21). The recurrence risk is that of the primary lesion, which is usually low.

OBSTRUCTIVE UROPATHIES

Congenital obstruction of the urinary tract may occur at the UPJ, the ureterovesicle junction, or in the urethra. Functional obstruction where no physical blockage exists is also seen, but megacystis, hydroureter, and hydronephrosis result from functional impairment of the bladder and/or urethra. Pregnancy outcome is generally governed by the volume of amniotic

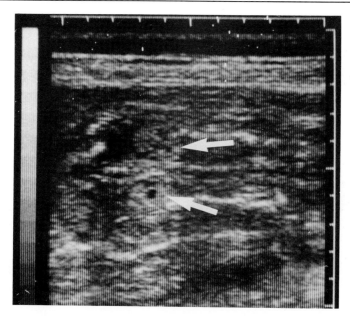

Figure 13-19 Urethral atresia is typically associated with small, echodense kidneys (arrows) that develop cystic dysplasia as gestation progresses.

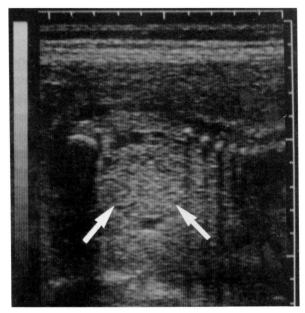

Figure 13-20 Later in gestation, the small, echodense kidneys of Figure 13-19 become enlarged (arrows), and small cysts may be seen within the parenchyma.

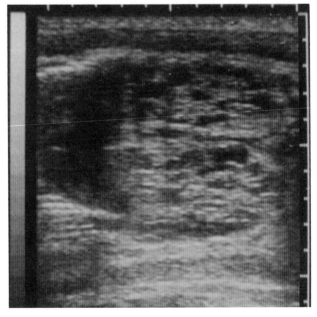

Figure 13-21 Near term, the cystic dysplastic kidney has grown large and filled with parenchymal cysts of variable size.

fluid. If the obstruction is bilateral or central and results in severe, long-standing oligohydramnios, then Potter's syndrome is likely and neonatal survival is not. If the obstruction is unilateral but results in extreme enlargement of the affected side, then polyhydramnios can result and threaten the pregnancy with prematurity. Antenatal intervention has been considered in the care of a variety of obstructive uropathies but has generally proved helpful in very few.

General Neonatal Management of Urinary Tract Obstruction

As noted above, early complete urinary tract obstruction in the fetus results in renal dysplasia, whereas obstruction later in gestation results in hydronephrosis and progressive loss of functioning nephrons. Increasing duration of obstruction and vesicoureteral reflux adversely affect developing renal parenchyma. Early relief of urinary tract obstruction in the neonate theoretically maximizes functional renal development and ultimate renal recovery. Improving the glomerular filtration rate (GFR) may ameliorate tubular dysfunction such as renal tubular acidosis, decreased concentrating ability, and sodium wasting. Recovery of GFR consistently occurs in infants less than 6 months old at the time of treatment. However, some of these children still have impaired renal acidification and maximal urinary concentrating abilities following definitive surgical treatment. Early control of vesicoureteral reflux and hypertension is also crucial for optimal recovery of renal function. Prevention of renal insufficiency also enhances the chances for appropriate somatic growth.

Ureteropelvic Junction Obstruction

Ureteropelvic junction obstruction is an uncommon but not rare malformation that may be partial or complete and is most often unilateral but may be bilateral. The prenatal sonographic appearance depends on the degree of obstruction. Mild cases of fetal renal pelvis dilatation are common and in most cases of no significance. If the sonologist measures the anteroposterior dimension of the fetal renal pelvis and finds it to be less than 5 mm, no clinical significance is indicated (Figure 13-22). If the dimension is 5 to 10 mm, then clinical significance is possible but not likely. If the fetal renal pelvis is over 10 mm in anteroposterior diameter, a clinically significant fetal UPJ obstruction is suggested, and serial observation and neonatal follow-up are indicated.

Partial obstruction at the UPJ generally causes dilatation of the renal pelvis and variable caliectasis (Figure 13-23). Complete obstruction leads to severe enlargement of the renal pelvis and progressive severe caliectasis (Figures 13-24 and 13-25). In many cases of complete or severe obstruction, a perirenal

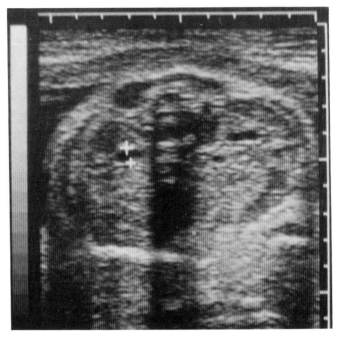

Figure 13-22 The normal fetal renal pelvis measures 5 mm or less in the anteroposterior axis, as seen here.

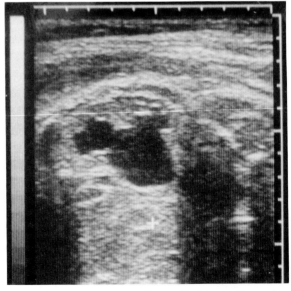

Figure 13-23 The moderate enlargement of the renal pelvis seen here, along with moderate caliectasis, indicates a significant ureteropelvic junction obstruction. In this case, the need for neonatal surgical intervention cannot be confidently predicted.

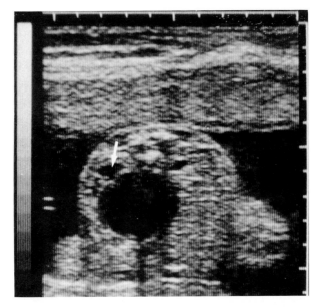

Figure 13-24 The discrete, circular, anechoic mass seen on this transverse midabdominal scan is the renal pelvis of a kidney with complete ureteropelvic junction obstruction at 24 weeks. Note the caliectasis (arrow).

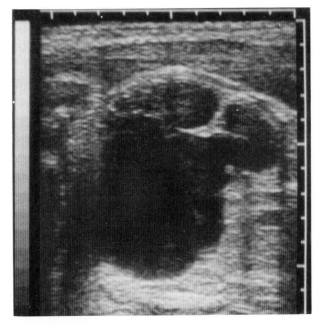

Figure 13-25 Near term, in the case of the infant in Figure 13-24, the renal pelvis and caliectasis had grown to huge proportions.

retroperitoneal urinoma is formed that may in fact be protective as a low-pressure recipient of urine from the affected kidney (Figure 13-26). These result from the progressive increase in pressure within the affected system, when a structurally weak area begins to dilate, accepting greater volumes of urine under relatively lower pressures. In general, intact survival is to be expected in the case of unilateral UPJ obstruction, whether partial or complete. In the rare case, the affected side grows to sufficient size to promote polyhydramnios on a size basis, but in general these do not alter obstetrical management (Figure 13-27). Often, the enlarged kidney is not palpable after birth, and only on neonatal ultrasound is the obstruction identified. It is important to delay the neonatal ultrasound for at least 24 to 48 hours because the profound neonatal intravascular volume shifts that normally occur immediately after delivery usually result in transient oliguria that might obscure the renal lesion.

Neonatal Care of Ureteropelvic Junction Obstruction

Congenital UPJ obstruction is the most common unilateral obstructive nephropathy in newborn children. The etiology of the majority of UPJ obstructions remains unknown. Hydronephrosis is frequently bilateral. The frequency of bilaterality approaches 25% to 30% of cases of hydronephrosis

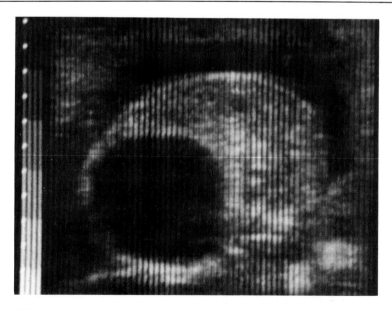

Figure 13-26 A perirenal or retroperitoneal urinoma is typically a discretely outlined anechoic mass, eccentric to the affected side and found in the dorsal midabdomen, as illustrated here. *Source*: Reprinted from *Practical Obstetrical Ultrasound* (p 145) by JW Seeds and RC Cefalo, Aspen Publishers Inc, © 1986.

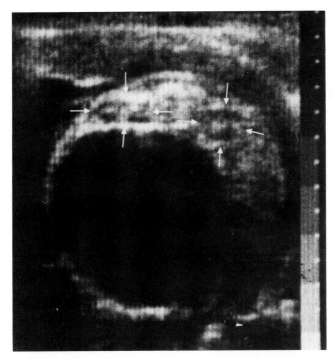

Figure 13-27 Perirenal cysts can actually be protective of the kidney on the affected side. This huge perirenal cyst was associated with preserved kidney structure and function. Both kidneys are seen on this scan (arrows).

in infants diagnosed at less than 6 months of age. There is a significant incidence of multicystic dysplasia in the contralateral kidney in these children. Clinical complications in neonates with UPJ obstruction include infection and deteriorating renal function. Up to 5% of children with hydronephrosis develop renal stones. Furthermore, hypertension is more common in infants with solitary kidney and UPJ obstruction.

Management and Prognosis

Although ultrasound and radionuclide studies are extremely useful in identifying the extent and location of the obstruction, radionuclide studies cannot predict the extent of recovery following surgical repair. If the progression of hydronephrosis or renal functional deterioration can be demonstrated by sequential diuretic renal scans or a dimercaptosuccinic acid Tc 99 scan urinary tract decompression via surgical or percutaneous techniques is indicated. When poor renal function is associated with unchanged hydronephrosis, pressure flow studies (Whitaker's test) may be indicated. If the infant is not in generally good condition, a nephrostomy catheter can be left in place. With significant obstruction, pyeloplasty is effective in relieving symptoms and resolving the radiographic features of UPJ obstruction (Figure 13-28). Pyeloplastic techniques vary with the pathological anatomy. The dismembered pyeloplasty is particularly useful when an aberrant crossing renal vessel is contributing to the obstruction (Figure 13-29A). Alternatively, a pyeloplasty in continuity is preferred when the UPJ is dependent or there is a narrowing of the upper ureter (Figure 13-29B). The anastomosis is performed with absorbable sutures with or without ureteral stents, depending on the surgeon's preference. The primary goal of management in this type of patient is preservation of total renal mass. Radiographic improvement can be seen as early as 6 months postpyeloplasty. Current reported success rates are in the range of 93% to 95%. Renal radionuclide studies have demonstrated superior functional improvement in infants with severe preoperative renal impairment. King documented that small infants had 150% improvement in renal function after relief of obstruction, compared to only 18% improvement in renal function in children older than age 5.

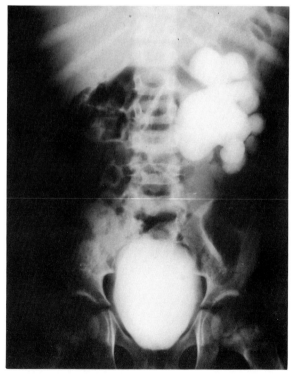

Figure 13-28 Intravenous urography demonstrates congenital unilateral ureteropelvic junction obstruction with characteristic hydronephrosis and calyceal blunting.

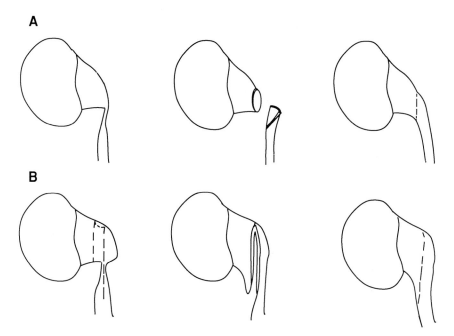

Figure 13-29 A, The upper sequence of drawings illustrates the dismembered pyeloplasty technique for the repair of ureteropelvic junction obstruction. **B**, The lower sequence of drawings shows a pyeloplasty in continuity, which is the preferred technique when the ureteropelvic junction is dependent or there is narrowing of the upper ureter. A flap based on the renal pelvis is developed to reconstruct the upper ureteral region.

Ureterovesicle Junction Obstruction

Rarely, obstruction occurs at the ureterovesicle junction. Most often unilateral, these are usually associated with duplication of the collecting system on the affected side and with the formation of a ureterocele within the bladder (Figure 13-30). The obstructed collecting system results in hydronephrosis in only one pole of the kidney (Figure 13-31). There are normal bladder filling and normal amniotic fluid volume.

Urethral Obstruction

The urethra may be obstructed primarily, as in the case of urethral atresia and the cloacal plate malformation, or secondarily, as in the case of posterior urethral valves. The appearance at birth of these various malformations may be similar, with severe distention of the fetal abdomen, respiratory failure, and neonatal death in a majority of cases. The appearance in early pregnancy,

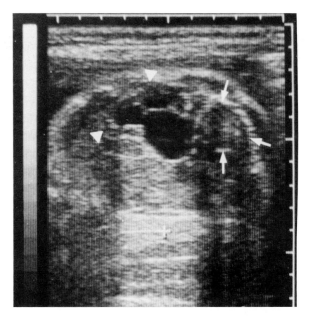

Figure 13-30 The lower pole of this kidney (triangle) is affected by hydronephrosis, while the upper pole (arrows) is not. Duplication of the collecting system was found, with ureterovesicle junction obstruction.

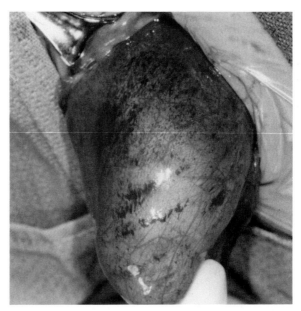

Figure 13-31 This surgical specimen represents massive hydroureter and hydronephrosis due to ureterovesicle junction obstruction.

however, is different due to the different times in gestation when these lesions become effective obstructions to the flow of urine.

Urethral Atresia

In the case of urethral atresia, early sonographic features include a large dilated bladder, ascites, diminishing amniotic fluid, and small, echodense kidneys (Figures 13-32 and 13-33).

As gestation progresses, the ascites disappears as the bladder enlarges to fill and distend the abdomen, and the amniotic fluid disappears (Figure 13-34). Later in pregnancy the kidneys begin to enlarge and are replaced by subcortical and parenchymal cysts of variable size, typical of cystic dysplasia (see discussion above of cystic dysplasia). Even technically effective efforts to divert urine from the bladder to the amniotic cavity in the case of urethral atresia have not resulted in survival. The pulmonary hypoplasia that characterizes these infants appears to be set in place in very early pregnancy, even before the loss of amniotic fluid, perhaps by distention of the abdomen and elevation of the diaphragm.

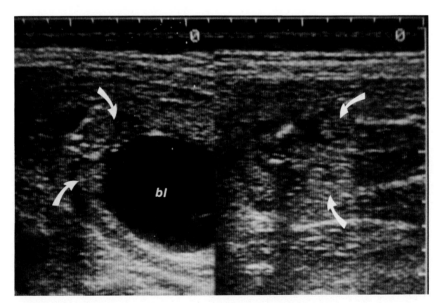

Figure 13-32 On the left side of this sonogram at 15 weeks' gestation of a fetus with urethral atresia, the large bladder (bl) and kidneys (arrows) are seen. A coronal view of the kidneys (arrows), on the right, confirms the small, echodense appearance consistent with dysplasia.

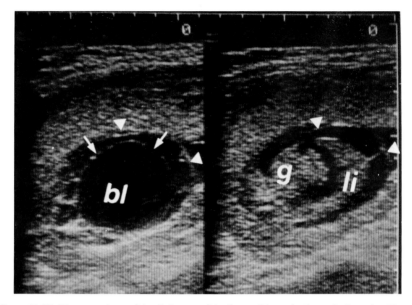

Figure 13-33 Alternate views of the abdomen of the fetus with urethral atresia show the dilated bladder (bl) within the distended fetal abdomen (triangles) and ascites. On the right side, the liver (li) and gut cluster (g) are seen within the ascites.

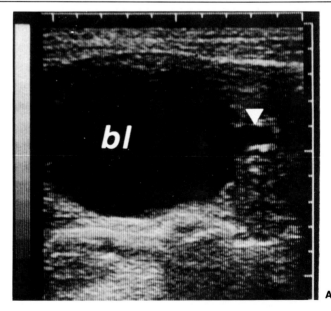

Figure 13-34 A, By 20 weeks' gestation, the bladder (bl) has grown to fill the abdomen, and the ascites is gone. The pelvic bladder (triangle) is as large as the normal fetal bladder at this age gets. **B,** This fetus with urethral atresia at 20 weeks has been irreversibly damaged, with renal agenesis and pulmonary hypoplasia.   ▶

Posterior Urethral Valves

Posterior urethral valves (PUVs) occur as a sporadic malformation almost exclusively in males. They vary in the degree of obstruction and in the gestational age at which the obstruction becomes effective. Although a few reported cases of proven valves have been discovered before 20 weeks, typically they become clinically apparent in the second half of gestation. The appearance is that of severe oligohydramnios, an extremely enlarged bladder, and enlarged, severely hydronephrotic kidneys (Figure 13-35). It is the appearance of the kidneys that sonographically differentiates this syndrome from that of urethral atresia. The hydronephrosis and caliectasis can be severe (Figure 13-36). Imaging of the enlarged bladder in the case of urethral valves may be done in a coronal or sagittal scanplane, with the posterior urethra seen only on the sagittal plane (Figure 13-37). The successful antenatal diversion of urine from the bladder of a fetus with posterior urethral valves

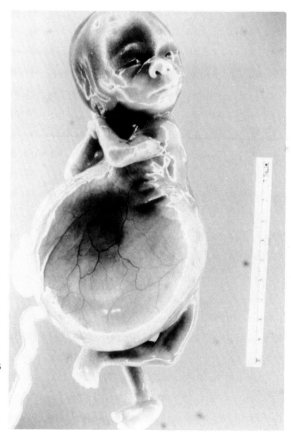

B

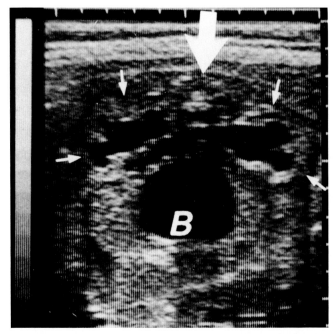

Figure 13-35 A large bladder (B) and severe hydronephrosis (arrows) are typical of posterior urethral valves discovered late in pregnancy. *Source*: Reprinted from *Practical Obstetrical Ultrasound* (p 148) by JW Seeds and RC Cefalo, Aspen Publishers Inc, © 1986.

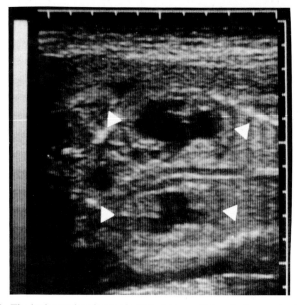

Figure 13-36 The hydronephrosis seen in these kidneys (triangles) suggests obstruction after the midpoint in gestation.

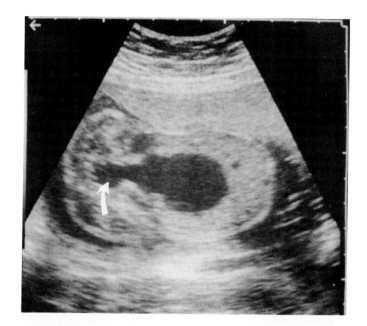

A

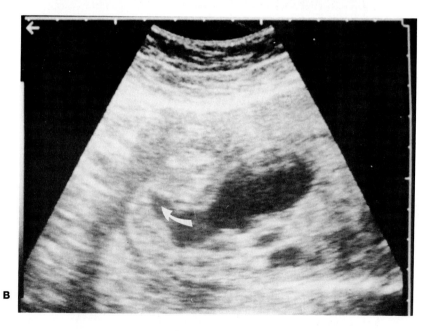

B

Figure 13-37 A, A coronal view of an obstructed bladder, with the pelvic portion to the left (arrow). This is not the posterior urethra, which is not in this plane at all. **B,** The sagittal scan of the same fetus does show the posterior urethra (arrow) extending anteriorly from the pelvic bladder.

early in the evolution of the syndrome can lead to reversal of many of the typical features and to intact survival. Late intervention is of less clear benefit.

Neonatal Care of Posterior Urethral Valves

Prevention of renal failure is the most important goal in the management of patients with PUV. The effects of intrauterine bladder outlet obstruction on renal development are progressive and depend on the length of time of effective obstruction . The high mortality that is seen for neonates with PUV is due mainly to pulmonary hypoplasia from extended development in an environment of severe oligohydramnios. Neonatal renal failure is a common feature in the survivors, and both dialysis and transplantation have been used effectively in such cases. If the GFR is less than 50% of normal for age at the time of diagnosis, chronic renal failure often occurs regardless of early relief of obstruction. Early postnatal surgical intervention favors preservation of renal mass by limiting renal injury and the development of irreversible functional changes. Preservation of renal function greater than 30% of normal during the first 2 years of life optimizes somatic growth. Loss of growth potential during this period may never be regained.

The use of prenatal ultrasound has resulted in the early diagnosis of PUV and in some cases has enabled the treatment to begin before the onset of infection, electrolyte abnormalities, and renal failure. Renal function can be roughly evaluated in utero by examining the amount of amniotic fluid present. It would be rare for a fetus with normal amniotic fluid volume to proceed to renal failure, and conversely, the fetus with severe oligohydramnios rarely does well.

Management

Following birth these infants can deteriorate rapidly, particularly those with pulmonary compromise or poor renal tubular function. The infant without antenatal diagnosis and with good pulmonary function at birth can escape detection until renal dysfunction becomes apparent. When the diagnosis has not been made, at birth infants may present with failure to thrive, associated acidosis, dehydration, and electrolyte disturbances. Although the diagnosis of PUV can be suggested by ultrasonography, a voiding cystourethrogram (VCUG) is the definitive test. It not only diagnoses the lesion but documents the presence or absence of vesicoureteral reflux (Figure 13-38). The majority of these infants benefit from placing a urethral catheter to facilitate bladder drainage. This is particularly important in infants with azotemia, dehydration, and electrolyte abnormalities or urinary tract infection. Occasionally a suprapubic cystostomy catheter is required when a urethral catheter cannot be passed. Fluid and electrolyte management can be complex in these infants. After early aggressive medical management, definitive surgical treatment should be undertaken as soon as possible.

Several operative procedures are used in treating PUV in neonates. Currently most surgeons perform either primary valve ablation or a vesicostomy and subsequent valve ablation. Although the risk of stricture is less than 1%, urinary incontinence is a frequent occurrence after valve ablation and is related to a number of other problems, including poor bladder emptying, previous bladder neck surgery, uninhibited contractions, and small bladder capacity. In the presence of infection that does not clear with bladder drainage or when renal function fails to improve after primary treatment, high urinary diversion (cutaneous pyelostomy or loop ureterostomy) have been used for renal salvage.

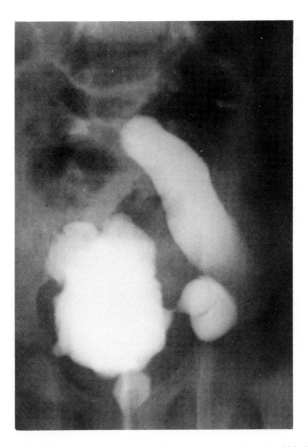

Figure 13-38 This voiding cystourethrogram demonstrates a trabeculated bladder, proximal urethral diverticulum, and severe left vesicoureteral reflux in this infant with posterior urethral valves.

CLOACAL PLATE SYNDROME

The failure of the urorectal septum to divide the urogenital sinus from the rectum is typically associated with failure of the anal and urogenital membranes to cannulate, resulting in persistence and distention of the cloaca. The result is a large anechoic mass in the lower fetal abdomen that is markedly irregular in outline due to its multisystem origin, and severe oligohydramnios (Figure 13-39). The kidneys often resemble those seen in urethral atresia in being small and echodense early in gestation and enlarged by variably sized cysts later. The prognosis for infants with this malformation is very poor, with Potter's deformities and pulmonary hypoplasia being the rule. Antenatal diversion would not be expected to improve this outcome.

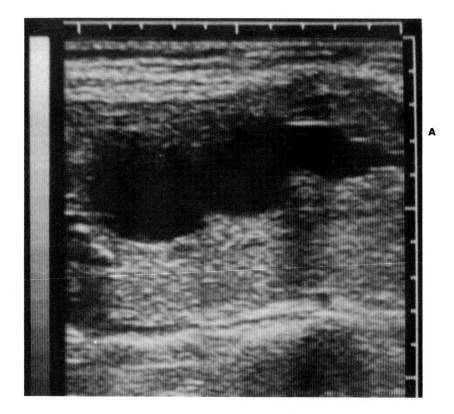

Figure 13-39 A, The irregular anechoic mass filling the abdomen of this fetus, combined with severe oligohydramnios, is characteristic of a cloacal plate malformation. **B,** Another example of the irregular anechoic mass typical of the cloacal plate syndrome. **C,** This somewhat oblique view of another fetus with a persistent cloaca (clo) again emphasizes the irregularity of the outline of the anechoic mass.

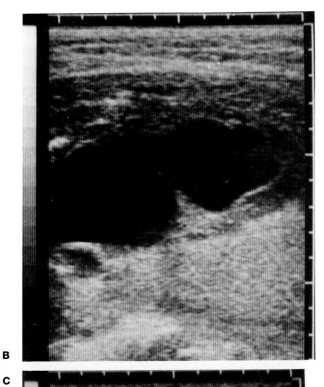

B

C

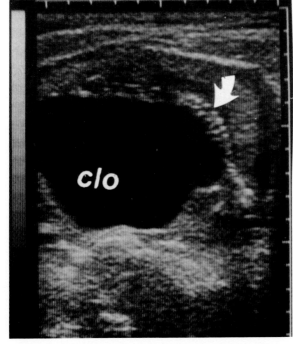

PRUNE BELLY SYNDROME

The appearance of any baby at delivery who is the victim of a bladder outlet obstruction is similar to that of the prune belly syndrome: There is an extremely distended abdomen that deflates with drainage of the bladder. The true prune belly syndrome, however, does not necessarily involve a physical obstruction of the urethra but rather a functional atony of the ureters and bladder so that urination does not occur until sufficient pressure results in overflow urination. The sonographic appearance is that of megacystis, hydroureter, and severe hydronephrosis, but amniotic fluid volume is normal or even increased (Figures 13-40) unless fetal renal failure has occurred. Hydroureter is sometimes severe (Figure 13-41). Pulmonary hypoplasia does not characterize prune belly syndrome unless oligohydramnios is present as a result of renal failure. Antenatal intervention is not indicated. Low-resistance diversion shunting would not correct the atonic dysfunction and would represent only an unneeded intervention.

Neonatal Care of Prune Belly Syndrome

The classic triad of prune belly syndrome includes a deficiency of the abdominal wall musculature combined with generalized urinary tract dilatation and undescended testes. There is a wide spectrum in this disorder, ranging from mild appearances requiring no definitive therapy to severe involvement and death in early infancy. The embryological defect that is responsible for this set of anomalies is still not known. Although the classic appearance of a severely distended neonatal abdomen that deflates to simulate the appearance of a prune often accompanies bladder outlet obstructions, obstruction is not a necessary component of this syndrome (Figure 13-42). There may be a defect in the lateral mesenchyme so that thoracic somite buds fail to differentiate into myeloblasts. These myeloblasts are responsible for the ventral and caudal migration to form the abdominal wall. Amniotic fluid volume is typically normal or increased in prune belly syndrome, although oligohydramnios does occur with some fetuses, perhaps due to terminal renal failure. In these cases pulmonary hypoplasia, orthopedic anomalies, and Potter's facies can be seen. The prognosis is not dependent on the degree of urinary tract dilatation but on the degree of renal dysplasia. The dilated bladder, renal pelves, and ureters are a result of the smooth muscle deficiency, not usually obstruction (Figure 13-43). The distal ureters are most severely affected. Typically the ureters are elongated, tortuous, and dilated, and peristalsis is ineffective. Approximately 75% of the patients will have free vesicoureteral reflux. Intravesicle pressure often is very low in these children. The bladder has an exceptionally large capacity and thickened walls, but there is no hypertrophied muscle.

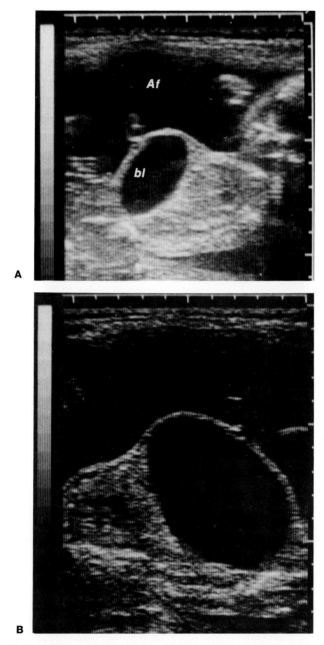

Figure 13-40 **A**, This sagittal sonogram of a fetus with prune belly syndrome at 20 weeks' gestation emphasizes the distended bladder (bl) but the presence of normal or even increased amniotic fluid (Af). **B**, Late follow-up of the fetus with prune belly syndrome shows the massively distended bladder that is possible, but again, the preservation of amniotic fluid. This fetus did very well after birth.

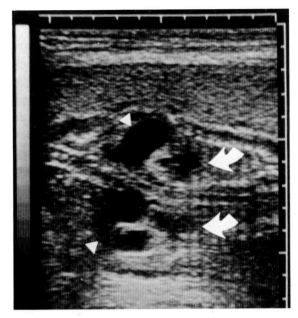

Figure 13-41 The sometimes massive hydroureter (triangles) and hydronephrosis (arrows) that accompany prune belly syndrome are shown on this coronal scan of both kidneys.

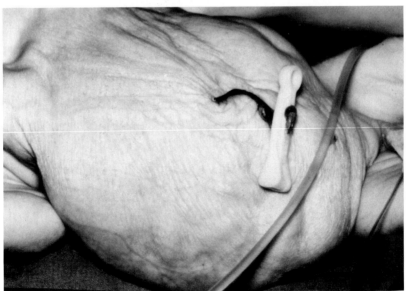

Figure 13-42 A, This newborn presents the typical appearance of prune belly syndrome. The abdominal musculature is absent, contributing to the lax appearance of the abdominal wall. **B**, The somewhat older child with prune belly syndrome. Cutaneous ureterostomies were constructed in this patient as a last resort to salvage renal function.

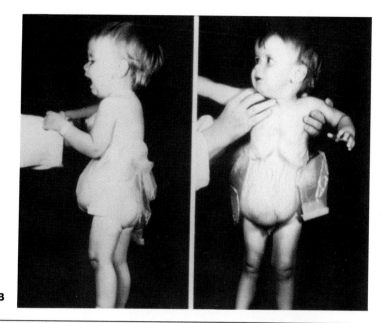

B

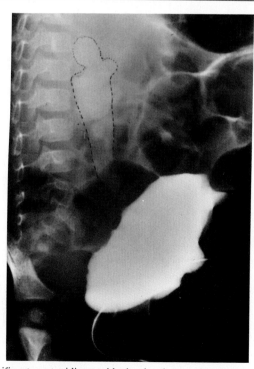

Figure 13-43 Significant postvoiding residual urine is seen in this infant with grade III vesicoureteral reflux and prune belly syndrome.

Management

Monitoring the serum levels of blood urea nitrogen (BUN), creatinine, and electrolytes in the first few days is clearly very important. Avoiding infection and placing the child on antibiotics will help reduce the chance of infection. A complete evaluation of the genitourinary tract with ultrasound and VCUG is warranted. A diuretic renal scan and intravenous pyelogram can be performed later. Despite the urinary tract dilatation and poor bladder function, surgical intervention should be limited to patients with progressive deterioration of renal function. Injudicious diversion procedures such as nephrostomy, ureterostomy, and vesicostomy may convert a balanced urinary tract into one that requires extensive reconstruction. If the creatinine and BUN rise during the first week to 10 days, this provides an ominous prognosis for normal function. If renal function deteriorates, vesicostomy should be used when diversion is needed. Reimplantation and tapering of the ureters may be required in some patients. Reduction cystoplasty may improve bladder emptying in selected patients. Abdominal wall reconstruction may improve the child's appearance and abdominal wall function during Valsalva maneuvers. To date there is no evidence that antenatal therapy is of benefit to these patients.

URINARY ASCITES

Urinary ascites may occur early in the case of urethral atresia, as illustrated above, or late in the course of urinary tract obstruction due to the rupture of some component of the dilated urinary tract. The appearance is that of severe ascites, outlining the intraperitoneal organs, and particularly a thick-walled urinary bladder in the lower abdomen (Figure 13-44).

Antenatal Intervention

Multiple reports have demonstrated the technical feasibility of placing a small diversion catheter into the fetal bladder to divert its contents to the amniotic cavity. There have been technical difficulties with the locational stability of these catheters, but multiple successes have been recorded. The greatest difficulty has been the selection of the fetus with the potential to benefit from the diversion. Fetuses with urethral atresia and those with a persistent cloaca have not been shown to benefit from diversion even when the procedure is technically successful. The renal and pulmonary sequelae in these infants that result from the primary obstruction appear to be irreversible. The vast majority of cases of unilateral UPJ obstruction would not benefit from intervention; survival without intervention is the rule, as is salvage of the affected kidney. Intervention carries risks of infection, preterm labor, and premature rupture of membranes that are not justified without serious expectation of benefit. In the rare case where a large perinephric cyst is causing polyhydramnios via intestinal or gastric compression or distortion and premature labor, it may be appropriate to consider antenatal intervention, but only if such consequential events are of serious significance. It is in the case of PUV detected between 20 and 30 weeks with severe oligohydramnios and progressive hydronephrosis that an argument for antenatal diversion catheterization may be made. The hydronephrotic changes in the kidneys may be reversed with low-resistance diversion, if they are of limited duration, and pulmonary hypoplasia may be prevented. Unfortunately, the discovery of such a case at just the right time is unusual. A late-discovered case of severe oligohydramnios with megacystis and severe hydronephrosis is a less convincing candidate for diversion. In all cases of bladder outlet obstruction, it is appropriate to submit either amniotic fluid or fetal urine for fetal karyotype. The probability of aneuploidy in the case of urinary tract malformation has been variably reported but is likely to approximate 10%.

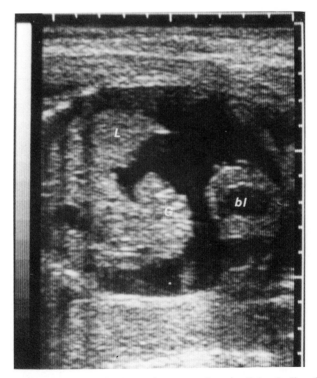

Figure 13-44 Urinary ascites is typically massive, as seen here, outlining the liver (L), gut (G), and the thick-walled urinary bladder (bl).

In the case of a possible candidate for antenatal diversion, it is never possible to precisely predict final respiratory or renal outcome at the time of diversion. Although some observers have established a rough relationship between fetal urinary osmolality and renal function, the ability to predict renal function given low-resistance diversion 10 to 15 weeks in the future is not available. In a similar way, although the comparison of fetal chest dimensions to a normative chart does allow the ability to predict pulmonary hypoplasia to some extent when delivery is to occur in the near future, it does not allow the precise prediction of fetal pulmonary hypoplasia at the time of urinary diversion. Therefore, the patient must accept some imprecision when she elects to request intervention. At the time of diversion, warmed normal saline may be injected to create a temporary amniotic cavity within which to place the catheter. A sample of this injected saline can be sent for karyotype after a period of time for cells to become suspended. After the catheter is in place within the bladder but before removal of the operative cannula, the fetal urine is removed, and the urine itself can provide the basis for a successful karyotype. Also, a portion of the urine may be tested for electrolyte concentrations and osmolality. Despite the prognostic limitations, it would be reassuring to note normal results in these tests.

GENERAL NEONATAL CARE OF GENITOURINARY MALFORMATIONS

Clinical Evaluation

In the case of antenatal diagnosis of a urinary tract anomaly, neonatal evaluation can be prompt and relatively specific. However, the majority of congenital urinary tract diseases remain undiagnosed antenatally. Significant abdominal masses are detected in approximately 1% of all neonates. Nearly 60% of these masses originate from the genitourinary tract. Furthermore, at least 50% of the neonates who present with ascites have a urologic disorder responsible for the ascites. Infants with major genitourinary anomalies are more likely to have specific dysmorphic features, such as those listed in Table 13-2. Severe oligohydramnios is often found in the case of poor fetal renal function and is usually associated with lethal pulmonary hypoplasia.

Postnatal Evaluation

Suspected genitourinary malformations in the neonate require careful postnatal evaluation for accurate diagnosis and appropriate treatment. Since renal physiology varies with gestational age, laboratory tests need to be interpreted in relationship to the adjusted gestational age of the infant.

Table 13-2 Dysmorphic Features of Genitourinary Malformations

Low-set ears
Ambiguous genitalia
Anorectal malformations
Vertebral anomalies
Cardiac defects
Tracheoesophageal fistula
Anterior abdominal wall defects

Plasma creatinine levels at birth reflect maternal creatinine concentration. Plasma creatinine falls from approximately 1 to 0.5 mg/dL at 5 days to 0.3 mg/dL at 9 days of age. Since the GFR is significantly lower in the preterm neonate, creatinine is not cleared as fast. It may be weeks before the plasma creatinine falls to a normal level. The GFR remains very low until 34 weeks' gestation, when it has been measured at 1 mL/min/kg. At birth the GFR increases to only 3 mL/min/kg but then doubles by 2 weeks of age. Although GFR at adult levels is not reached until age 2 years, the maturation of GFR occurs at the same rate in infants of the same gestational age, either in utero or ex utero.

Renal tubular function also varies with gestational age. Compared to the term neonate, the premature infant has increased sodium excretion from the distal tubule and decreased sodium resorption from the proximal tubule. Maximal concentrating ability is limited, especially in preterm infants who can achieve a maximal osmolarity of 500 to 600 mOsm/L. At term neonates can concentrate their urine only to 600 to 700 mOsm/L compared with 1200 mOsm/L for the older child or adult. Furthermore, a markedly lower renal threshold for bicarbonate combined with a diminished ability to handle acid loads is present in neonates.

The BUN may be a useful indicator of renal function in the neonate. If the BUN is greater than 20 mg/dL or rises over 5 mg/dL per day, this is reasonable evidence of renal insufficiency. However, severe catabolic stress, increased protein intake, or sequestered blood in the tissues can be associated with elevations in BUN without renal failure.

Changes in renal function that occur during the transition from fetal to postnatal life influence the choice of diagnostic imaging procedures used for these infants. Intravenous pyelography is not usually helpful in neonates because of their limited ability to concentrate urine, along with the difficulty they have excreting a highly osmolar load. On the other hand, postnatal ultrasonography is invaluable as a noninvasive study to determine the size and location of the kidneys, ureters, and bladder. Ultrasonography has proven to be an optimal screening test for obstructive uropathy and is also helpful in differentiating cystic from solid renal masses (Figure 13-45). The

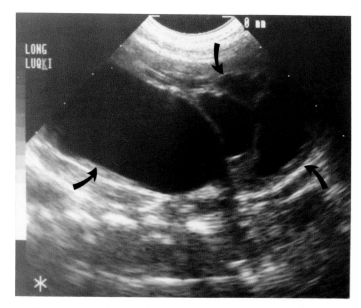

Figure 13-45 This abdominal ultrasound demonstrates severe hydronephrosis and hydroureter in a neonate with an obstructed, duplicated collecting system.

VCUG is indicated for any infant with hydronephrosis. A VCUG may define the etiology of suspected obstructive uropathy (e.g., posterior urethral valves) and is essential for diagnosing vesicoureteral reflux (Figure 13-46). Diuretic renography using injected radioisotopes such as diethylene triamine penta-acetic acid Tc 99 may be useful in addressing function or obstruction (Figure 13-47). Unfortunately, diuretic renography appears to have some serious limitations in the neonate, because if GFR is low, extraction of the radioactive tracer is low. Furthermore, since concentrating ability is limited, the washout phase may not show a response to diuretic injection and therefore simulate obstruction. Although the functional immaturity of the kidneys may be sufficient to interfere with testing for up to 2 months after birth, there is some usefulness to this test when there is one normal kidney and the function of the two sides can be directly compared.

FURTHER READING

Adzeck NS, Harrison MR, Flake AW, Laberge JM. Development of a fetal renal function test using endogenous creatinine clearance. *J Pediatr Surg.* 1985; 20:602.

Arger P, Coleman B, Mintz M, et al. Routine fetal genitourinary tract screening. *Radiology.* 1985; 156:485-489.

Baker ME, Rosenberg ER, Bowie JD, Gall S. Transient in utero hydronephrosis. *J Ultrasound Med.* 1985; 4:51-53.

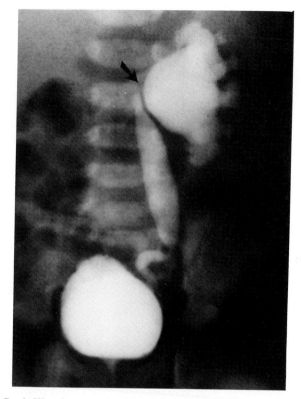

Figure 13-46 Grade III vesicoureteral reflux and congenital ureteropelvic junction obstruction (arrow) are demonstrated in this voiding cystourethrogram.

Beck AD. The effect of intrauterine urinary obstruction upon the development of the fetal kidney. *J Urol.* 1971; 105:784-789.

Bowie JD, Rosenberg ER, Andreotti RF, Fields SI. The changing sonographic appearance of fetal kidneys during pregnancy. *J Ultrasound Med.* 1983; 2:505.

Duckett JW. Prune belly syndrome. In: Welch KJ, Judson GR, Ravitch MM, O'Neal JA, Rowe MI, eds. *Pediatric Surgery.* 4th ed. Chicago: Yearbook Medical Publishers; 1986: 1193-1203.

Gardner S, Burton BK, Johnson AM. Maternal serum alphafetoprotein screening—A report of the Forsyth County Project. *Am J Obstet Gynecol.* 1981; 140:250.

Glick PL, Harrison, MR, Golbus MS, et al. Management of the fetus with congenital hydronephrosis, II: Prognostic criteria and selection for treatment. *J Pediatr Surg.* 1985; 20:376-387.

Glick PL, Harrison MR, Noall R. Correction of congenital hydronephrosis in utero, III: Early mid-trimester ureteral obstruction produces renal dysplasia. *J Pediatr Surg.* 1983; 18:681-687.

Golbus MS, Harrison MR, Filly RA, et al. In utero treatment of urinary tract obstruction. *Am J Obstet Gynecol.* 1982; 142:383-388.

Harrison MR, Golbus MS, Filly RA, et al. Fetal surgery for congenital hydronephrosis. *N Engl J Med.* 1982; 306:591-593.

Hendren WH. A new approach to infants with severe obstructive uropathy: Early complete reconstruction. *J Pediatr Surg.* 1970; 5:184.

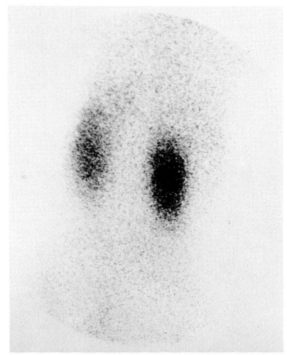

A

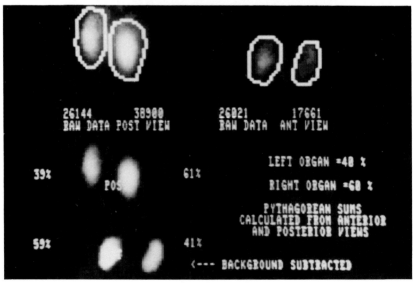

B

Figure 13-47   Differential renal function can be accurately estimated using diethylene triamine penta-acetic acid Tc 99 scanning techniques, as demonstrated in A and B. **A**, This raw image reveals differential function between the two kidneys. **B**, Computer enhancement shows that the right kidney provides 60% and the left kidney 40% of the total renal function.

Hobbins J, Romero R, Grannum P, Berkowitz R, Cullen M, Mahoney M. Antenatal diagnosis of renal anomalies with ultrasound. *Am J Obstet Gynecol.* 1984; 148:868–877.

Kelalis PP, Culp OS, Stickler GB, et al. Ureteropelvic obstruction in children: Experiences with 109 cases. *J Urol.* 1971; 106:418.

Kim MS, Mandell J. Renal function in the fetus and neonate. In: King LR, ed. *Urological Surgery in Neonates and Young Infants.* Philadelphia: WB Saunders Co; 1988.

King LR, Coughlin PWF, Bloch EC. The case for immediate pyeloplasty in the neonate with ureteropelvic junction obstruction. *J Urol.* 1984; 132:725.

Kirkinen P, Jouppila P, Tuononen S. Repeated transabdominal renocenteses in a case of fetal hydronephrotic kidney. *Am J Obstet Gynecol.* 1982; 142:1049–1051.

Koontz WL, Seeds JW, Adams WJ, et al. Elevated maternal serum alphafetoprotein, second trimester oligohydramnios and pregnancy outcome. *Obstet Gynecol.* 1983; 62:301.

Mandell J, Kinard HW, Mittelstaedt CA, Seeds JW. Prenatal diagnosis of unilateral hydronephrosis with early postnatal reconstruction. *J Urol.* 1984; 132:303.

Manning FA, Harman CR, Lange IR, et al. Antepartum chronic fetal vesicoamniotic shunts for obstructive uropathy: A report of two cases. *Am J Obstet Gynecol.* 1983; 145:819–822.

Nimrod C, Davies D, Stanislaw I, Harder J, Persuad D, Nicholson S. Ultrasound prediction of pulmonary hypoplasia. *Obstet Gynecol.* 1986; 68:495.

Potter E. Bilateral absence of ureters and kidneys. *Obstet Gynecol.* 1965; 25:3–12.

Seeds JW, Bowes WA. Ultrasound-guided fetal intravascular transfusion in severe Rhesus immunization. *Am J Obstet Gynecol.* 1986; 155:818–819.

Seeds JW, Cefalo RC, Herbert WNP, Bowes WA. Hydramnios and maternal renal failure: Relief with fetal therapy. *Obstet Gynecol.* 1984; 64(suppl):26S.

William DI. Male urethral obstruction. In-Williams DI, Johnston JH, eds. *Pediatric Urology.* 2nd ed. London: Butterworth & Co; 1982: 259–262.

ADDITIONAL RESOURCES

Manning FA. International Fetal Surgery Registry, 59 Emily Street, Winnipeg, Canada, R3E OW3.

Chapter 14

Nonimmune Hydrops

Hydrops fetalis is a pathologic condition of the fetus including generalized skin edema combined with serous effusions of the pleural, peritoneal, and/or pericardial cavities. Hydrops is often associated with fetomaternal blood group incompatibilities, leading to maternal isoimmunization and fetal hemolytic disease, but nonimmune hydrops fetalis (NIHF) refers to the occurrence of hydrops without hematologic evidence of fetomaternal blood group incompatibility. The reported incidence of nonimmune hydrops is estimated to be 1 in 2500 to 1 in 3500 neonates. Nonimmune hydrops has very poor fetal and neonatal prognosis, with perinatal mortality rates ranging from 50% to 98%.

DIAGNOSIS

Prenatal detection of fetal hydrops is reliably accomplished with ultrasonographic visualization of the fetus. The minimum criteria to establish the diagnosis include generalized skin thickening and/or two or more of the following: placental enlargement greater than 6 cm, ascites, pleural fluid, and pericardial fluid (Figures 14-1 and 14-2). The condition may be apparent early in pregnancy (Figure 14-3) or not be detected until late. The peritoneal fluid is seen to outline the abdominal viscera, including the falciform ligament and liver (Figure 14-4). Typically, generalized hydrops produces roughly proportional effusions of the chest and abdomen (Figure 14-5) and is associated with a markedly thickened placenta (Figure 14-6). Once the sonographic diagnosis of hydrops fetalis is made in a fetus or infant, a methodical search for the etiology of the hydrops must be made.

Rh isoimmunization should be excluded by performing antibody screening on the mother. If blood group incompatibilities are excluded, further evaluation should progress, using the least invasive tests first. Table 14-1 lists recommended studies to facilitate the diagnosis of hydrops.

Amniocentesis or fetal blood sampling should be considered to exclude aneuploidy as an etiology. Pulmonary maturity studies may be performed on amniotic fluid and may help with obstetric management if the fetal lungs

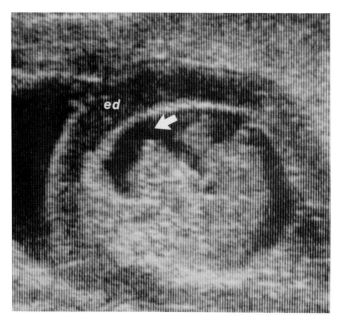

Figure 14-1 This transverse scan of the fetal abdomen shows the skin edema (ed) and ascites (arrow) present in a case of nonimmune hydrops.

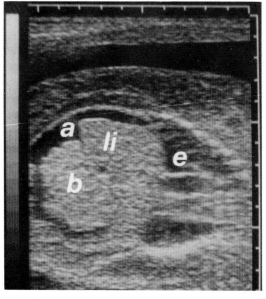

Figure 14-2 A longitudinal view of the same fetus shown in Figure 14-1 shows the ascites (a), the pleural effusion (e), the liver (li), and the bowel cluster (b).

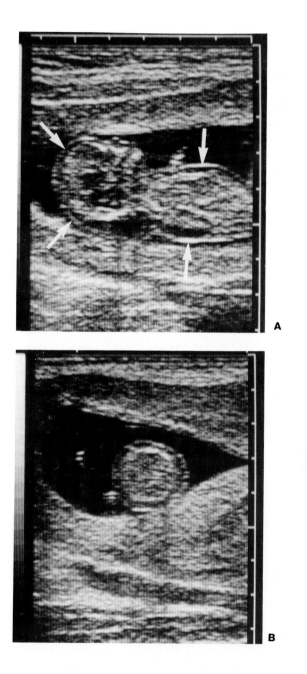

Figure 14-3 A, This sagittal view of a 14-week fetus with hydrops shows the skin edema (arrows). **B,** A transverse view of the same fetus emphasizes the skin edema.

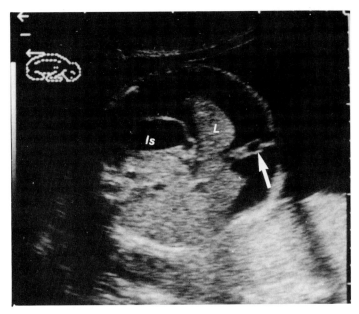

Figure 14-4 The liver (L), the lesser sac (ls), and the falciform ligament are nicely highlighted by ascitic fluid (arrow) in this fetus with hydrops.

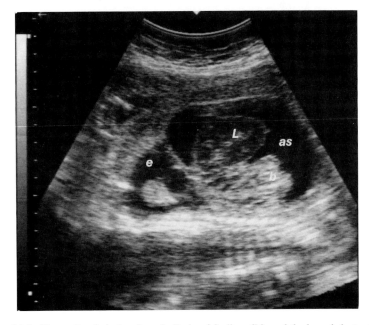

Figure 14-5 The ascites (as), the pleural effusion (e), liver (L), and the bowel cluster (b) are seen on this sagittal scan of a hydropic fetus.

Table 14-1 Prenatal Evaluation of Nonimmune Hydrops

Complete maternal blood count
Kleihauer-Betke screen
Hemoglobin electrophoresis
TORCH titers
VDRL
Parental glucose-6-phosphate dehydrogenase and erythrocyte pyruvate
  kinase studies
Glucose tolerance evaluation
Detailed real-time ultrasound
Fetal echocardiography

prove to be mature. It is also possible to sample the serous fluid collections with fetal paracentesis or thoracentesis for biochemical and microbiologic evaluation. Cell culture and karyotype have been successfully performed on a variety of fetal fluids, including serous effusions of the chest and abdomen.

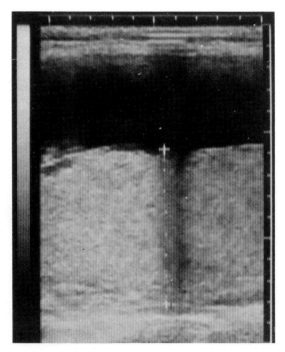

Figure 14-6 The typically thickened placenta seen in cases of nonimmune hydrops is illustrated here. Any time placental thickness exceeds 6 cm, it is considered abnormal.

ETIOLOGY

Three possible pathophysiologic mechanisms for NIHF have been proposed: severe anemia, congestive heart failure, and decreased colloid oncotic pressure.

Severe anemia may lead to fetal tachycardia with resultant high-output cardiac failure. Severe anemia may also cause decreased colloid oncotic pressure, with transudation of intravascular fluid to the extravascular spaces on an osmotic basis. Finally, the fetal tissues may become hypoxic secondary to the decreased oxygen-carrying capacity, and one of the pathologic responses to tissue hypoxia is capillary leakage, with transudation of fluid out of the intravascular spaces on this basis.

Congestive heart failure is probably the cause of fetal hydrops in those fetuses with in utero dysrhythmias such as supraventricular tachycardia or heart block. Most structural congenital heart defects do not cause in utero congestive heart failure because the fetal circulation largely bypasses the left side of the heart. However, some structural defects will cause fetal heart failure. These include insufficiency of the atrioventricular valves, premature closure of the foramen ovale or ductus arteriosus, and intracardiac tumors such as rhabdomyomas.

In those fetuses with liver parenchymal distortion or hepatic dysfunction, or in those fetuses who are losing a significant portion of their plasma proteins to serous fluid collections, reduced colloid osmotic pressure is probably an important contributing factor.

Table 14-2 is a list of conditions that have been associated with NIHF, although some of these have appeared as isolated case reports only. In as many as 45% of fetuses, the etiology of hydrops will remain unknown even after the birth of the infants.

CARDIAC ANOMALIES

The next largest group of patients with other than idiopathic hydrops are those fetuses with structural abnormalities of the heart or rhythm disturbances, comprising 12.5% and 4.0% of cases, respectively. This high frequency of cardiac abnormalities in association with NIHF mandates careful scrutiny of the fetal heart. Although most of these anomalies are discussed in greater detail in Chapter 9, a brief review here is appropriate. Fetal congestive heart failure, with resultant hydrops fetalis, can occur from either tachy- or bradydysrhythmias. Complete heart block in the fetus can occur as a result of several pathologic processes. As many as 25% of infants with congenital heart block have a structural abnormality of the heart, commonly endocardial fibroelastosis and transposition. Diagnosis of fetal complete heart block in the presence of fetal hydrops has a very poor prognosis.

Table 14-2 Hydrops-Associated Conditions

1. Cardiac
   Premature closure of the foramen ovale
   Anomalies of the tricuspid or pulmonary valves
   Severe atrial septal defect
   Severe ventricular septal defect
   Hypoplastic left heart
   Ebstein's anomaly
   Aortic valve stenosis
   Subaortic stenosis
   Dilated heart
   Atrioventricular canal defect
   Single ventricle
   Tetralogy of Fallot
   Subendocardial fibroelastosis
   Intracardiac tumors
   Transposition of the great vessels
   Complete heart block
   Fetal bradycardia
   Supraventricular tachycardias
   Atrial flutter with rapid ventricular response
2. Infections
   Fetal coxsackie or parvovirus infection
3. Hematologic
   Alpha-thalassemia
   Fetomaternal transfusion
   Twin-to-twin transfusion
   Glucose-6-phosphate dehydrogenase deficiency
   Vena caval, portal vein, or femoral thrombosis
4. Chest malformations
   Diaphragmatic hernias
   Congenital cystic adenomatoid malformation
   Pulmonary sequestration
   Pulmonary hypoplasia
   Pulmonary lymphangiectasia
   Mediastinal teratoma
   Hamartoma of the lung
   Congenital chylothorax
5. Chromosomal
   Turner's syndrome
   Trisomy 21
   Trisomy 18
   Triploidy
   Trisomy 13
6. Other congenital diseases
   Tuberous sclerosis
   Storage diseases (Gaucher's)
   Achondroplasia
   Osteogenesis imperfecta

Table 14-2 continued

7. Renal disease
    Congenital nephrosis
    Renal vein thrombosis
    Renal dysplasia
8. Gastrointestinal disorders
    Meconium peritonitis
    Gastrointestinal obstruction
    Tracheoesophageal fistula
    Small bowel volvulus
    Prenatal bowel perforation
    Duplication of gut
9. Disorders of multiple gestation
    Twin-to-twin transfusion
    Parabiotic twin syndrome
10. Placental and cord anomalies
    Chorioangioma of placenta or cord
    Chorionic vein thrombosis
    Placental and umbilical vein thrombosis
    Umbilical cord torsion
    True cord knots
    Angiomyxoma of cord
    Aneurysm of cord
11. Other causes of hydrops
    Congenital neuroblastoma
    Polysplenia syndrome
    Torsion of ovarian cyst
    Sacral teratoma
    Fetal trauma
    Amniotic band syndrome
    Maternal diabetes

On the other hand, there are numerous case reports of successful in utero cardioversion of supraventricular tachycardia and atrial flutter by administering various agents to the mother.

In the fetus remote from term with NIHF secondary to supraventricular tachycardia, chemical cardioversion should be attempted. Digoxin is usually the first therapeutic option. A loading dose of oral digoxin, 0.75 to 1.25 mg in divided doses, or intravenous loading is recommended. Often, larger loading doses are necessary in the pregnant woman to achieve therapeutic levels, due to the increased clearance of the drug. If after a reasonable period of therapeutic blood levels in the mother the fetus fails to respond, it may then be appropriate to try one of the other drugs.

HEMATOLOGIC DISORDERS

Of the hematologic disorders, the most common one that can be responsible for nonimmune hydrops is alpha-thalassemia. In populations in which a large proportion of patients are of Southeast Asian or Mediterranean origin, alpha-thalassemia can be a common cause of fetal and neonatal loss. The homozygous state for alpha-thalassemia is uniformly fatal, usually in the fetal period but occasionally in the immediate neonatal period. The mothers of these fetuses are likewise at risk for perinatal morbidity and mortality. Maternal risk is increased because of the common occurrence of severe preterm maternal pre-eclampsia and complications from retained placentas.

Eleven percent of the Southeast Asian population screened in this country carry alpha-thalassemia, and up to 39% of these patients have some inherited hemoglobin disorder. The initial screening procedure should be an evaluation of the maternal red blood cell indices and hemoglobin or hematocrit determination. If the mother has a microcytic anemia, then the father of the pregnancy should be evaluated for the same problem. If both parents have such an anemia, not secondary to iron deficiency, then hemoglobin electrophoresis should be performed on both parents. If they are heterozygous for alpha-thalassemia, one can offer prenatal diagnosis for their fetus using restriction endonuclease gene mapping on chromatin material from fetal cells from amniocentesis, or, where available, chorionic villus biopsy. If the mother presents late in her pregnancy with a fetus with hydrops, confirmation of the fetal hemoglobinopathy can be performed by amniocentesis. Since the homozygous state is uniformly fatal, this documentation allows the patient and her doctors to expedite delivery to avoid maternal morbidity secondary to pre-eclampsia, operative morbidity from an unnecessary cesarean birth, or hemorrhage from a retained placenta.

MISCELLANEOUS CAUSES

Congenital idiopathic hydrothorax in the fetus may cause nonimmune hydrops by increasing the intrathoracic pressure, with obstructed venous return. In the patient whose fetus is preterm, diversion catheters have been placed into the fetal chest to allow drainage of the effusion into the amniotic fluid, thus decompressing the chest and permitting improved cardiac return. In severe cases of congenital hydrothorax prior to 26 weeks' gestation, the fetus may have already suffered from a degree of pulmonary hypoplasia; however, the diagnosis of pulmonary hypoplasia can be made reliably only postnatally and should not be assumed antenatally.

DELIVERY

Frequent fetal assessments of well-being should occur. Serial ultrasound scans to follow the progression or remission of the hydrops and to continue searching for an etiology if none has yet been found are important. Weekly or biweekly nonstress testing of the fetus should be instituted around 30 weeks' gestation.

The timing of the delivery depends on evidence of maternal or fetal compromise. A progression in the severity of the hydrops or poor results on antenatal fetal well-being assessments are an indication to proceed with delivery. Maternal physiologic embarrassment or onset of pre-eclampsia may also necessitate early delivery. If the mother and hydropic fetus are stable, delivery is delayed as long as possible.

At the time of spontaneous labor (or indicated obstetrical intervention) the mother should be at a hospital with a neonatal intensive care unit. Hydropic infants are commonly depressed at birth, may have associated congenital anomalies requiring immediate medical or surgical care, and may have problems with chest expansion because of serous fluid collections.

A uterus massively distended by polyhydramnios and a severely hydropic fetus can compromise maternal respiratory and renal function. Conservative clinical care often involves hospitalization and bed rest, and the polyhydramnios may require either delivery or therapeutic amniocentesis for decompression of the uterus. When polyhydramnios is present, the uterus demonstrates poor contractility, and labor may be ineffective without drainage of some of the fluid. If amniotic fluid drainage is necessary to permit normal progression of labor, transabdominal drainage rather than amniotomy should be performed, so that the decompression of the uterus can proceed in a controlled fashion and the risks of placental abruption are minimized.

There may be a limited role for prenatal aspiration of fetal pleural or ascitic fluid to facilitate lung expansion at the time of delivery. If such fetal fluid aspiration is planned, it should be done as soon as possible prior to the delivery, as these fetal effusions commonly reform rapidly.

The large, edematous placenta associated with NIHF has little respiratory reserve and may not provide adequate fetal support during labor, often making cesarean delivery the method of choice. These edematous fetuses, likewise, are at risk for shoulder dystocia and soft tissue trauma. Postpartum hemorrhage from the large placenta is an additional hazard of vaginal delivery.

NEONATAL MANAGEMENT

The hydropic neonate admitted to the intensive care nursery is extremely ill. The primary concern is usually ventilation. The fetus may experience respiratory distress from prematurity, external compression of fetal lungs from ascites, pleural effusions, pulmonary edema, or secondary pulmonary hypoplasia. Thoracentesis and paracentesis early in neonatal life may be lifesaving but should be undertaken cautiously as they can cause rapid fluid shifts from the intravascular compartment to the extravascular one.

Congestive heart failure, anemia, and intravascular fluid depletion may be present, and exchange transfusion, pressor support, and diuretics may be required.

Routine care of the neonate with NIHF is also important. Because of the severe edema, the neonate's skin may break down. Adequate nutrition to obtain positive nitrogen balance in infants who are hypoproteinemic may require total parenteral nutrition. Intensive ventilatory support is required, and chest tubes are often needed to drain the pleural effusions or air leaks.

PARENTAL COUNSELING

Many of the conditions associated with NIHF have a genetic basis, although the majority are multifactorial or sporadic. The parents of an affected infant should be counseled regarding the chance of recurrence in a future pregnancy as well as the possibilities for prenatal diagnosis. As chromosomal analysis and restriction endonuclease technology improve, the likelihood of early accurate prenatal diagnosis of conditions causing NIHF will increase.

Although in some instances NIHF is genetic, most cases are idiopathic or multifactorial, and the risk of a recurrence in a subsequent pregnancy is very small. However, there are reported cases of recurrences of idiopathic NIHF in siblings, so careful surveillance of subsequent pregnancies is recommended.

FURTHER READING

Ambramowicz J, Jaffe R, Altaras M, Ben-Aderet N. Fetal supraventricular tachycardia: Prenatal diagnosis and pharmacological reversal of associated hydrops fetalis. *Gynecol Obstet Invest.* 1985; 20:109–112.

Anderson HM, Hutchison A, Fortune D. Non-immune hydrops fetalis: Changing contribution to perinatal mortality. *Br J Obstet Gynaecol.* 1983; 90:636–639.

Davis CL. Diagnosis and management of nonimmune hydrops fetalis. *J Reprod Med.* 1982; 27:594–600.

Etches PC, Lemons JA. Nonimmune hydrops fetalis: Report of 22 cases including three siblings. *Pediatrics.* 1979; 64:326–332.

Evron S, Yagel S, Samueloff A, Margaliot E, Burstein P, Sadovsky E. Nonimmunologic hydrops fetalis: A review of eleven cases. *J Perinat Med.* 1985; 13:147–151.

Fleischer AC, Killam A, Boehm F, et al. Hydrops fetalis: Sonographic evaluation and clinical implications. *Radiology.* 1981; 141:163–168.

Graves GR, Baskett TF. Nonimmune hydrops fetalis: Antenatal diagnosis and management. *Am J Obstet Gynecol.* 1984; 148:563–565.

Guntheroth WG, Cyr D, Mack L, Benedetti T, Lenke R, Petty C. Hydrops from reciprocating atrio-ventricular tachycardia in a 27 week fetus requiring quinidine for conversion. *Obstet Gynecol.* 1985; 66 (suppl):29S-33S.

Guy G, Coady D, Jansen V, Snyder J, Zinberg S. Alpha-thalassemia hydrops fetalis: Clinical and ultrasonographic considerations. *Am J Obstet Gynecol.* 1985; 153:500–504.

Hirsch M, Friedman S, Schoenfeld A, Ovadia J. Nonimmune hydrops fetalis—a rational attitude of management. *Eur J Obstet Gynecol Reprod Biol.* 1985; 19:191–196.

Holzgreve W, Holzgreve B, Curry C. Nonimmune hydrops fetalis: Diagnosis and management. *Semin Perinatol.* 1985; 9: 52–67.

Hutchison AA, Drew J, Yu V, Williams M, Fortune D, Beischer N. Non-immunologic hydrops fetalis: A review of 61 cases. *Obstet Gynecol.* 1985; 59:347–352.

Iliff PJ, Nicholls JM, Keeling JW, Gough JD. Non-immunologic hydrops fetalis: A review of 27 cases. *Arch Dis Child.* 1983; 58:979–982.

Im SS, Rizos N, Joutsi P, Shime J, Benzie R. Nonimmunologic hydrops fetalis. *Am J Obstet Gynecol.* 1984; 148:566–569.

Lanham JG, Walport MJ, Hughes GV. Congenital heart block and familial connective tissue disease. *J Rheumatol.* 1983; 10:823–825.

Macafee CAJ, Fortune DW, Beischer NA. Non-immunologic hydrops fetalis. *J Obstet Gynecol Br Comm.* 1972; 77:226–237.

Machin GA. Differential diagnosis of hydrops fetalis. *Am J Med Genet.* 1981; 9:341–350.

Mahoney B, Filly R, Callen P, Chinn D, Golbus M. Severe nonimmune hydrops fetalis: Sonographic evaluation. *Radiology.* 1984; 151:757–761.

Maidman JE, Yeager C, Anderson V, et al. Prenatal diagnosis and management of nonimmunologic hydrops fetalis. *Obstet Gynecol.* 1980; 56:571–576.

Seeds JW, Bowes WA. Results of treatment of severe fetal hydrothorax with bilateral pleuroamnionic catheters. *Obstet Gynecol.* 1986; 68:577–579.

Turkel SB. Conditions associated with nonimmune hydrops fetalis. *Clin Perinatol.* 1982; 9:613–625.

Index

.